# Cosmetic Dermatologic Surgery

# Cosmetic Dermatologic Surgery

Editor: Horatio Fowler

AMERICAN
MEDICAL PUBLISHERS
www.americanmedicalpublishers.com

AMERICAN
MEDICAL PUBLISHERS
www.americanmedicalpublishers.com

**Cataloging-in-publication Data**

Cosmetic dermatologic surgery / edited by Horatio Fowler.
p. cm.
Includes bibliographical references and index.
ISBN 979-8-88740-024-2
1. Skin--Surgery. 2. Surgery, Plastic. 3. Surgery, Operative.
4. Skin--Diseases--Treatment. I. Fowler, Horatio.
RD520 .C67 2023
617.477--dc23



American Medical Publishers,
41 Flatbush Avenue,
1st Floor, New York,
NY 11217, USA

ISBN 979-8-88740-024-2 (Hardback)

# Contents

# Preface

Cosmetic dermatologic surgery is a type of surgery that is done to improve a person's appearance, self-esteem and self-confidence. It can be done on any part of the body or face. Facial profile of a person can be improved by using face-lift techniques, which are the most frequently used procedures in cosmetic dermatology. Thread and closed suture lifting is a minimally invasive face-lifting surgery that lifts and reposits ptotic soft tissue that develops with age. This technique has become increasingly popular as an alternative to traditional surgical rhytidectomy or neck lifting. The use of thread-lift sutures for face augmentation is a low-risk procedure that the oral and maxillofacial surgeons can use to provide patients an alternative to or in conjunction with other facial aesthetic procedures, including facial filler treatment and neuromodulator treatment, or surgical procedures. This book provides comprehensive insights into the field of cosmetic dermatologic surgery. It presents researches and studies performed by experts across the globe. Surgeons, students and experts actively engaged in this field will find this book extremely insightful.

Various studies have approached the subject by analyzing it with a single perspective, but the present book provides diverse methodologies and techniques to address this field. This book contains theories and applications needed for understanding the subject from different perspectives. The aim is to keep the readers informed about the progresses in the field; therefore, the contributions were carefully examined to compile novel researches by specialists from across the globe.

Indeed, the job of the editor is the most crucial and challenging in compiling all chapters into a single book. In the end, I would extend my sincere thanks to the chapter authors for their profound work. I am also thankful for the support provided by my family and colleagues during the compilation of this book.

**Editor**

Section 1

# Transcutaneous Suture Lifts and Suspensions

# 1

# Serdev Sutures® in Lower Face and Neck

Nikolay Serdev

## 1. Introduction

The concept of lower face SMAS lift via sutures, through skin punctures alone (or by hidden incisions in the retro-lobular fold), explains how to re-structure and re-position the lower face, associated facial elements and neck, without visible pre- and retro-auricular scars. The author uses the specially designed, curved elastic Serdev® needles with lengths of 60 mm, 100 mm and 140 mm and prefers the Bulgarian semi-elastic, polycaproamide (Polycon) surgical suture USP 2, with long delayed absorption durability.

## 2. Lower face and neck lift by sutures, with skin perforations only or by using a hidden 2.5 cm retro-lobular incision

The first methos is a closed approach suture method of lower SMAS face and neck lift. The author uses skin punctures alone to introduce the needle and suture, in order to capture, lift and fix loose lower face and neck SMAS to stable structures like periosteum, without tissue undermining. Colli fascia, mastoid or occipital periosteum are used as anchor points to fix and elevate the lower SMAS, enabling lower face and neck lifting.

In the second method, the author uses limited undermining of 3-4 cm in front of the tragus, via retro-lobular incision. The fold behind the earlobule is the only place to hide the incision and at the same time obtain the optimal approach to cheek SMAS and platysma in front of the tragus. Usually, the retrolobular fold permits a 1.5-2.5 cm long incision. Thus, lifting the SMAS restores aesthetic angles, shape and proportions, which is the basis for beautification and rejuvenation.

### 2.1. The concept

Ptosis and laxity of the "subdermal facial mask" - the SMAS - in lower face and neck reflects the signs and appearance of lower face aging. The concept of using the closed approach semi-elastic sutures with delayed absorption, is to tighten and elevate the lower face and neck, without unnecessary incisions. It is a fact that soft tissue and skin are attached to the SMAS. Accordingly, lifting and fixing the SMAS into a more favourable position enables repositioning of soft tissue facial structures as well. Loose SMAS and skin laxity imparts a heavy, hanging, sad and tired facial expression. In young patients without genuine ptosis, heavy facial features, poorly expressed cheekbones and jaw lines, flawed proportions and angles, as well as sad appearance should be corrected. In many patients heavy subdermal fat and fat pad should be removed simultaneously.

Classic face lifts can not avoid some visible scars or an "operated-on" appearance, secondary to skin and SMAS rotation and pull. The concept of the suture lift of lower face and neck SMAS is to achieve immediate results and to avoid trauma, visible pre- and retro-auricular incisions, excisions and scars.

As subdermal and submental fat in the lower face is superficial to SMAS, it cannot be lifted with the SMAS lift. If necessary, it should be reduced concurrently or prior to lifting. The author uses ultrasound assisted liposculpturing in the lower face and neck since 1994 (SMEI Sculpture and later - VASER) as a best option for atraumatic fat removal and tightening of skin.

### *2.1.1. Definition*

The two methods, described by the author, represent lower face and neck SMAS suspension, tightening or duplication, using elastic sutures durable through extended absorption delay, via needle perforations alone or via hidden retro-lobular incision, where SMAS-platysma is lifted and fixed to the mastoid, and in some selected cases - to occipital periosteum.

### *2.1.2. Objective*

The primary goal in lower face and neck closed approach suture lifting technique is the straightening and repositioning of the subdermal facial mask - the SMAS/platysma - with the perspective of refreshing the facial appearance and obtaining rejuvenation and beautification, corresponding to aesthetic angles, proportions and anatomic position, typical for youth. It is used for sculpturing the jaw line, softening the nasolabial fold and beautification, mostly in minor and medium jowling, submental laxity. It is ideal in cases of beautification, associated with early or medium facial ptosis. In cosmetic surgery it is very important to respond to patient's requirements for immediate beautification, to avoid visible scars, as well as to give patients the chance to promptly resume work and social activities, without long recovery period.

For this objective, the author's methods were created to be minimally invasive, without trauma and scars.

### *2.1.3. Anatomy*

Face droops with age, due to gravity, atrophy and loosening of the facial ligaments. Jowling is caused by displacement of the SMAS and skin aging. The neck is a face related area. The sagging neck is an important part of the aging face.

The SMAS is a fibro-muscular layer that connects platysma and galea and acts as a suspension for the overlying facial skin. The continuity between the facial SMAS and the platysma is an anatomical fact, useful in performing facelift surgery.

Subdermal plexus of vessels is superficial to SMAS. Motor nerves and facial muscles lie deep to SMAS. SMAS provides a suspensory sheet, which distributes the forces of facial expression. The concept that lifting this layer leads to better long-term suspension of overlying skin has become universally accepted.

SMAS continues inferiorly towards the platysma and represents aponeurotic connections between mimetic musculature and the overlying skin.

SMAS overlies the parotid gland in mandibular angle and tends to be substantial and easy to handle, because the parotid gland, zygomaticus major and minor muscles protect underlying facial nerve branches. With regard to protecting the facial nerve structures, we can accept that lower SMAS-platysma face-lift "by sutures only" or "with a retro-lobular incision" is done in a fairly secure area. The suture lift should protect the parotid gland and for this reason is performed only in the mobile superficial layers to capture the facial SMAS and platysma.

## 2.2. Surgical technique

The scarless lower face and neck SMAS-platysma lift by sutures takes about 10 minutes per side and is done under local anaesthesia and i.v. sedation.

### *2.2.1. METHOD I: using skin perforations only*

**1. Lower face SMAS lift by suture (A-C)**

**First Pass A-C**

a) Perforate points A, B, and C with a No. 11 scalpel blade, only skin deep. Position the blade in direction of Langer's lines.

**NB!** Stay away from deep mastoid penetration (at point A), stay away from parotid gland (located deeper at point C), and submandibular gland (located more medially, could be near point B).

b) Enter the needle perpendicularly through the skin perforation at point A (without fixation of any dermal tissue), then **tangentially** through the mastoid periosteum at the anterior mastoid border.

**NB!** Do not push needle perpendicularly into mastoid - it is very soft and can be easily perforated (be aware of mastoid and inner ear anatomy). Do not push the needle - twist it gently forwards or backwards.

c) Proceed through fascia colli and superficial subcutaneous tissue from A to C. Proceed parallel to the skin - place the needle tip laterally. The handpiece concavity shows the needle tip position in the tissue. The pass should be superficial and below the skin. However, if too superficial - dimpling will appear above the needle. Avoid this by twisting the needle backwards and then forwards again, a little deeper (but still in a superficial plane). A deeper pass will produce a bulging effect.

**NB!** Stay superficial. Never introduce the needle into or below the sternocleidomastoid muscle (vascular nerve bundle, a. and v. jugularis interna). Stay away from external jugular vein as well.

d) Just before exiting at point C, SMAS (platysma) is captured. To capture SMAS, turn needle tip downwards, progress a bit and twist needle tip upwards.

**NB!** Stay in superficial mobile layer, away from the parotid gland (just below mobile SMAS).

e) Pass through perforation point C.

Do not push through skin perforation point C. Place skin perpendicular to needle tip, twist the needle softly and progress gently and easily. The tip should appear at perforation point C, without resistance in front. Perforation or resistance indicates engagement of dermis, resulting in a dimple that is difficult to remove. Free the needle tip and repeat the movement until the tip appears without the feeling of resistance.

f) The needle tip is threaded and is pulled out through the needle pass in line C-A.

**Second Pass A-C**

The second parallel needle pass goes through the same skin perforations and tissue plane, 2-3 mm away from the first one. Platysma has to be engaged again. Appearing in perforation point C, the needle is threaded with the second end of the suture that is withdrawn through the second needle pass C-A. The suture loop dives in the subdermis at point C. The knot is made under medium elastic tension. Possible skin dimples should be managed by pulling the skin away from the suture, using a mosquito instrument. Thus, the first suture of lower face SMAS fixation to mastoid (or to occipital periosteum – rare and mostly in men to hide the swelling bulging) is fulfilled (Fig. 1, 2).

**PROCEDURE Video**
http://www.youtube.com/watch?v=zpDvCxC9hDg

Inject local anesthesia into points A, B, and C and also into the tissue corridor to be used for the needle passes.

The points of skin perforations should be planned in advance:

**Point A** - fixation at mastoid periosteum

**Point B** - fixation of lateral border of platysma to be lifted to A. A-B direction is to cervico-mandibular angle.

**Point C** - fixation of check SMAS and lateral border of platysma to be lifted to A. A-C direction is to the chin.

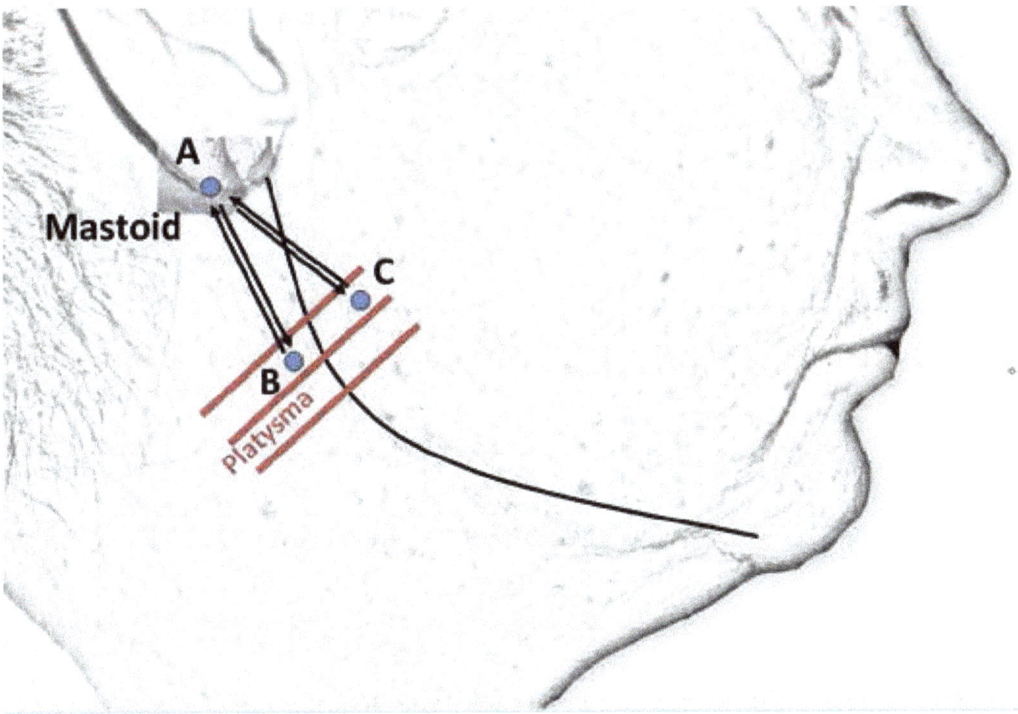


**Figure 1.** Lower face and neck SMAS lift, using Serdev Suture®

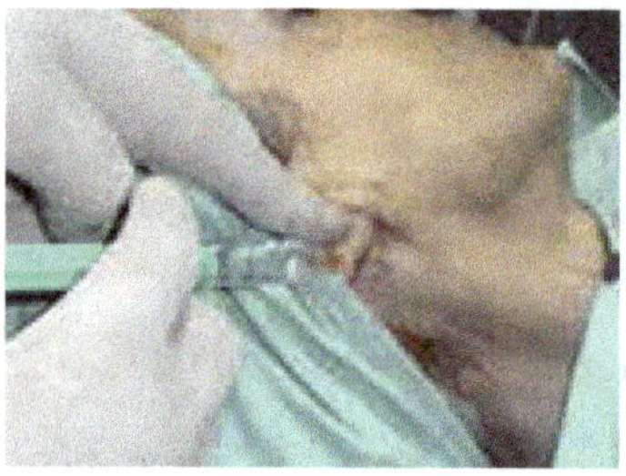
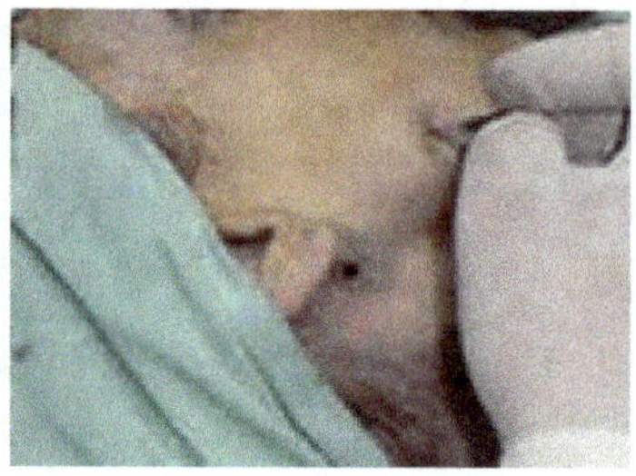
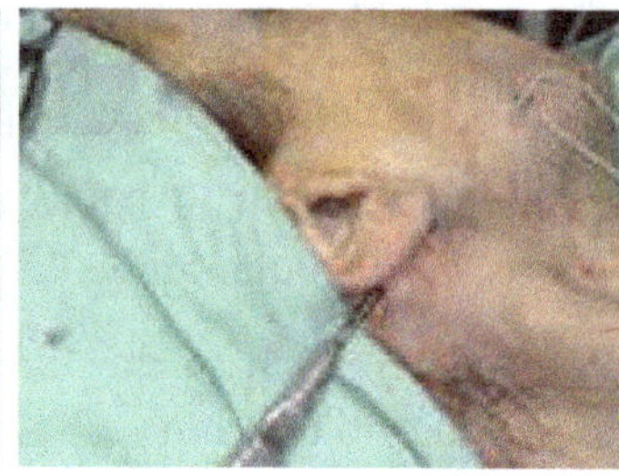

A. B. C.

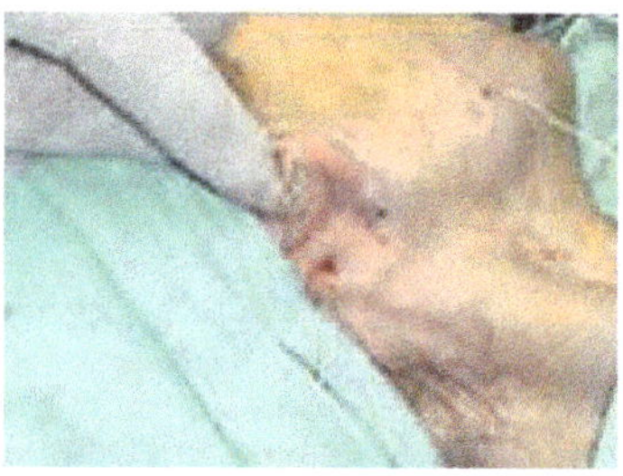
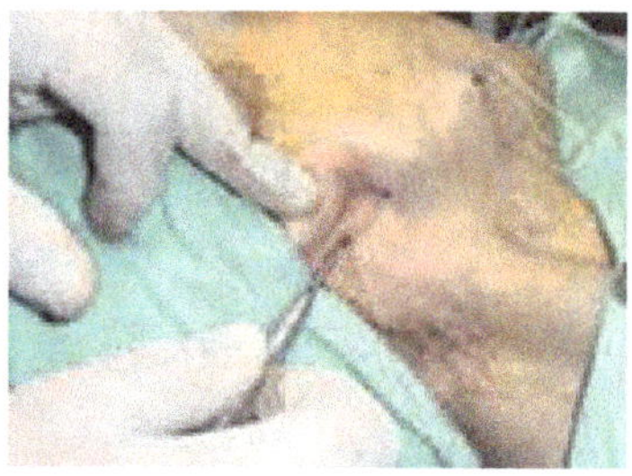
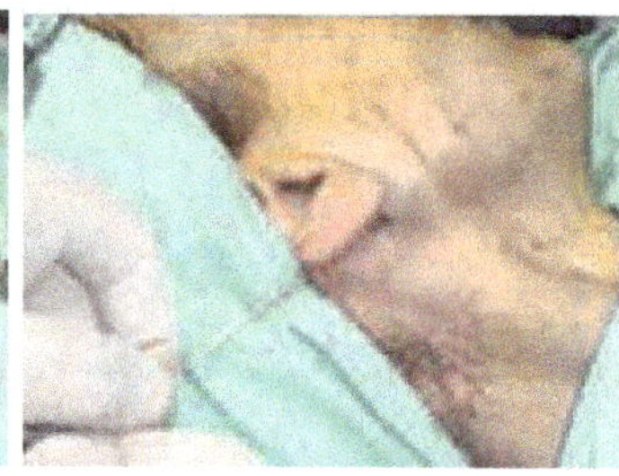

D. E. F.

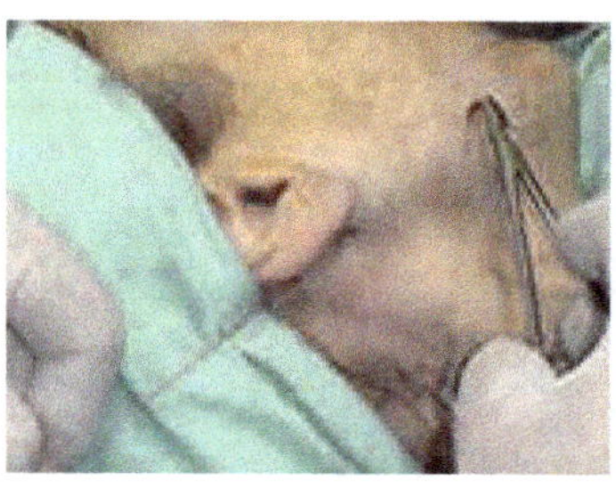
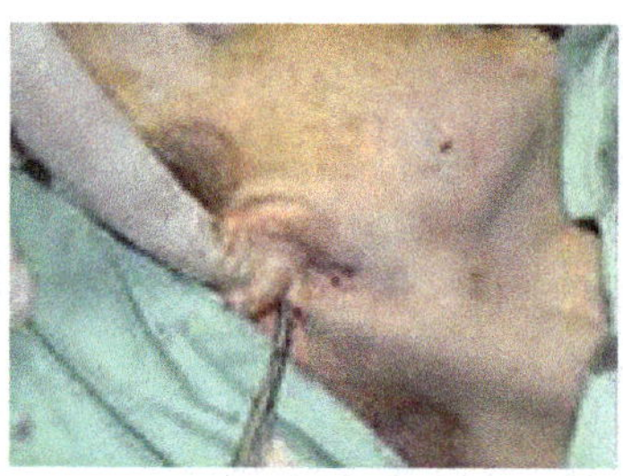

G. H.

**Figure 2. A.** Lidocaine infiltration of the mastoid periosteum, colli fascia and SMAS at perforation points A, C, and along the line A-C , **B.** Scalpel blade No 11 skin perforation in the selected points, **C.** The needle is introduced through skin perforation A, then **tangentially** through the mastoid, superficial subdermal through colli fascia, SMAS/platysma and perforation point C. No dimpling should be visible above the needle., **D.** The suture is introduced through the needle pass C-A, **E.** Second pass of the needle following the same plan 2-3 mm away from the first pass, the needle eye is threaded, no dimpling is visible above the needle, **F.** The second end of the suture is introduced through the second needle pass C-A. The suture circle is fulfilled. The pull on the suture lifts the cheek SMAS, **G.** Skin dimpling has been removed by releasing the skin from attachments using a mosquito instrument., **H.** Skin is released at point A. Nice jaw line is visible.

## 2. Neck lift (A-B)

The second suture is done in the same manner, from point A to point B.

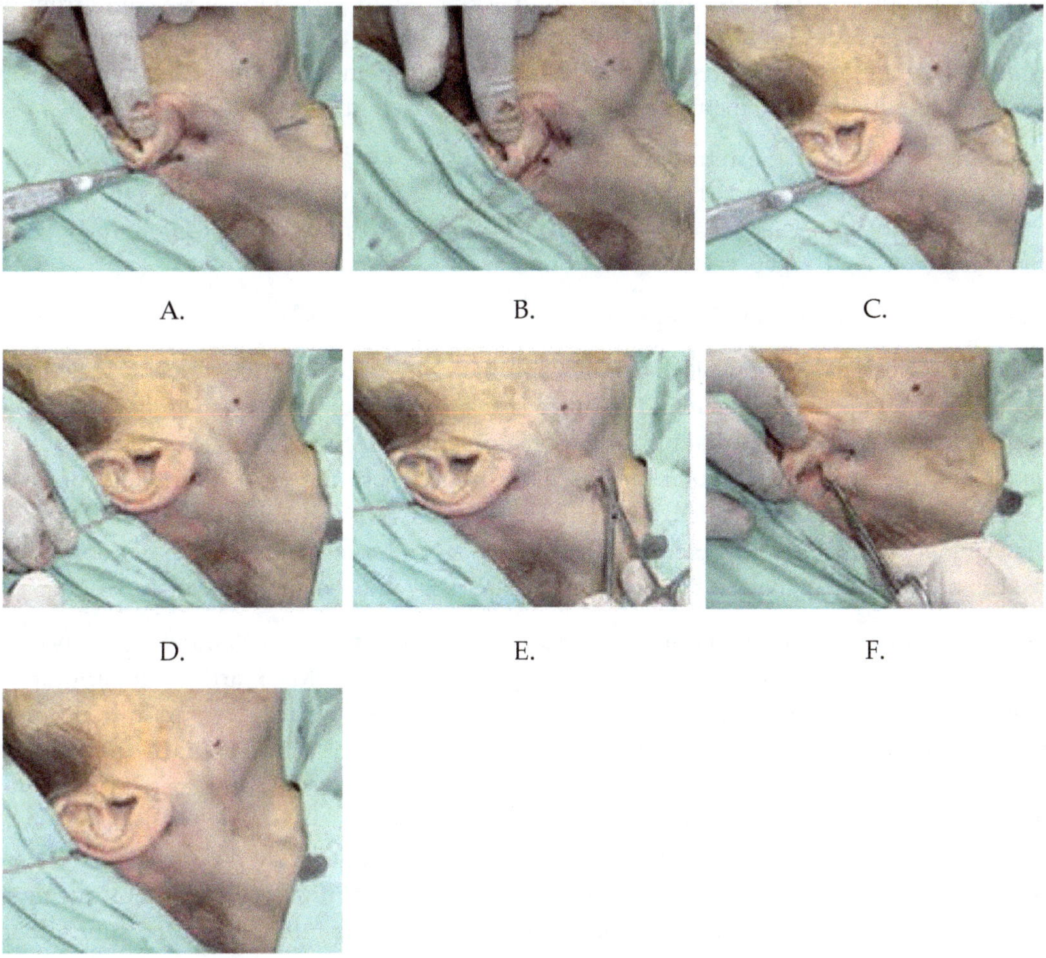

A. B. C. D. E. F. G.

**Figure 3. A.** The needle is introduced through the skin perforation point A, then **tangentially** through the mastoid, **superficial** subdermal through colli fascia, **above the sternocleidomastoid muscle**, through platysma and perforation point B in the direction of the cervico-mandibular angle, **B.** The suture is introduced through the needle pass B-A, **C.** Second pass of the needle following the same plan, 2-3 mm away from the first one, **D.**The second end of the suture is introduced through the second needle pass, suture loop dives into the skin perforation point B and the suture circle is fulfilled. The pull on the suture lifts the platysma, **E.** Skin dimpling at skin perforation point B is removed by releasing the skin from attachments, using a mosquito clamp, **F.** Skin dimpling at skin perforation point A is removed by releasing the skin from attachments using a mosquito clamp, **G.** The knot is made and the result of neck lift and cervico-mandibular angle is immediately visible.

At the other side, lifting is performed by suture in the same fashion.

### 2.2.2. *METHOD II: using a 2.5 cm retro-lobular incision*

The author has found that the only place to hide the incisions and at the same time have a very good approach to cheek, lower face and neck SMAS in a distance of 3-4 cm in front of the tragus, is the fold behind the ear lobule. It usually permits a 1.5 to 2.5 cm long incision, which is enough to elevate pre-auricular SMAS and retromandibular platysma into the skin incision line and to suture them to the colli fascia and mastoid.

Infiltration is done in the retro-lobular fold and 3-4 cm in front of tragus. 1.5 to 2.5 cm incision in the fold is done and a blunt subcutaneous undermining is performed through the retro-lobular opening in a radius of 3-4 cm from the earlobe in direction to: 1. oral commissure, 2. chin, and 3. cervico-mandibular angle.

After undermining there are **2 options:**

**Option 1**. Cheek SMAS and platysma are captured with a mosquito instrument, pulled out into the wound opening and sutured to colli fascia and mastoid. In this manner the lower face and neck SMAS lift is developed from the preauricular SMAS (at the level of the earlobule) and platysma (at the mandibular angle), and attached posteriorly to the mastoid process. Medium elastic tension is applied, providing a lower face SMAS backward & upward lift and platysma upward lift (Fig. 1). Skin is closed in one layer. Gauze dressings are not obligatory but can be used overnight or for some hours. Sutures are removed after 7 days.

**Option 2.** After the retrolobular incision and undermining is done, a 60 mm Serdev® needle is introduced in the undermined subdermal space and biting SMAS, arrives in perforation point C in lower face (or B in neck). After threading the needle, the surgical suture is introduced into the incision. Then, from skin perforation point A, **tangentially** through the mastoid, the needle arrives in the retrolobular incision and takes the suture end, introducing it at skin perforation point A. The suture is located in the line A-C in the lower face (or A-B in the neck area) fixing mobile SMAS (platysma) and immobile mastoid periosteum. Second pass is subdermal again taking the second suture end at point C (or B) and introducing it into skin perforation point A. Thus, the circle of the suture is fulfilled and the suture loop dives in point C (or B in neck). The knot is tied at Point A. Skin dimpling at points C and B is removed by traction of the skin perforation points C or B and the suture in opposite directions. One or two stiches are placed, in order to close the wound.

Both Serdev Suture® techniques of lower face and neck SMAS lift are quicker and safer than classic invasive face lift techniques. Mobile SMAS is lifted behind the ear lobule and sewn down to stable bone and periosteal structures. This technique gives an aesthetic and normal "non-operated on" appearance to the face, without scars and totally covers patient's expectation.

It is also possible to combine lower SMAS lift with other procedures such as fat pad removal, ultrasonic assisted liposculpturing of lower face and neck, medial platysma suturing, skin resurfacing, rhinoplasty, etc. Only a small number of patients need additional platysma sewing at the midline. In double chin cases, most important is to remove the fat collection. In authors hands, ultrasonic assisted liposuction is the best method to obtain a good cervico-mandibular angle of the neck and to tighten the skin in such cases.

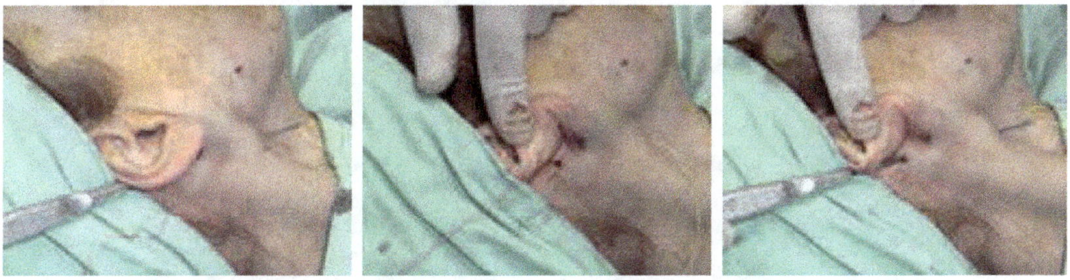

A. B. C.

**Figure 4. A.** After Lidocaine infiltration, retrolobular incision and about 3 cm blunt dissection of the preauricular and subauricular zones, the platysma is fixed with the needle in point B and the needle is threaded, **B.** The suture is introduced from the skin perforation point B into the opening of the retrolobular incision. A tangential bite of the mastoid from point A and suture end is introduced from the incision to point A. **C.** The needle is introduced again from skin perforation point A subdermally to perforation point B and the needle is threaded. Introduction of the suture in line B-A follows, the suture loop will dive in perforation point B and the suture circle will be finalized. The suture will be knotted, dimples removed. Closure of the retroauricular incision follows.

## 2.3. Results

530 patients have been operated with Method I during the period 1994-2011. Method II was performed in 386 patients. The result in these cases was immediate and optimal: there are no limitations to postoperative activities; no "operated-on" appearance, no visible scars and no real signs of operative intervention. The moderate facial tension generally imparts a pleasant sensation for the patient. Neither haematomas, nor infections have been observed. Bruising is rare.

In method I, in very loose skin cases, it is possible to obtain some swelling (bulging) effect at the sternocleidomastoid site that adapts and disappears in 2-3 weeks and could be easily covered by hair in female patients. In method II, skin undermining prevents from bulging or folding.

In method I, the skin punctures disappear in 2-3 days. In method II, the skin scar in the retrolobular fold is invisible and, additionally, there is no skin tension.

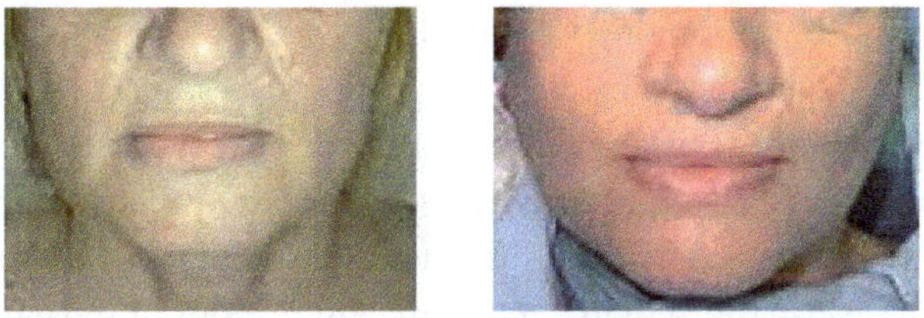

**Figure 5.** Visible change in the lower face appearance after lower SMAS lift by sutures with skin punctures only.

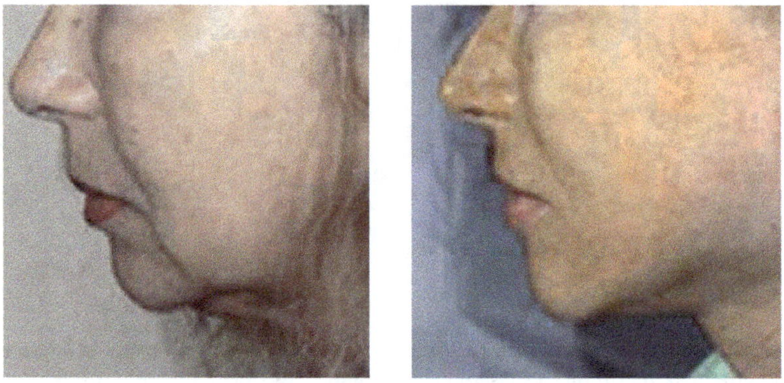

**Figure 6.** Result, immediately after surgery in the OP theatre. Immediate total change in the lower face after temporal, brow lift and a lower SMAS lift, using sutures with skin punctures alone.

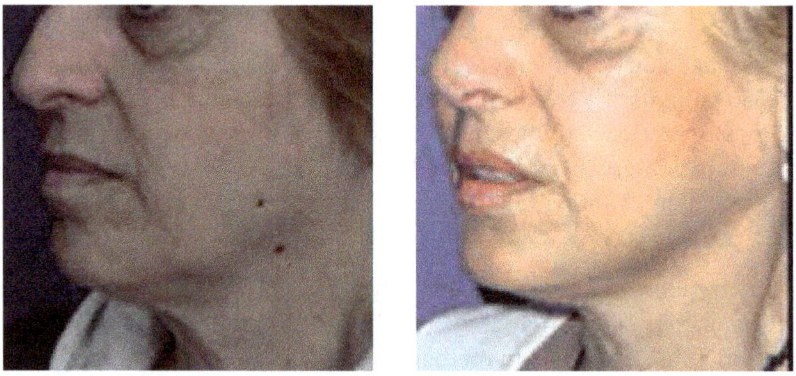

**Figure 7.** Before and after temporal SMAS, brow, and lower SMAS lift using sutures with skin punctures alone, combined with rhinoplasty. The change pleases the patient. Rejuvenation of the face.

In one case, when method II, option one was used, upper lid ptosis occurred during fixation of the pre-auricular SMAS. Immediate release of the suture solved this "complication" on the spot and another suture was performed without further complication. In one 63 year old patient, in line with her aesthetic requirements, an additional pre-auricular skin excision (S-lift) was performed 3 years after the suture lift. Due to the previous SMAS lift using method II, it was not possible to excise more than 2 to 3 mm skin in front of the ear.

No other complications or complaints have been observed in this period.

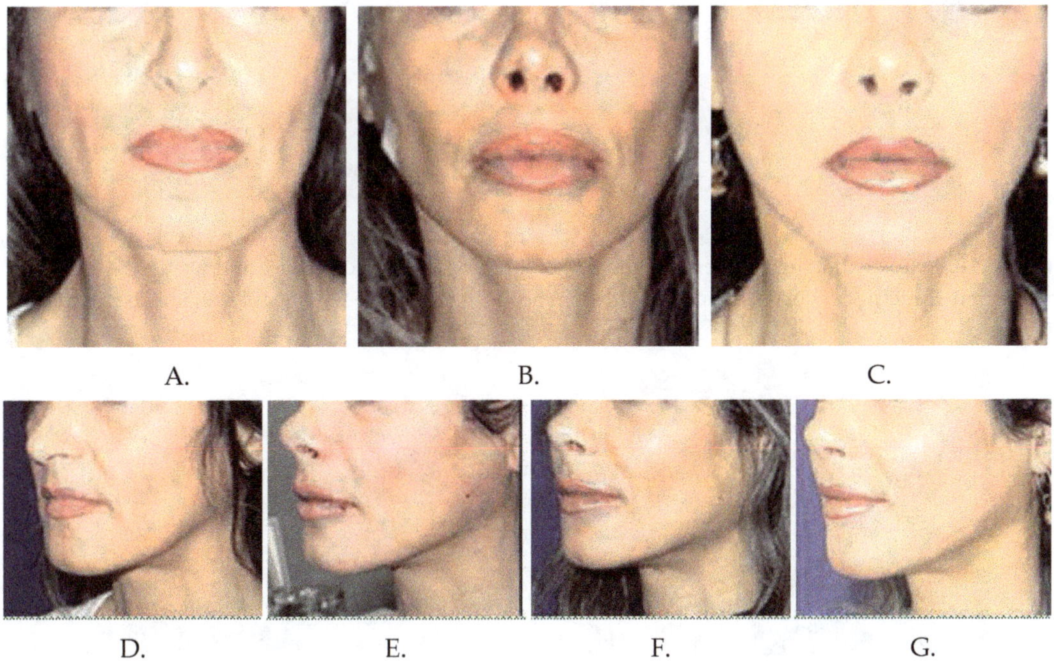


**Figure 8.** **A, D.**Before, **B, E.** Immediately after simultaneous temporal, medial and lower SMAS face lift by sutures using skin punctures only, brow lift by sutures, rhinoplasty, and lip augmentation. The skin punctures for the lower SMAS lift by sutures are visible (E), **F.** the day after surgery.**C, G.** After 3 days with make-up.

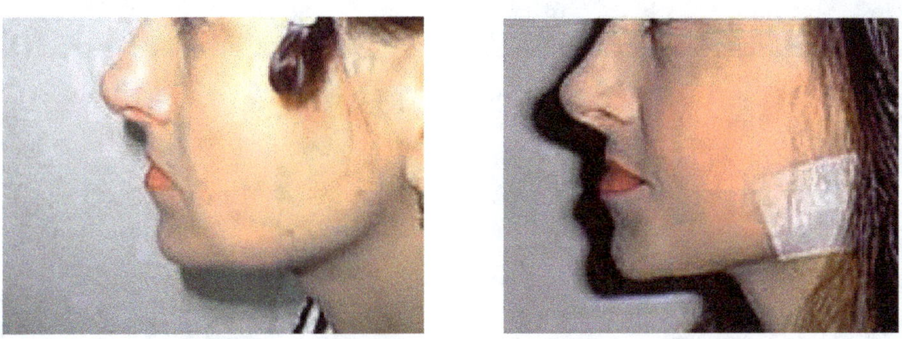

A. B.

**Figure 9.** **A.** Before and **B.** immediately after surgery in an 37 years old patient. A pleasant result in the lower face and jaw line. The bandage covering the skin punctures stays for overnight only. Patients usually return to work in a day or two.

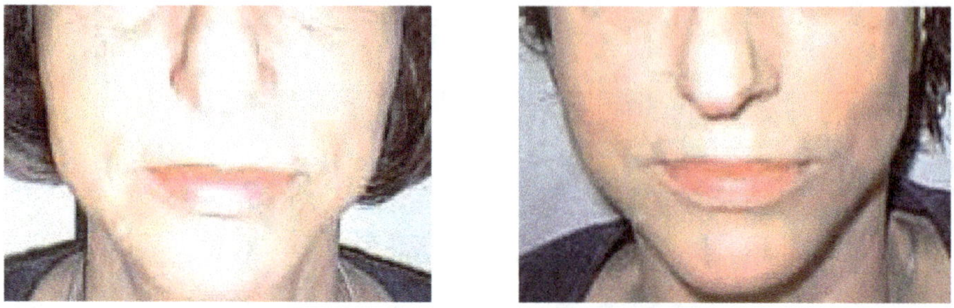

A. B.

**Figure 10.** Rejuvenation in an elderly patient. **A.** Before and **B.** after lower face and neck SMAS lift with retro-lobular incisions. Very good result with skin beautification. The SMAS and skin attached to it is tightened.

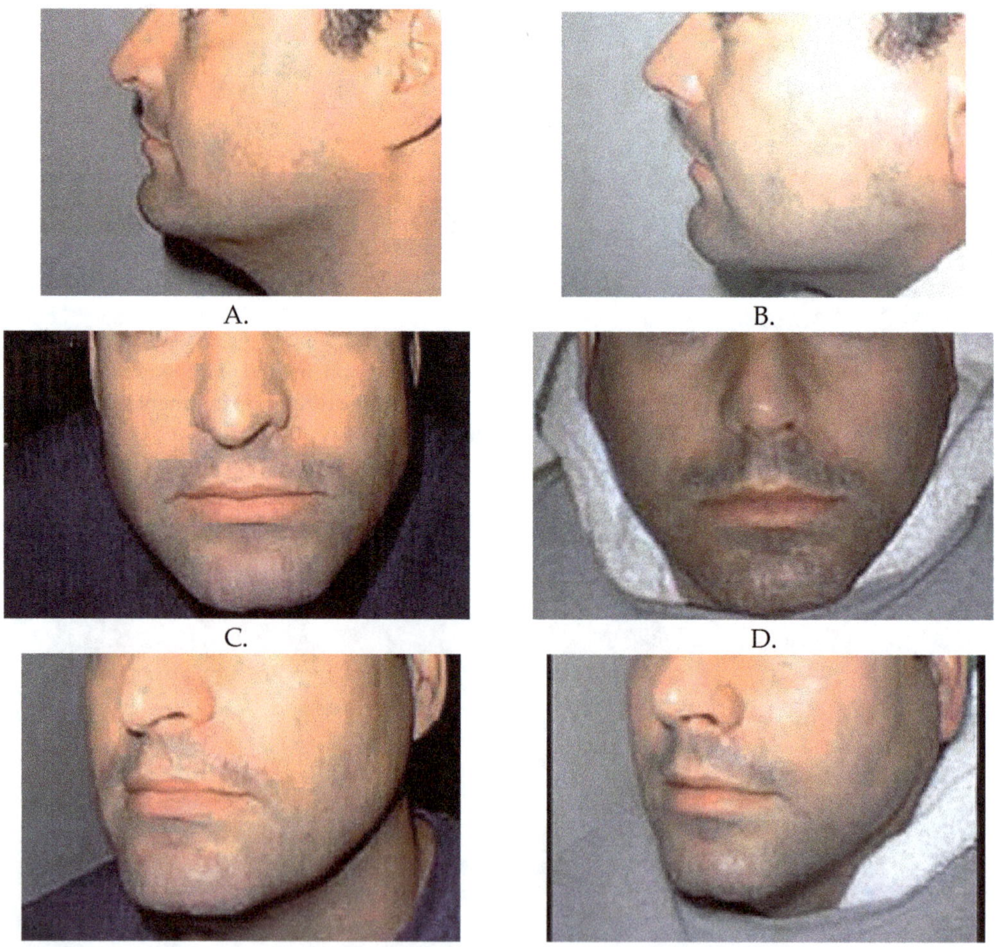

A. B. C. D. E. F.

**Figure 11.** **A, C, E.** Before. **B, D, F.** After lower face SMAS lift with retro-lobular incisions in a 40 years old man, plus T-excision and columella sliding rhinoplasty. No signs of an operated-on appearance. Defined cervico-mandibular angle post op.

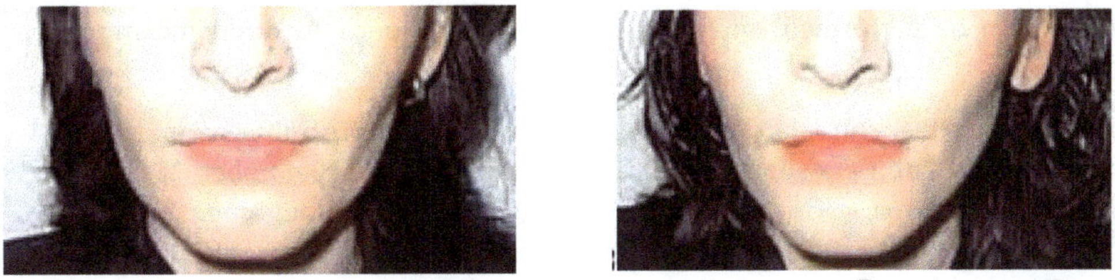

A. B.

**Figure 12.** **A.** Before. Thin and loose skin in the lower face. Gravity effect on the soft tissue and skin is visible in different positions. **B.** After lower SMAS-platysma lift with retro-lobular incisions in a 37 years old female patient. The SMAS, attached soft tissue and skin are tightened. No signs of gravity on the soft tissue and skin are visible in any position after surgery. Lovely tightened youthful "hungry cheeks", pleasing the patient.

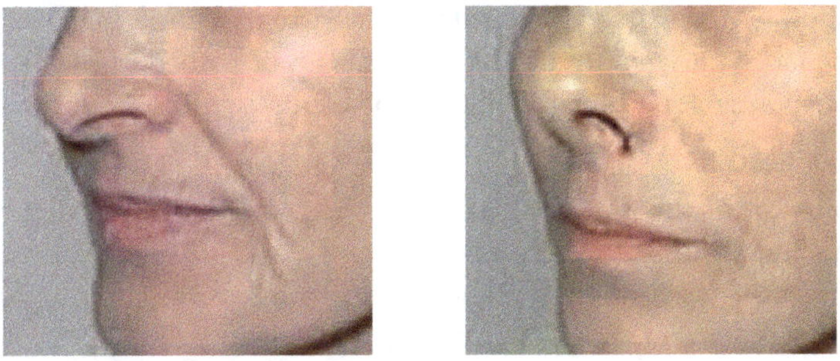

A. B.

**Figure 13.** **A.** Before, **B.** Effect on the nasolabial and marionette folds in a 53 years old patient after lower SMAS lift, rhinoplasty and allar base narrowing.

## 2.4. Complications

Minimal and very rare problems have occurred with the suture technique in some patients. As described above, one case of taking a facial nerve branch in the suture during performing method II led to ptosis of the upper lid and was solved immediately by removing of the suture. It is a rare complication, because the facial nerve runs a little higher, just below the tragus and immediately after that penetrates deep into the parotid gland. Sutures can be easily removed and placed again at any time with nearly no downtime.

In method I, the needle penetrates the tissue much lower and we have had no cases of facial nerve insertion in the suture. Three patients described some loss of sensation in the ear lobe for a couple of weeks. The trauma of involving the great auricular nerve in the suture, provoked by a lateral traction, adapts in some weeks. Swelling and bruising are rare.

## 2.5. Discussion

Beautification and immediate social activity are the first and most important aspect of patients' requirements. The author's experience indicates that his specific methods of lower

SMAS lift can be performed safely with minimum complications and maximum patient satisfaction.

Solely stretching the skin is an obsolete concept. Excision SMAS lifts, extended SMAS lift, deep plane, and sub-periostial face-lifts are associated with a number of complications, including haematoma, pixie ear, nerve injury, and skin sloughing. Deep-plane and composite techniques achieve a deeper suspension, but the risk of facial nerve injury is higher. Post-operative care is longer and pre- and retro-auricular incisions are not the patient's best contemporary option.

The author's suture methods are performed to obtain and preserve a youthful lower face and neck through fixing lower face and neck SMAS to mastoid (or very rarely to occipital periosteum). These techniques of "scarless lower SMAS face and neck lift" provide a safe alternative to other face lifts using preauricular skin incisions and elevation, platysmal and subplatysmal flaps, SMAS dissections, submental surgery, deep plane or composite face lifts. Injury to the facial nerve in rhytidectomy has been described in less than one percent of the cases, and a spontaneous return of function results within 6 months in more than 80 percent of these injuries.

With the introduction of the author's technique, performed without aggressive platysmal and subplatysmal flaps and SMAS dissections, the risk of injury to facial nerve branches has decreased significantly. Nevertheless, the operating surgeon must follow up the patient's reactions carefully for signs of facial palsy during operation.

The scarless lower face and neck SMAS lift by sutures, using skin needle perforations only or hidden retro-lobular incision, provides a safe and effective ambulatory method for beautification and rejuvenation of early and medium sagging face. It is an effective method that addresses problems of jowling or submental laxity. A nice and youthful shaped jaw, acute cervicomandibular angle and straightened cervical skin are the most desirable effects. The results fully correspond to patients' desires. The effect is immediate and without visible scars.

The lower SMAS lift is a bidirectional lower face and neck lift that gives a harmonious, strong lifting effect on the sub-zygomatic area and jaw and creates an acute cervicomandibular angle. It achieves partial correction of the nasolabial folds and submental area laxity.

In author's patients, the lower SMAS-platysma lift is very often combined with temporal, mid-face SMAS lift and brow lift by sutures, in order to obtain a "total SMAS lift". Generally, SMAS lifts by sutures are nice and easy ambulatory weekend procedures.

## 3. Chin enhancement and form correction

The primary goal of facial aesthetic (cosmetic) surgery is beautification, achieving balance and harmony. The mental area must be addressed to the complete synthesis of the face. The concept of augmenting, correcting and adjusting the chin position has evolved so significantly that it is now an important procedure in face beautification. Various autogenous implants for chin augmentation have been in use for over 100 years. The advent of synthetic materials has given rise to various types of alloplastic implants with their advantages, disadvantages and complications.

The author's technique of chin soft tissue suspension, using a simple durable suture with extended absorption delay, is indicated to correct microgenia, to obtain the necessary projection and to adjust chin symmetry. It is ideally suited for correction of most chin disproportions, such as: profile deficiencies, aging (witch) chin, asymmetries, disharmonies, and is used for beautification and rejuvenation of the entire face as a single or combined operation, with very satisfying cosmetic results.

## 3.1. Introduction

The importance of the chin in face beautification is determined by the fact that the chin is a part of the lower third of the face. Aesthetically it has to fit to the straight line of the noble profile, to the "beauty triangle" of the lower face, and the facial golden section rule of 3 proportionally equal parts. Chin prominence gives the essence of visage character.

Profile deficiencies are due to congenital, traumatic and aging factors with different degrees of deformity. Loss of volume or a genetically small mandible affect the aesthetics and expression of the face, mouth, chin, and neck. Disharmony between the skeletal support and the soft tissue envelope is a common cause of aesthetic concerns.

Although standards of beauty evolve over time, classical facial features such as symmetry, straight profile, good chin projection and proportions remain as rules. A comprehensive beautification (including rejuvenation of the chin) depends on accurate analysis of the lower face with attention to the contours and underlying structures.

Many surgical options are available to restore the definition of the chin region. A large variety of materials are used by surgeons for augmentation purposes, although the search for the perfect implant continues.

The author's surgical suspensory procedure, using a simple suture, has the aim to return the chin's soft tissue to a more aesthetic and youthful position and to meet patients' demands for immediate result, fast recovery and beatification without implanting foreign materials.

### *3.1.1. Anatomy*

Although the process of facial aging is predictable, the rate of changes varies from person to person. With aging, laxity develops in the skin and subcutaneous tissues, the result of which is an aesthetically incorrect projection and contour of the anterior mandible. The soft tissues are subject to gravity and undergo progressive atrophy. Aging (Witch) chin is an unpleasant aesthetic defect, characterized by ptosis of the premental tissue and a deep submental fold. Bone resorption and soft tissue atrophy are the most important components. Loss of bone volume leads to loss of support for the soft tissues of the face.

Aesthetic cosmetic rejuvenation of the face and neck involves repositioning of poorly supported soft tissues. The effect of surgery in these cases aims to improve and restore a youthful appearance. This depends on the bone structure, amount and distribution of subcutaneous fat, as well as the interconnectedness of the superficial muscles to the overlying skin.

*3.1.2. The objective* of the author's specific technique is to suspend the loose and hanging soft tissue of the chin, to give natural height of the chin projection and to advance the submental skin in order to obtain a youthful jaw line. Avoidance of common problems associated with implantation of foreign materials is an additional goal.

### *3.1.3. Definition*

Suturing and suspending the loose chin soft tissue in front of the immobile menton in order to obtain volume, projection and a straight profile. Using the suture method, the chin could be positioned forward, up or down, left or right, thus obtaining proper aesthetic proportions and facial symmetry.

### *3.1.4. Surgical approach*

Two skin punctures to insert the needle.

## 3.2. Author's surgical technique

One or more Serdev Sutures® of the chin soft tissue could be used to obtain roundness and projection of the chin, where desired. The author uses only two skin perforation points (A and B) in the sub- and supra- mental folds to insert the needle and perform a suture, which, bulging the sutured fibrotic soft tissue, creates volume in front of the immobile menton. An additional option is the horizontal suture with 2 lateral skin perforation points.

Using different angles of needle positioning, the author has introduced the Serdev Suture® method for total or partial enhancement, augmentation and positioning of the chin up or down (to adapt facial aesthetic proportions), or left or right (to obtain symmetry). I.e. chin lift is created tridimentionally: up or down, forward, left or right. Creation of a dimple is another option with author's techniques.

The author prefers to start from the submental skin perforation point A. **Video**: http://www.youtube.com/watch?v=oqJreY-JsCM. If more tissue is necessary, the perforation point A is located in the submental fold. When positioning the needle in the skin perforation point, the submental perforation has to be moved forward anteriorly to the menton. **NB!** Do not perforate the muscles dorsal to the menton. If a "Witch" chin has to be lifted, the submental skin perforation point should be positioned much more anteriorly, so the projection will be higher. If the chin has to be projected downwards, the second perforation point B can be lower than the supramental fold and first point A should be maximally dorsal at the submental fold. The suture can be placed more lateral to project one side of the chin only (to equalize symmetry), or the central chin tissue can be fixed to the mental periosteum more laterally with the same result.

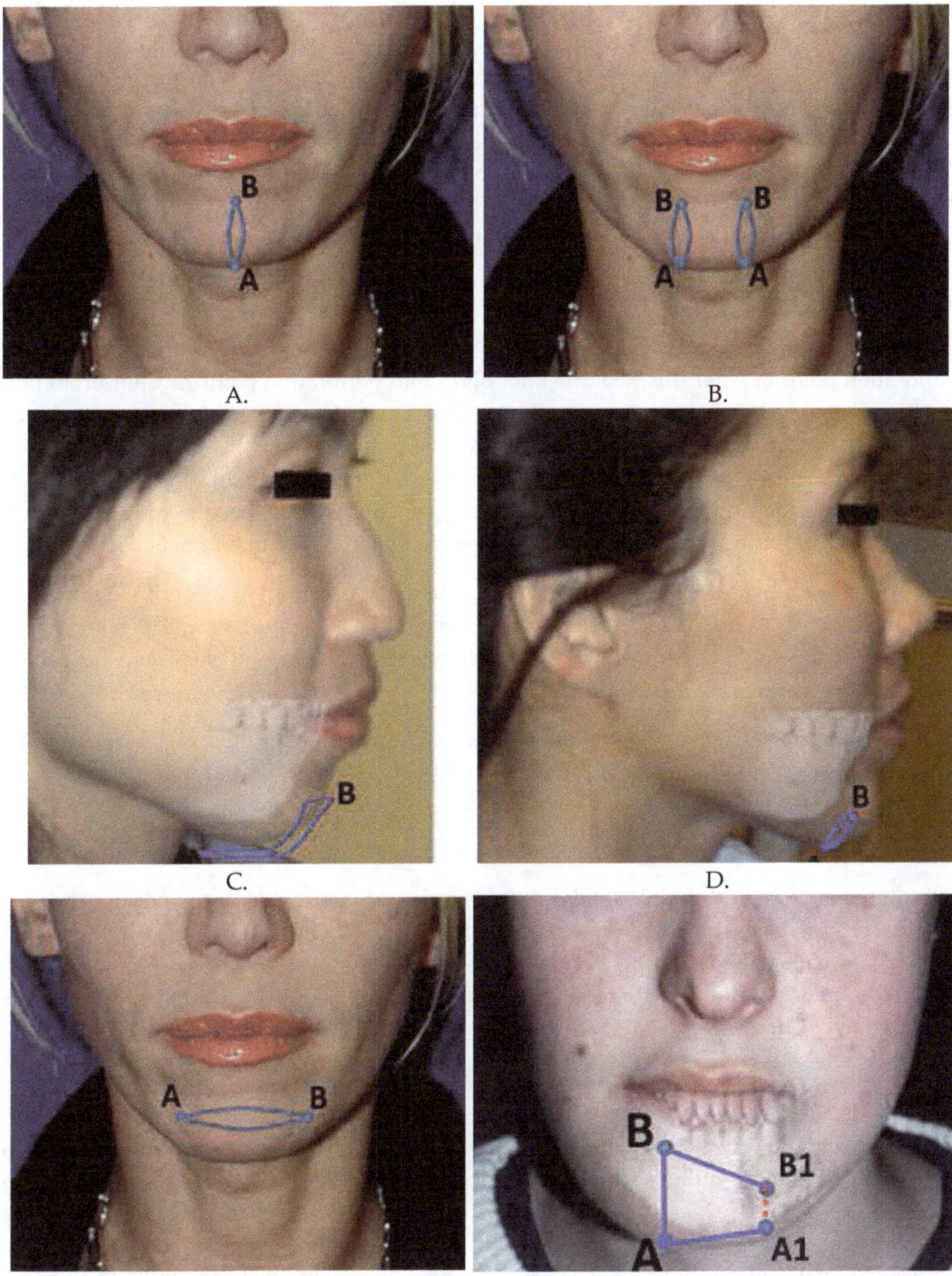


**Figure 14.** A, B, C, D, E, F. Different variations of fixation of the fibrotic soft tissue, with or without fixation to menton

### 3.3. Vertical chin suture

A 50 mm or 60 mm Serdev® needle enters through the submental skin puncture, then in front of the menton, slips along the anterior surface of the bone and exits through the other skin puncture at the supramental fold. After threading the needle with surgical suture USP 0, the suture is positioned in the deep first needle pass. Performing the second pass, the needle re-enters through point A, then medium deep through the soft tissue, and exits through point B to take the second suture end and introduce it in the second pass. **NB!** When performing the medium deep pass it should not be superficial. If skin dimpling appears above the needle, the pass is too superficial and should be repositioned deeper.

Thus, the suture circle is finalized and when pulling the suture, the suture loop dives in perforation point B. After it is tied, the knot dives into perforation point A. Chin projection is immedially visible. Then, any dimpling and skin attachment to the suture should be removed using a mosquito clamp. **NB!** If the needle pass does not engage dermis, removal of dimpling at the skin perforation points is easy. If dermis is caught, dimple removal is impossible and the suture procedure should be repeated. Twist the needle softly forward or backward to find its way through the skin perforation openings without fixation of dermis.

Performing such a suture, the available chin soft tissue is projected in front of the immobile menton and enhancement/augmentation is obtained. The angle of needle position gives direction of the enhancement - up, down, left or right. In cases of persistent deep chin dimple, 2 sutures are possible both sides.

If the projection is not sufficient, an additional horizontal suture can be added. The horizontal suture has 2 perforation points laterally and 2 passes should be done – the first one deep near the menton and the second - middle deep.

The number of sutures could be more than two, in order to obtain the necessary projection.

This ambulatory procedure takes only a few minutes. No dermal closure and no bandages are used. Facial wash should be done on the following day. The skin puncture in the supra-mental fold could be visible for 2-3 days and patients may use make up. The early post-operative period swelling is almost invisible and patients can return to their social life as soon as they wish.

### 3.4. Results

1095 patients underwent the above-described procedures for ambulatory suture chin augmentation in the author's clinic and abroad, between 1993 and 2012. Patients were followed up between 2 and 11 years and have reported excellent clinical success. No complications have been observed. There has been no aesthetic disappointment, no seromas, no haematomas and no infection. The soft tissue enhancement has been observed to be an average of 8.0 mm (range 4.1 to 11.8 mm). No asymmetry has been observed. On the contrary, this particular technique has been used to solve problems with asymmetry of the face. The author frequently leaves a bit of dimpling at the lower submental perforation area that defines the lower chin line better and enhances the Caucasian appearance that is very much appreciated by patients. Straight line of the profile has been obtained satisfactorily. Sometimes, additional 2-3 mm of chin prominence are required. In order to reach a straight profile line, a second suture enhancement has been done in 21 cases and in one case of pronounced retrogenia and small amount of soft tissue, the enhancement was done in 3 steps.

The obtained chin projection enhances the "beauty triangle" of the "chin and checkbone complex". The neckline becomes more slender and youthful. These visual criteria measure the degree of success in fashioning of chin aesthetics. We now believe that by using this soft tissue suture technique, with the exception of extreme cases, it is possible to satisfy the above-mentioned criteria in most patients.

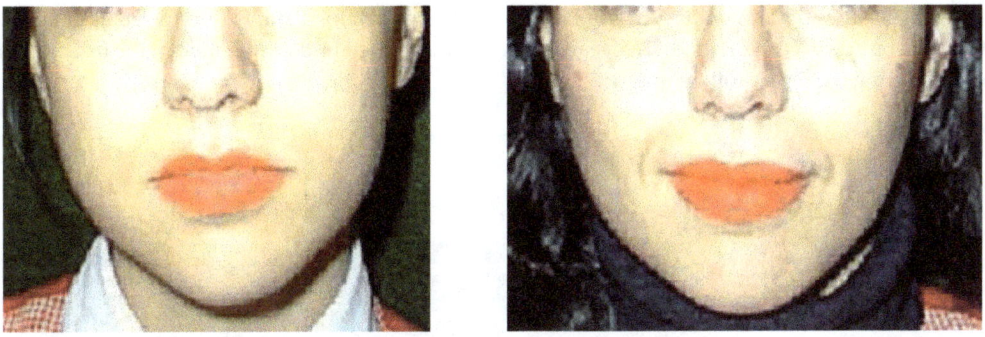

A. B.

**Figure 15.** **A.** Before and **B.** after chin correction and enhancement along with lower face ultrasonic liposculpture to obtain the beauty triangle of chin and cheekbones. The additional upper lip augmentation is a part of the face proportion adjustment and beautification.

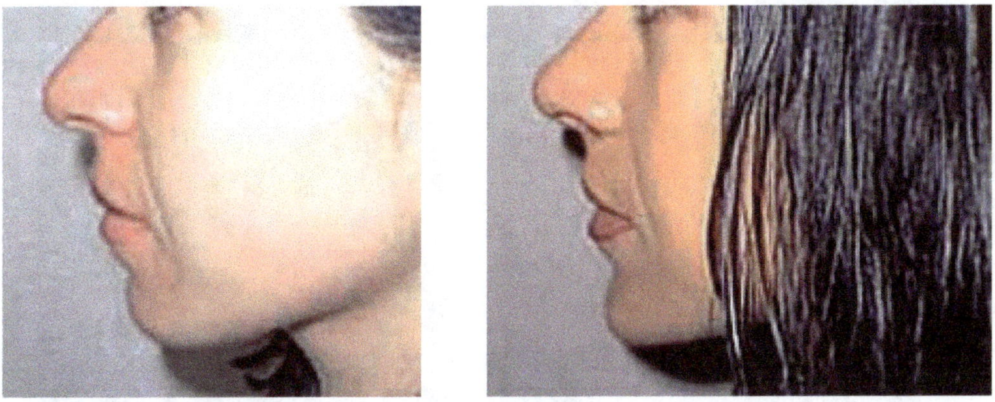

A. B.

**Figure 16.** **A.** Before and **B.** after chin enhancement to obtain straight line of the profile and define the jaw line, and good proportions with 3 equal parts of the face. Simultaneous rhinoplasty – T-excision and columella sliding for nasal tip rotation and projection.

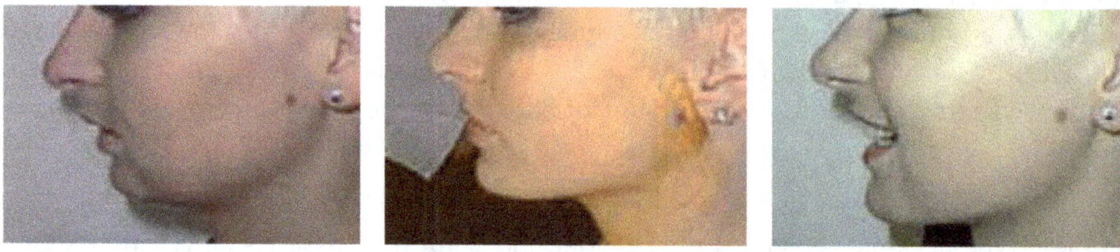

A. B. C.

**Figure 17.** **A.** Before, **B.** immediately after chin enhancement and tip rhinoplasty (T-excision and columella sliding) to obtain a straight profile and aesthetic proportions of the face (intra-op Betadine desinfection still not washed off). A slender neckline, due to skin lift forward (when moving the submental skin perforation point A in front of the menton) is obtained and is recognized as an attractive feature of youth with this method. **C.** 5 years later. It is difficult to find any change in the operated chin position during the 5 year follow up.

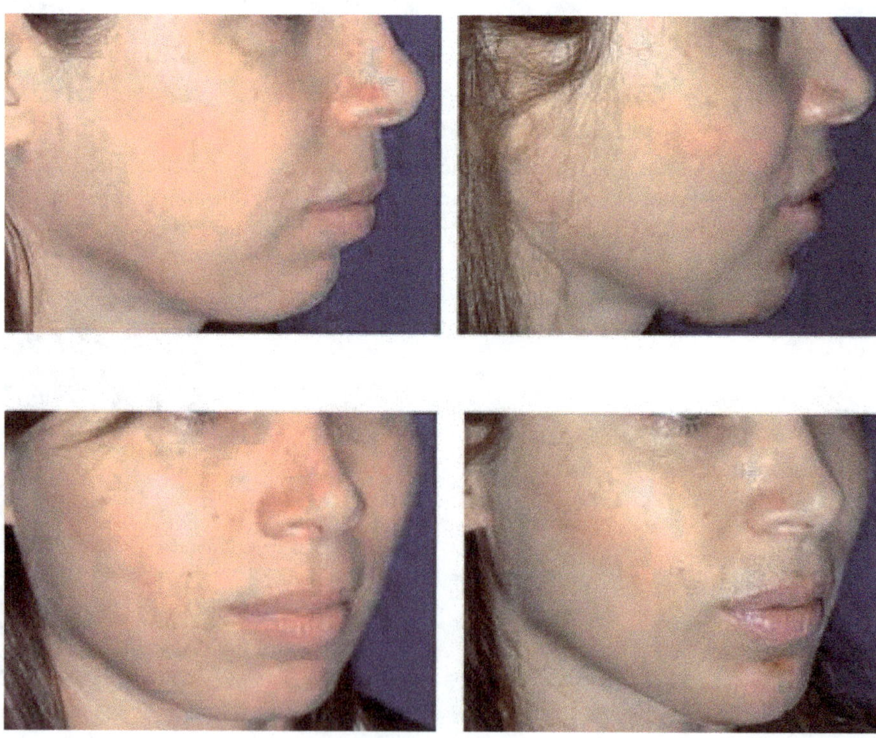

**Figure 18.** Better chin position is visible from all angles

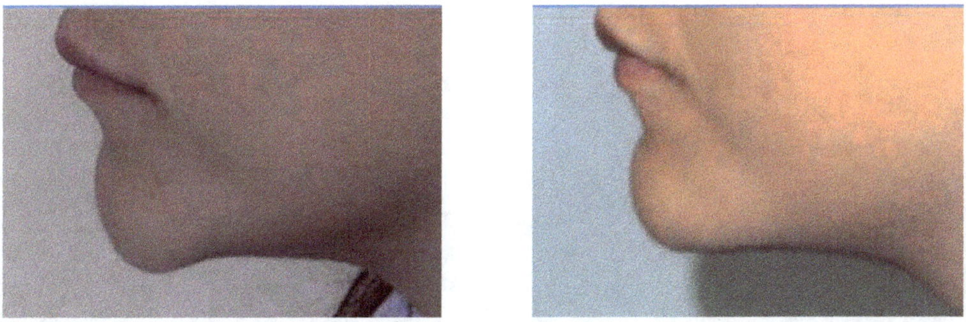

A. B.

**Figure 19.** **A.** Before – A witch chin in a young patient. **B.** After chin enhancement in front, suturing the tissue higher.

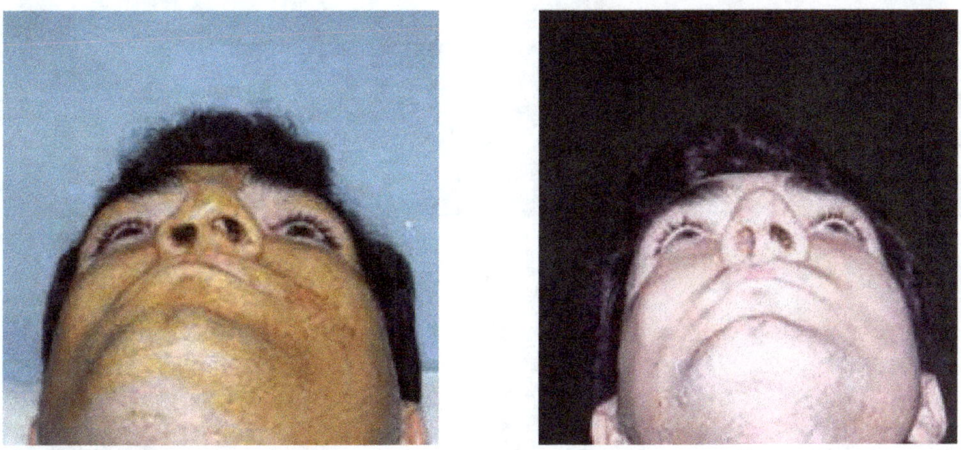

A. B.

**Figure 20.** **A.** Before (Betadine disinfected) and **B.** After correction of the chin position and nose deformity in one session. The chin is sutured to the left.

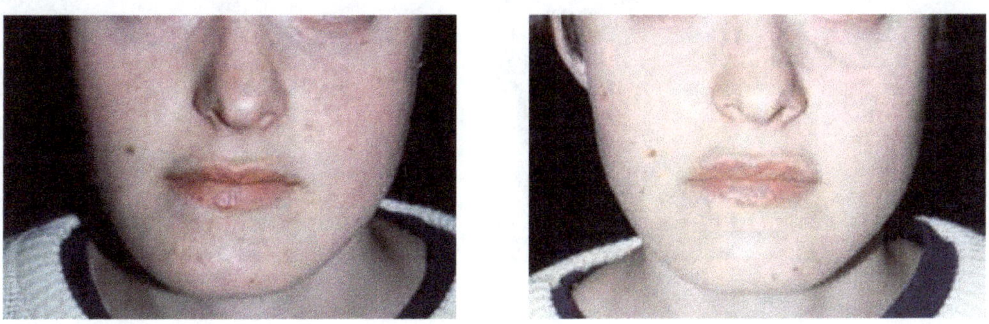

A. B.

**Figure 21.** **A** Before, **B.** After chin suture to the left to correct the deformity of the face.

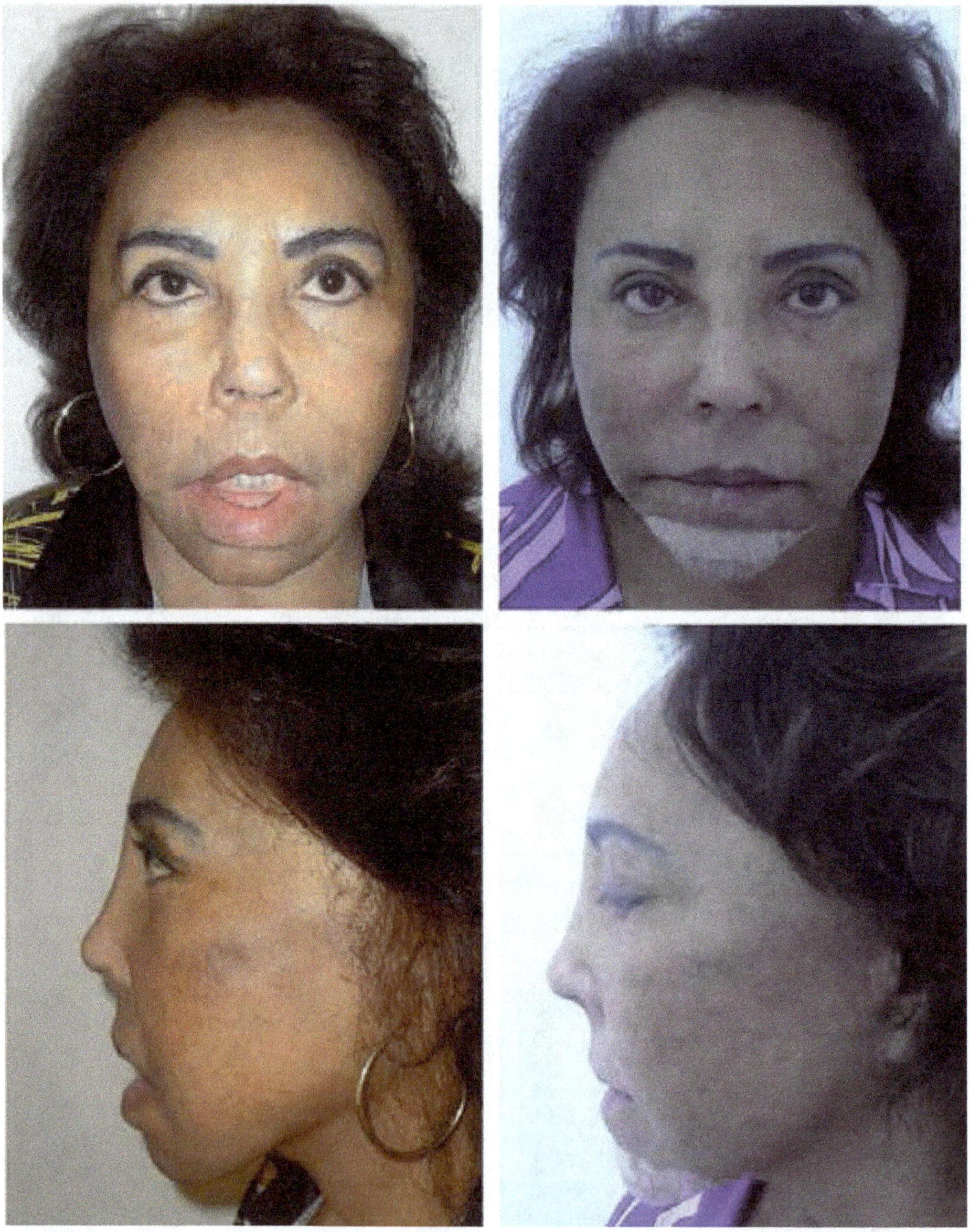

A. B.

**Figure 22.** **A.** Too much plastic surgery. Hanging chin/lower lip complex after removal of infected chin implant. **B.** Immediately after fixation of the chin fibrotic tissue to periosteum by suture.

The longevity of any technique depends on the stage and progression of aging, i.e. atrophy of the soft tissue and skeleton. The author has had a satisfactory longevity of results in his patients and secondary chin enhancement after years was necessary only in 5 cases. Using serial photography during the follow up period he has not noticed remarkable changes in the result.

The chin soft tissue suture technique for anterior adjustment and form correction provides a soft, natural facial appearance and it continues to be the method of choice for form correction, augmentation and beautification of the chin. All patients have rejected implantation techniques.

### 3.5. Chin dimple

Dimple formation is easy and consists of dermis fixation to periosteum by Serdev Suture® scarless closed approach. In such case, 2 points at the 2 ends of the dimple are used to capture the dermis between them. For this reason, the author may or may not use additional perforation points. It depends on what the patient wants – a dimple solely or with additional chin enhancement, and/or chin form correction.

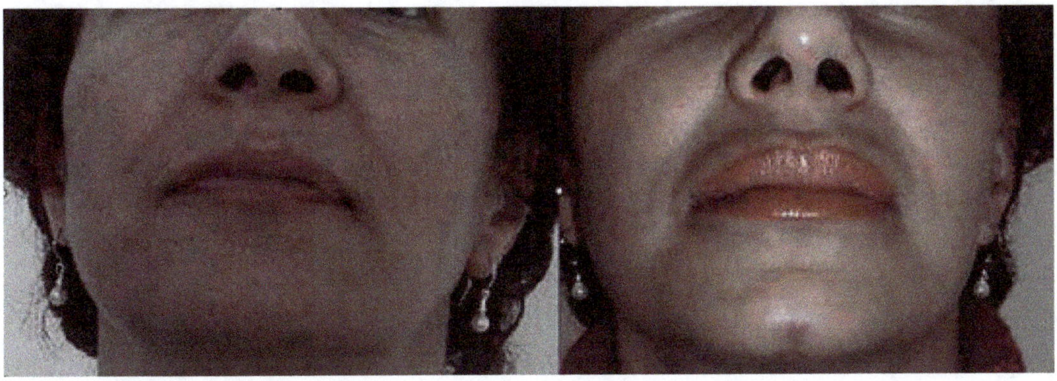

A. B.

**Figure 23.** Immediate result after scarless chin dimple formation by suture.

### 3.6. Discussion

For the past several decades, various materials have been developed to improve the appearance of the chin as one of the important subunits of the face. Initially, autogenous tissue grafts, such as: removed nasal hump, described by Aufricht in 1934, autogenous skeletal and cartilage transplants, ear cartilage grafts, rib cartilage grafts, fat, fascia, tendon, bone and dermal fat grafts have been used. Additional options became available with the development of a variety of alloplastic materials for augmentation genioplasty. Polymers are used primarily for bone deficiency substitution. Mersilene mesh introduced in 1950, silicone and silicone bag-gel inplants, Gore-Tex, Medpor, Supramid, Silastic, injectable collagen, expanded polytetrafluoroethylene (e-PTFE), high-density polyethylene (HDPE), polydimethylsiloxane (PDMS), Proplast I (PI), Proplast II (PII), porous block hydroxyapatite (PBHA) are available for correction of microgenia. Placed through an anterior oral sulcus incision or a submental incision with a screw fixation, many of these implants have good organotrophic characteristics, allowing tissue ingrowth. Available in a variety of block, sheet, and preformed shapes, they can be easily modeled and maintained. Antibiotics, irrigation, and closure of the incisions are performed. A lot of absorbable injectable materials came into the market in the last decade. Reviews of biomaterials used for mandibular implantation prove that although today's armamentarium of implant materials is vast, the search for the perfect implant continues.

Risks and complications with foreign materials: We address general considerations of toxicity relevant to all biomaterials. Investigations and overviews present data from a large number of clinical series on incidence of complications for materials used in this specific application. Although few, there are results that show infection, displacement, temporary paresthesias, incidences of absorption, rejection, or extrusion, implant migration, etc. Complications are manageable: these include implant displacement, infection has been treated with irrigation, closed system suction, etc. Most often infection requires a re-operation to remove the implant. Other complications such as internal and external soft tissue erosion, indentation, slippage, asymmetry and late bone resorption under the implant have been seen. Wound repair around implants is achieved through capsule formation. Fibrous capsule formation can be interrupted by infection, immune reaction, implant migration, or extrusion. No implant can be perfect for every face.

Due to the search of simpler techniques and based on his own experience, the author proposes an operation without implants, using only a suture of the chin soft tissue, suitable for chin enhancement, beautification and form correction. The author followed up 527 patients with chin augmentation and chin form correction for 2 and more years of whom no one had a complication. 398 of them had combined face beautification operations done.

As a single procedure or simultaneously with other facial rejuvenation operations, the chin suture of the soft tissue is ideally suited for correction of most chin aesthetic disharmonies in patients with a congenitally small mandible, patients requesting facial beautification and rejuvenation as well as correction of asymmetry. Simplicity and immediate return to social life are the major benefits of this procedure. It provides a natural, "non-operated-on" look that is largely sought after by patients today.

As implants are foreign bodies with some limits of longevity, they are mostly not accepted in the author's selection of patients and his technique became a method of choice, minimizing the tissue trauma. It appears to be an attractive alternative to other chin augmentation techniques.

## 4. Total face beautification using Serdev Sutures®

Beautification is the main goal in cosmetic surgery. Both words "cosmetic" in Latin and "aesthetic" in Greek language mean "beautification". Cosmetic and aesthetic surgery are wrongly understood as rejuvenation, anti aging, restoration, reconstruction etc., if no beautification is obtained.

It has been found that certain points in a face composition automatically attract the observer's attention. Many objects and scenes with certain proportions please us automatically.

### 4.1. Aesthetic proportions

Aesthetics as a science has been first established in ancient Greece and is based on aesthetic proportions, angles and volumes. Those aesthetic rules are intransient and are a persistent base for the understanding of beauty in all ethnic groups and cultures. It is studied in "History of Art".

In face aesthetics, the main proportion guidelines are given by **the Golden Section Rule** – the face is divided into 3 equal parts. Ancient Greeks have found that distance between columns has to be equal, to give an aesthetic perspective from different points of view. Leonardo da Vinci investigated the principle that underlies our notions of beauty and harmony and called it the Golden Section. Long before Leonardo, Babylonian, Egyptian, and ancient Greek masters also applied the Golden Section proportion in architecture and art.

Another golden rule is **the Golden Ratio** of 1.6 (1.6180339887…) that is an important rule in human body and extremity proportions. It is attracting our attention so much that credit cards have been created using the golden ratio.

#### *4.1.1. Aesthetic angles*

As face ptosis affects the lateral face, angles should be positioned higher (laterally) to create the beauty of youth, corresponding to the mask of comedy in ancient theatre, unlike the mask of tragedy. So, the lifting effect on face should be lateral.

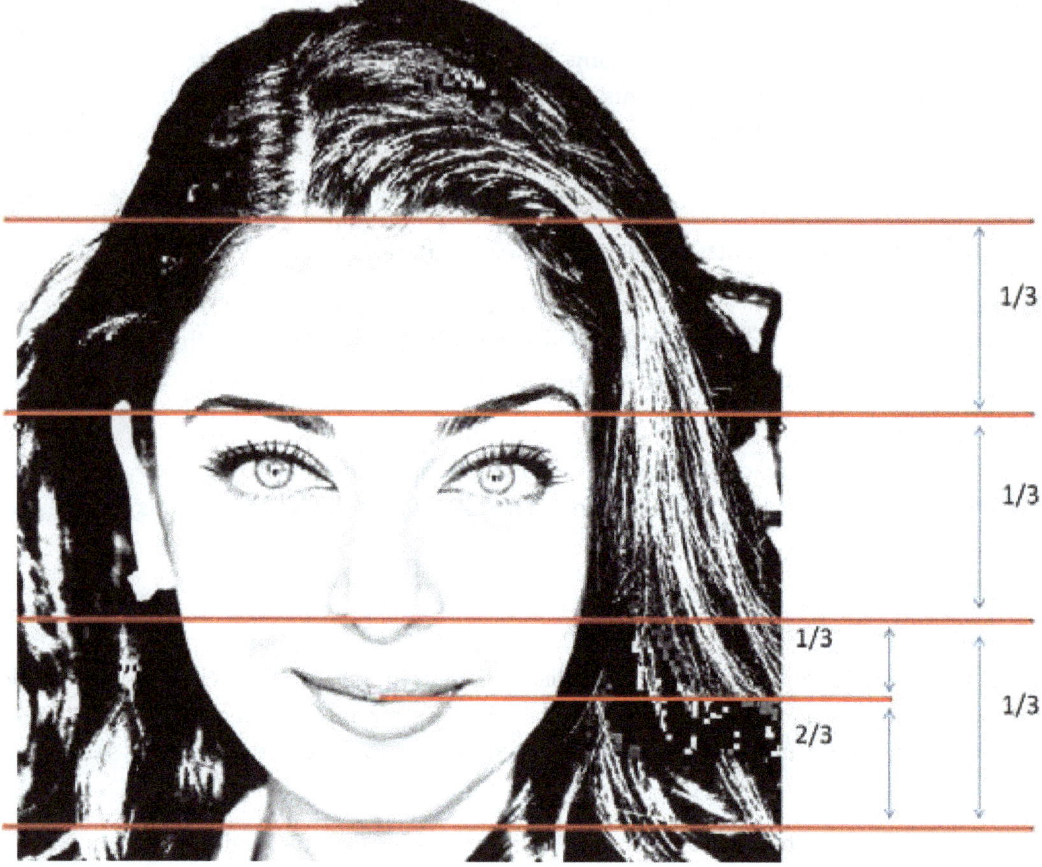


**Figure 24.** The Golden Section Rule permits precise examination of the face and its proportions

### *4.1.2. Aesthetic volumes*

In the face, the "beauty triangle" visualizes apparent chin and cheekbones. Higher cheekbones represent youth.

The straight profile line is a noble sign.

As people look each other in the eyes when communicating, our first goal is to open and give light to the eyes and never modify them into an "operated-on" appearance.

Considering patient faces we can recognize unaesthetic signs. Following aesthetic rules, regardless of age, we can add beauty to a face.

The main goal of Serdev Sutures® is to create the appropriate aesthetic proportions, volumes and angles in face and body.

## 4.2. Some clinical cases

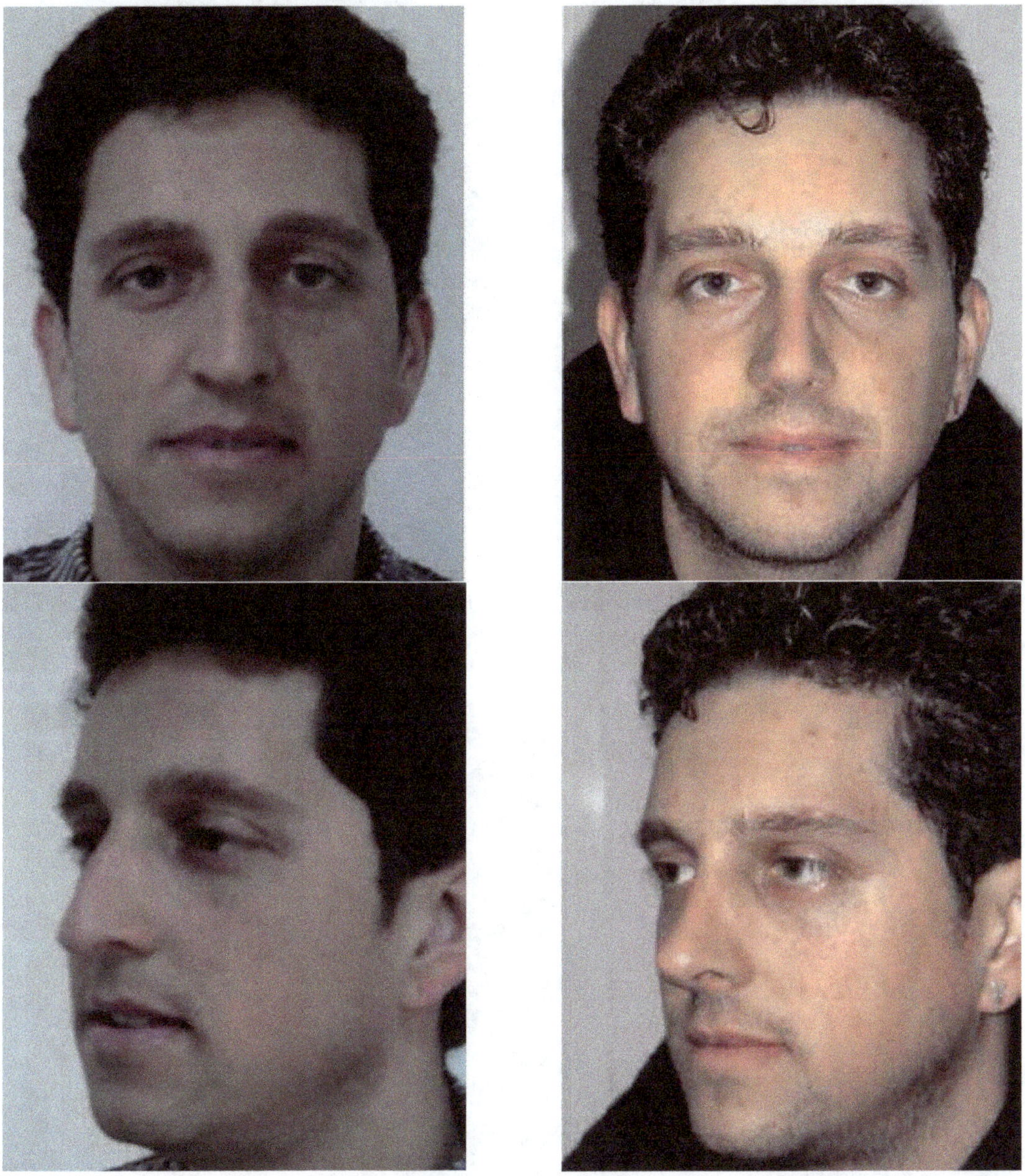

A. B.

**Figure 25. A.** Before: Low eyebrows give darkness to the eyes; unaesthetic proportions – the Golden Section Rule of the face is not present; nobleness is not present - retrograde chin, profile line is not straight. The proportion ratio in the lower third of the face is 1:3 instead of 1:2. **B.** After: Brow lift to open the eyes. Their color is finally visible; Rhinoplasty to create the 3 equal thirds (golden section rule), chin enhancement to create more visible beauty triangle (in men, the cheekbones should not look "sweet"), straight profile and proper lower face third ratio of 1:2. The result is **total face beautification**. "Playboy" ear pendant serves to demonstrate patient's self-confidence after surgery.

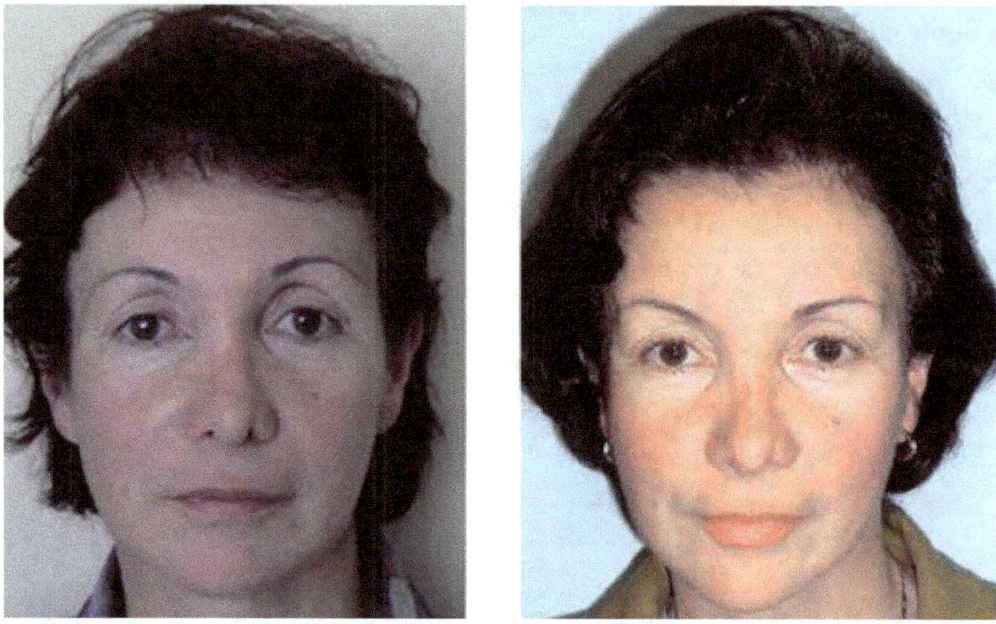

A. B.

**Figure 26.** **A.** Before: Brow ptosis, hollow eyes, gradual facial ptosis. Sad appearance. **B.** After Temporal and Brow Serdev Suture® lifts: eyes and face are full of light. See the color of the eyes. The Golden Section Rule is apparent. The lower face is changed from heavy and square into fresh and oval.

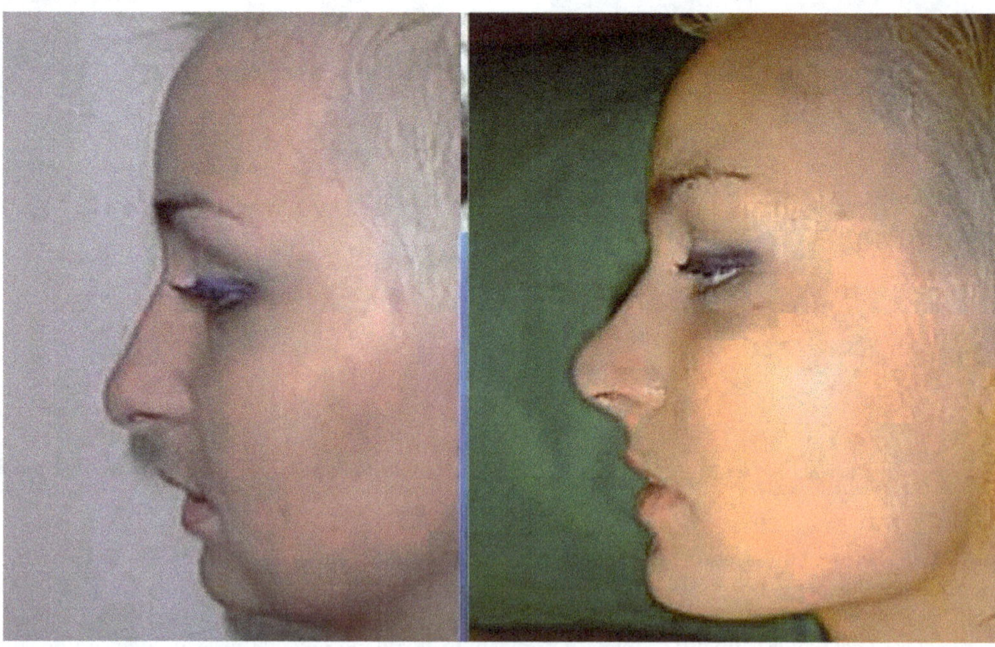

A. B.

**Figure 27.** **A.** Before. Nice young lady, but with longer nose, small chin; disrupted golden section rule, lower face proportion and the line of straight profile. **B.** Immediate beautification results in the operating theater after temporal lift by suture to lift the facial angles laterally and repositioning the cheekbone soft tissue; rhinoplasty to obtain the 3 equal parts of the face (golden section rule) - author's T-excision for tip rotation and columella sliding for tip projection, and chin enhancement to obtain the straight profile, beauty triangle and proper proportion ratio 1:2 in the lower third of the face. Suturing the chin in front has defined the jaw line. Skin still not cleaned from the Braunol. No operated-on appearance, immediately after 3 operations (including 2 suture lifts).

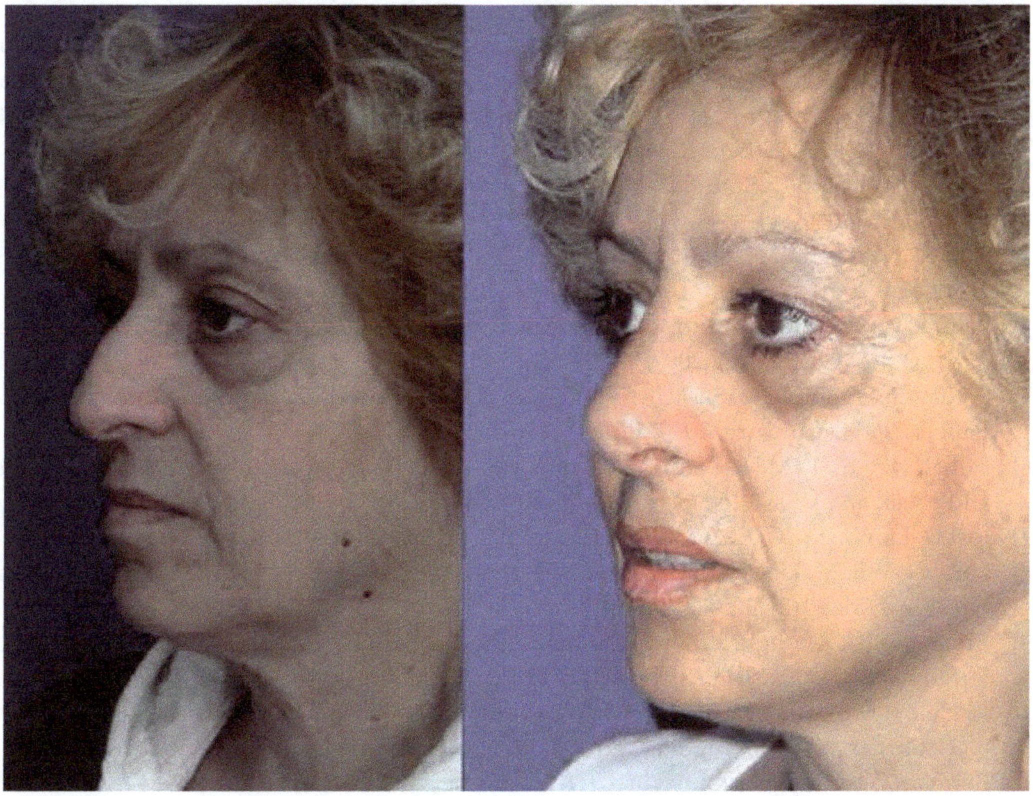

A. B.

**Figure 28. A.** Before: aging face, disproportions and lack of aesthetics in all proportions, volumes and angles. **B.** After scarless closed approach suture Brow, Temporal, Mid-face, Lower face and neck lift, Chin enhancement and Rhinoplasty. Fresh No operated-on appearance and open eye look, sparkling radiation, proper proportions are present, straight profile, angles lifted laterally, volumes, beauty triangle, defined jaw line and cervico-mandibular angle are present. Better skin texture. Blepharoplasty and cheekbone lift could be added, if and when patient decides.

## 5. Conclusion

In a way, cosmetic surgery as a multidisciplinary science is a fine art, inherently combining knowledge of architecture, sculpture, painting, design, fashion and even poetry. Scarless closed approach Serdev Suture® lifts, suspensions and tissue volumizing serve to create beauty on the basis of a proper understanding of anatomy, aesthetics as a science, ideal proportions, angles and volumes.

## Author details

Nikolay Serdev
*New Bulgarian University, Sofia, Bulgaria*

## 6. References

[1] Serdev, N.P. Year 1994, Suture Suspensions For Lifting Or Volume Augmentation In Face And Body (English version), presented at the 2nd Annual Meeing of the National Bulgarian Society for Aesthetic Surgery and Aesthetic Medicine, Sofia, 18 March 1994, Int J Aesth Cosm, 2001,1:1, 2561-2568

[2] Serdev NP. Serdev Suture Techniques Lower SMAS Face Lift, Original Papers, Int J Cosm Surg, 2009, 9:4, 1 - 2

[3] Serdev NP.Ambulatory temporal SMAS lift using minimal hidden incisions. IJACBS, 1(2):17-24, 2001.

[4] Serdev NP. Serdev Suture Techniques Lower SMAS Face Lift (Bulgarian), Original Papers, Int J Cosm Surg, 2009, 9:4, 1-12

[5] Serdev NP. SERDEV SUTURE TECHNIQUES - Lower SMAS Face LIFT, Original Papers, Int J Cosm Surg, 2010, 10:1, 1-2

[6] Mitz V, Peyronie M. The superficial musculo-aponeurotic system (SMAS) in the parotid and cheek area. Plast Reconstr Surg 58: 80-88, 1976.

[7] Jost G, Lamouche G. SMAS in rhytidectomy. Aesthetic Plast Surg 2: 69-74, 1982

[8] Larabee WF, Makielski KH, Cupp C. Facelift anatomy. Facial Plastic Surgery Clinics of North America 1(2): 135-52, 1993.

[9] Brennan HG. Rhytidectomy: Mandibular and submandibular contouring. Facial Plastic Surgery Clinics of North America 1(2): 181-96, 1993.

[10] Kridell RWH, Covello LV. The aging face (rhytidectomy). In BJ Bailey (ed.): Head & Neck Surgery – Otolaryngology, 2nd edition. Lippincott – Raven, 1998, pp. 2693-716.

[11] Berman WE. Rhytidectomy. In CJ Krause (ed.) Aesthetic Facial Surgery. Lippincott, 1991, pp 513-31.

[12] Dedo DD. The aging neck. In BJ Bailey (ed.): Head & Neck Surgery – Otolaryngology, 2nd edition. Lippincott – Raven, 1998, pp. 2717-32.

[13] Baker DC, Conley J. Avoiding facial nerve injuries in rhytidectomy. Anatomical variations and pitfalls. Plast Reconstr Surg 6: 781-95, 1979

[14] Seckel BR. Facial Danger Zones: Avoiding Nerve Injury in Facial Plastic Surgery. Quality Medical Publishing, St. Louis, 1994.

[15] Webster RC, Smith RC, Papsidero MJ, et al. Comparison of SMAS plication with SMAS imbrication in face lifting. Laryngoscope 92: 901-12, 1982.

[16] Lewis JR. Multiple-tiered deep support of cheeks in meloplasty and rhytidectomy. Aesthetic Plast Surg 1: 21-5, 1983

[17] Owsley JQ. SMAS-platysma facelift. A bidirectional cervicofacial rhytidectomy. Clin Plast Surg 3: 429-401, 1983

[18] Randall P,Skiles MS. The "SMAS sling": an additional fixation in face lift surgery. Ann Plast Surg 1:5-9, 1984
[19] Webster RC, Smith RC, Smith KF. Face lift, Part 4: Use of superficial musculoaponeurotic system suspending sutures. Head Neck Surg 3: 780-91,1984
[20] McCoullough EG, Perkins SW, Langsdon PR. SASMAS suspension rhytidectomy. Arch Otolaryngol Head Neck Surg 115: 228-34, 1989.
[21] Hamra ST. The deep-plane rhytidectomy. Plast Reconstr Surg 86: 53-61, 1990.
[22] Hamra ST. Composite rhytidectomy. Plast Reconstr Surg 90:1-13, 1992.
[23] Ramirez OM. The subperiosteal rhytidectomy: The third-generation facelift. Ann Plast Surg 28: 218-232, 1992.
[24] Beeson WH. Extended posterior rhytidectomy. Facial Plastic Surgery Clinics of North America 1(2): 197-216, 1993.
[25] Serdev, N.P. Chin form correction and augmentation using simple suture. Int J Aesth Cosm Beauty Surg IJACBS 2001, 3 (1), 42-66
[26] Serdev, N.P. Chin Form Correction And Augmentation Using A Simple Suture, Presentations, Int J Cosm Surg, 2003, 3:3, 1-36
[27] Serdev, N.P. Chin Enhancement And Form Correction Using A Suture Of The Soft Tissue, Original Papers, Int J Cosm Surg, 2002, 2:1, 1-10
[28] Serdev, N.P. Chin augmentation using simple suture. Int J Cosm Surg 2001, 2 (1) 42-66
[29] Mottura AA. Chin augmentation with nasal osteocartilaginous graft. Plast Reconstr Surg 2002 Feb;109(2):783-7
[30] Karras SC, Wolford LM. Augmentation genioplasty with hard tissue replacement implants. J Oral Maxillofac Surg. 1998 May;56(5):549-52
[31] Cox AJ 3rd, Wang TD. Skeletal implants in aesthetic facial surgery. Facial Plast Surg 1999;15(1):3-12
[32] Hwang K. Chin augmentation with a bone graft from the mandibular region. J Craniofac Surg 2000 Nov;11(6):543-6
[33] Ramirez OM. Mandibular matrix implant system: a method to restore skeletal support to the lower face. Plast Reconstr Surg 2000 Jul;106(1):176-89
[34] Gubisch W, Kotzur A. Our experience with silicone in rhinomentoplasty. Aesthetic Plast Surg 1998 Jul-Aug;22(4):237-44
[35] Snyder GB, Courtiss EH, Kaye BM, Gradinger GP.A new chin implant for microgenia. Plast Reconstr Surg 1978 Jun;61(6):854-61
[36] Schoenrock LD, Chernoff WG. Subcutaneous implantation of Gore-Tex for facial reconstruction. Otolaryngol Clin North Am 1995 Apr;28(2):325-40
[37] Lewis RP, Schweitzer J, Odum BC, Lara WC, Edlich RF, Gampper TJ. Sheets, 3-D strands, trimensional (3-D) shapes, and sutures of either reinforced or nonreinforced expanded polytetrafluoroethylene for facial soft-tissue suspension, augmentation, and reconstruction. J Long Term Eff Med Implants 1998;8(1):19-42
[38] Singh S, Baker JL Jr. Use of expanded polytetrafluoroethylene in aesthetic surgery of the face. Clin Plast Surg 2000 Oct;27(4):579-93
[39] Gross EJ, Hamilton MM, Ackermann K, Perkins SW. Mersilene mesh chin augmentation. A 14-year experience. Arch Facial Plast Surg 1999 Jul-Sep;1(3):183-9

[40] Sclaroff A, Williams C. Augmentation genioplasty: when bone is not enough. Am J Otolaryngol 1992 Mar-Apr;13(2):105-8

[41] Kheir JN, Leslie LF, Fulmer NL, Edlich RF, Gampper TJ. Polydimethylsiloxane for augmentation of the chin, malar, and nasal bones. J Long Term Eff Med Implants 1998;8(1):55-67

[42] Yaremchuk MJ. Mandibular augmentation. Plast Reconstr Surg 2000 Sep;106(3):697-706

[43] Odum BC, Bussard GM, Lewis RP, Lara WC, Edlich RF, Gampper TJ. High-density porous polyethylene for facial bone augmentation. J Long Term Eff Med Implants 1998;8(1):3-17

[44] Dann JJ, Epker BN. Proplast genioplasty: a retrospective study with treatment recommendations. Angle Orthod 1977 Jul;47(3):173-85

[45] Qian Y, Fan Z, Yang Q. Application of MEDPOR surgical implant in the craniofacial reconstruction Zhongguo Xiu Fu Chong Jian Wai Ke Za Zhi 1998 Mar;12(2):71-3

[46] Jafar M, Younger RA. Screw fixation mentoplasty. J Otolaryngol 2000 Oct;29(5):274-8

[47] Rubin JP, Yaremchuk MJ. Complications and toxicities of implantable biomaterials used in facial reconstructive and aesthetic surgery: a comprehensive review of the literature. Plast Reconstr Surg 1997 Oct;100(5):1336-53

[48] Robinson M, Shuken R. Bone resorption under plastic chin implants. J Oral Surg 1969 Feb;27(2):116-8

[49] Maas CS, Merwin GE, Wilson J, Frey MD, Maves MD. Comparison of biomaterials for facial bone augmentation. 1: Arch Otolaryngol Head Neck Surg 1990 May;116(5):551-6

[50] Sclafani AP, Romo T 3rd. Collagen, human collagen, and fat: the search for a three-dimensional soft tissue filler. Facial Plast Surg 2001 Feb;17(1):79-85

[51] Constantinides MS, Galli SK, Miller PJ, Adamson PA. Malar, submalar, and midfacial implants. Facial Plast Surg 2000;16(1):35-44

[52] Moenning JE, Wolford LM. Chin augmentation with various alloplastic materials: a comparative study. Int J Adult Orthodon Orthognath Surg 1989;4(3):175-87

[53] Romo T 3rd, Baskin JZ, Sclafani AP. Augmentation of the cheeks, chin and pre-jowl sulcus, and nasolabial folds. Facial Plast Surg 2001 Feb;17(1):67-78

[54] Jones RH. The effects of zygomatic and chin augmentation on facial aesthetics. Ann R Australas Coll Dent Surg 1998 Oct; 14:114-8

# 2

# Percutaneous Suspension Sutures to Change the Nasal Tip

M. B. Des Fernandes

## 1. Introduction

Although a number of procedures have been described for placement of "shaping sutures" during open and closed rhinoplasty, scant attention is given to the possibility of percutaneous placement of sutures without dissection of the skin envelop. Periodically patients will present who want minimal changes to their nose because the tip is too bulky, not well defined and the nose is longer than ideal. Many of these patients have no concerns about the bridge width and do not have a dorsal hump. This is the perfect patient to consider using the operation that will be described.

Many other patients have had an attractive straight nose when they were young and as they have aged, the nose has become coarser, broader and tends to lengthen and lose support from the septum and then droops into becoming a hooked nose. The operation that will be described specifically addresses these changes and with this surprisingly simple operation, the nose can be restored to much closer to the original.

Other patients who have had a corrective rhinoplasty develop a typical "polly-beak" deformity. By elevating and rotating the nasal cartilages one can restore a normal nasal tip projection and a straight bridge.

## 2. Methods and instruments

The following instruments and materials are required:

1. 11 or 15 blade scalpel
2. 18 gauge (green) needle or a 22 (yellow) spinal needle.
3. Sharp pointed fine scissors
4. Fine dissector (optional)

5. Toothed Adson's forceps.
6. Fine needle holder to tie the knot.
7. Skin hook to free the skin from the buried thread
8. 4/0 or 5/0 non-absorbable suture. This could be an elasticised suture as described by Serdev.

The procedure is usually done in an office setting on an ambulatory patient under simple local anaesthetic usually without the need for any sedation.

The guide-line markings are made on the nose with the patient sitting up to assess the degree of droop of the nose and get an impression of the amount of lift and rotation of the tip of the alar cartilages that will be required to get the ideal result and then to feel how much more the nose may comfortably be lifted to exaggerate the immediate result.

## 3. Standard markings

1. A dot is placed to the right side of the dorsum of the nose immediately below the osteo-cartilagenous junction of the bridge of the nose, about 4 mm from the midline. This point is chosen so that when the anchoring transfixion suture goes through the cartilaginous septum, the tract will be anterior to the anterior nasal mucosal recess inside the nose.
2. Then a line is drawn on the side of the nose directed towards the lowest part of the columella (see Fig 1).

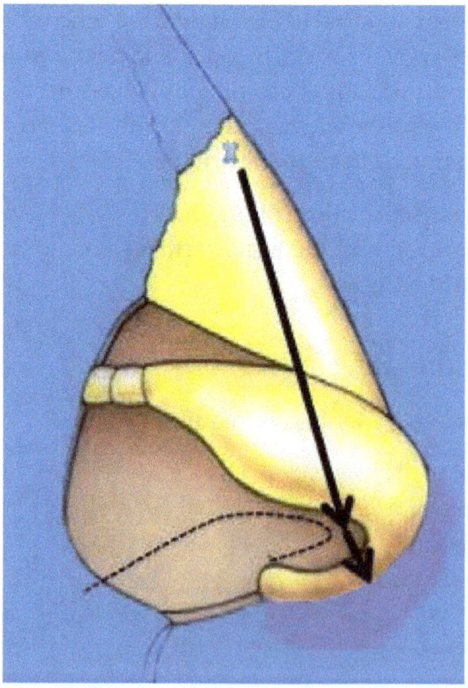

**Figure 1.** Showing the markins on the lateral side of the nose for the standard nose.

3. The line will traverse the soft triangle of the nostril as it courses towards the lowest part of the columella. Usually this is at the position where the columella changes angle in the "ideal" nose.
4. As one draws this line one has to take into account the shape of the lower lateral alar cartilages. (See Fig 2). Normally as seen from the front in figure 2, the line is straight downwards.

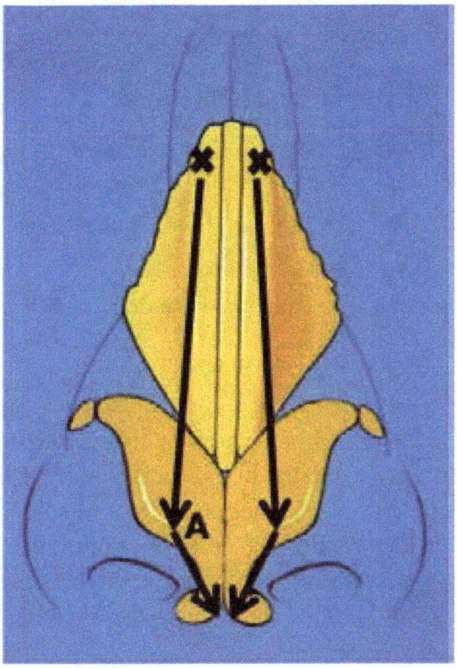


**Figure 2.** Showing the skin markings for the standard nose

5. However, if the cartilages are bulging and wide then one should deviate the line laterally towards the maximum width as seen from the frontal view. (See Fig 3) Generally if one presses on the lateral alar wings one can determine where this essential point is to apply medial pressure in order to narrow the nose tip. Its worth spending time familiarising yourself with these little details.
6. Then mark the midline of the columella with a vertical 3-4 mm line where the incision will be made. This incision is also dependant on where the columella will be lifted.
7. Similar markings are made on the opposite side.

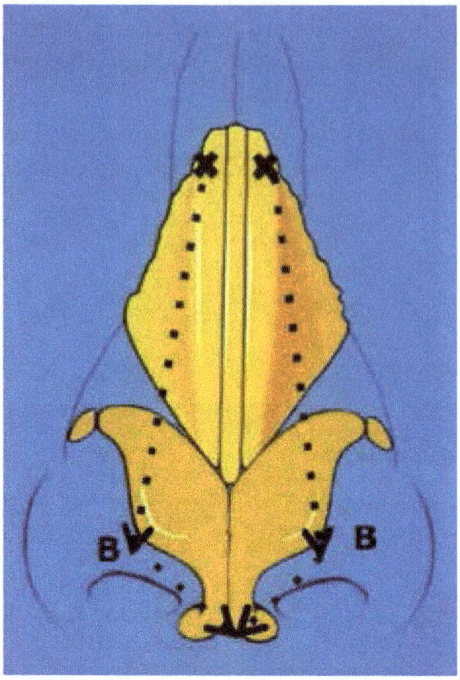


**Figure 3.** Showing the markings for a nose with broad alar dome cartilages.

## 4. Anaesthesia

An inferior orbital nerve block should be done first and in some people this gives excellent anaesthesia of the whole nose especially if the local anaesthetic is placed in the inferior orbital foramen. In other people it may be necessary to add specific block to the lateral nasal nerves as well as the nerves at the nasal spine to the columella. By blocking these nerves, anaesthesia is achieved easily and painlessly. It is advisable to check that the septal cartilage is numb by infiltrating across to the other side where the anchors will be placed.

## 5. Placement of the suspension sutures

1. Two stab incisions need to be made at the points marked X in figures 1 and 2 and then use the sharp pointed scissors to make sure to dissect the skin away from the cartilage that the skin is entirely free of the surrounding deep tissues. These holes should be as small as possible.
2. Make the incision on the columella and then dissect the skin away from the vertical alar cartilages in the area and extend the dissection area across into the "soft triangle" and even to the inferior edge of the lateral lower alar cartilages. By doing this one reduces the possibility of the needle passing into the nose as it is pushed across the "soft triangle" down towards the incision in the columella.
3. Insert the chosen needle perpendicularly through the incision on the right side of the nose

4. Once one reaches the layer just outside the upper lateral cartilage, change direction of the needle and point it down under the guidelines previously marked.
5. One has to distort the nose by pushing it medially and at the same time it is useful to put the Adson's forceps into the columella incision in order to retrieve the needlepoint. Make sure that the needle does not catch any tissue of the columella.
6. The needle is now positioned outside of the nasal cartilages and the non-absorbable thread (4/0 or 5/0) is passed up the needle until it protrudes through the hub at the end of the needle.
7. Pull back the needle until one reaches the entry point on the side of the nose, change direction to be perpendicular again and then push the needle through the septal cartilage to emerge through the opposite incision without catching any of the tissues attached to skin. This is the anchor so one has to be sure that the thread is not too close to the edge of the cartilage. It is easy to avoid the anterior nasal mucosal recess because it does not come into the sharp angle between the nasal septum and the upper lateral cartilages
8. Hold on to the thread and remove the needle. Most people expect that the bevel of the needle will cut the suture as it goes through the septum, but it generally never does. In doing this type of procedure for several thousands of times, the thread has been cut only twice. By this stage we have constructed more than half of the important loop that will eventually narrow, rotate and lift the alar cartilages.
9. The final stage is approached differently. The needle is now carefully inserted into the columella incision taking care not to catch any of the outer skin layer in the soft triangle of the left nostril and then pushed up to the stab incision on the left side of the nose.
10. By using the Adson's forceps one can guide the needle tip out through the stab incision without catching the surrounding soft tissue.
11. The thread is passed through the needle until it emerges from the needle hub before the needle is pulled out.
12. The suspension loop has now been created outside the upper and lower lateral alar cartilages and one can check what the nose looks like as one tightens the threads. The nose tip is lifted and the lower lateral alar cartilages are compressed towards each other medially and narrowed.
13. Examine the inside of the nostrils to be certain that the thread has not been accidentally placed medial to the alar cartilages. If this has been done and has not been detected, then it might cause a chronic infection and pain.
14. It is advisable to make two throws in the same direction so that the knot can be adjusted before the third throw which seals the knot. A double throw is recommended and altogether I recommend about six throws to ensure that the knot never slips. The knot is cut exactly on the knot so that the ends do not later protrude through the skin.
15. Always over-correct. In general it is unlikely that one over-corrects even though the nose tip is rather exaggeratedly lifted. Of course one should not over-correct too excessively. One major advantage of this operation is that it is easy to do and should one not over-correct sufficiently then the procedure is easy to repeat. The same is true should one over-correct.

16. Should you feel that the nose has not been adequately lifted a second suture can be inserted. I do not try and remove the first suture.
17. I suggest taping the nose with micropore for about two days to limit swelling and also to ensure immobility. The nose tip can be rather sensitive for the first few days.
18. Over the next three to six weeks the nose tip will drop down into a stable position. By 8 to 10 weeks one reaches a stable position.

## 6. Further modifications

In some patients the described procedure makes a difference but one does not achieve the refinement of the nose tip that is desired. In these cases one needs to add extra sutures. Experience has shown that generally these sutures need to be shorter.

1. If the suture designed above will not narrow the nose sufficiently then one needs to add a suture lower down on the nose with more direct pressure on the upper edges of the lower lateral cartilages. (See Figs. 5 and 6)

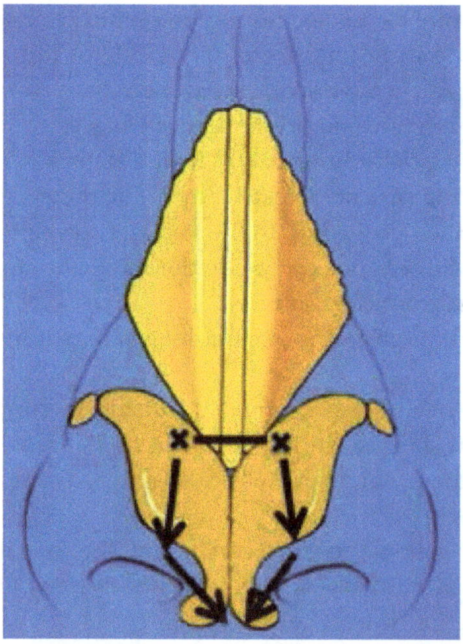

**Figure 4.** Showing the frontal view of the skin markings where one needs more pressure on the alar wings.

As one creates this suture in much the same way as described above, take care to ensure that the alar cartilages are not lifted anteriorly which will create a ridge on the lower nose instead of maintaining a straight bridge to the tip, or supra-tip bump. This suture is often important for creating a really fine nose tip.. A variant that can be done, depending on the anatomy, is the pass above the lower lateral alar cartilages through the septum and then around them to make a more defined cinched tip (See Fig 6 and 7).

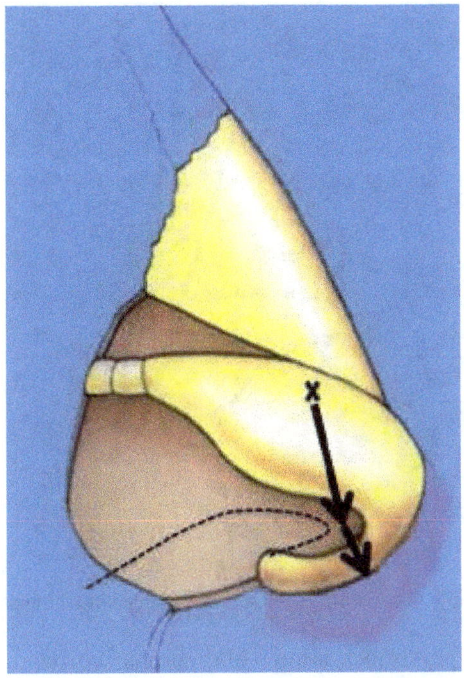

**Figure 5.** Showing the lateral marking for the shorter suture to compress the alar cartilages more directly.

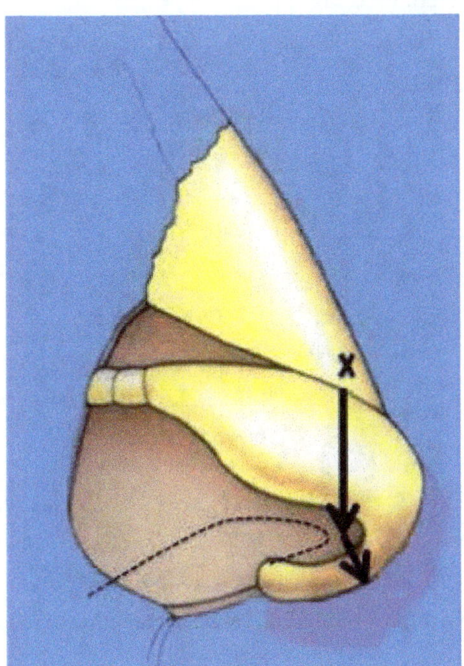

**Figure 6.** Showing the markings for a more pinched tip with the suture going through the septum only.

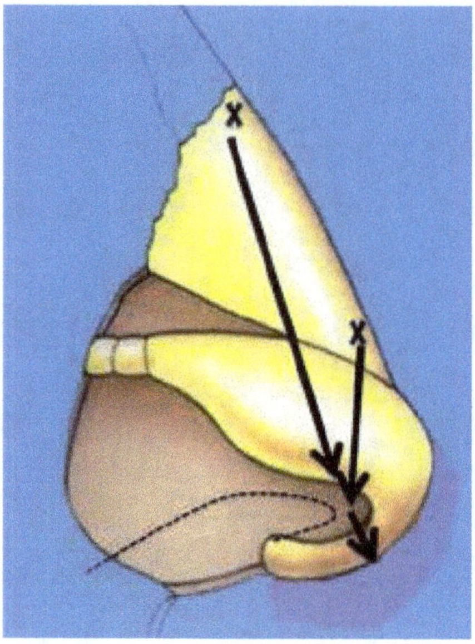

**Figure 7.** Showing the composite view of both longer and then a shorter cinching suture to the nasal tip.

2. In some cases with very bulky lateral alar wings we need to do a slightly different suture to get better compression. Here it is necessary to make four stab incisions on the alar cartilage in a design that allows more compression on the alar cartilage and compresses the tip as well. (See Fig. 8)

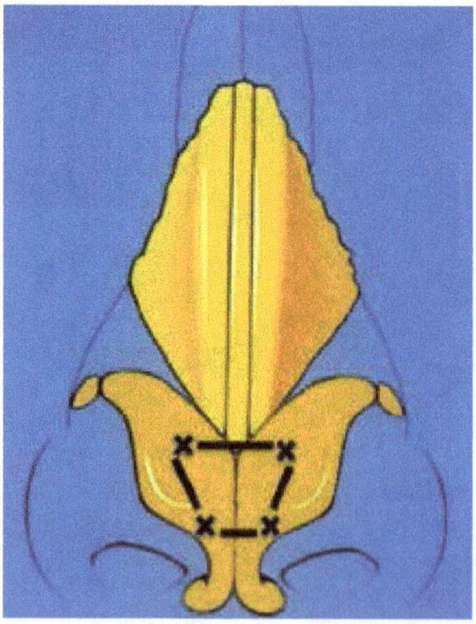

**Figure 8.** Showing the square suture combination in the upper edge of the medial wing of the lower alar cartilage.

Here we have to be cautious about not entering the nasal cavity. These sutures do not need to be anchored to the septum. I rarely use this suture.

3. In some cases the alar cartilages are not positioned evenly and one cartilage may be lower than the other. In this case the displaced cartilage can be lifted by a loop created in the same fashion as described above but one goes medial to the "normal cartilage so that the one thread of the suspension loop lies in between the alar cartilages and the other part lies exterior to the lower cartilage as shown in figure 9.

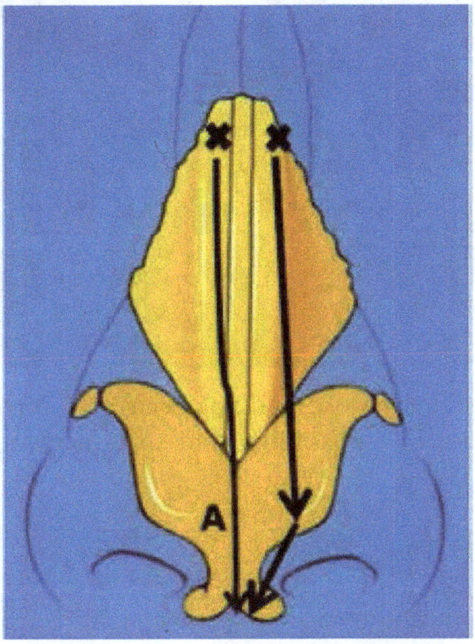


**Figure 9.** Showing the surface markings of the suture used to pull up the left alar cartilage. It would be the mirror image for the right side.

Tightening the loop will lift the alar cartilage to a matching position and then the suspension suture for both alar cartilages can be positioned. Do not expect that a simple loop will correct this type of asymmetry.

4. In cases of excessive bulk of the columella that hangs very low, then one should consider an elliptical excision of mucosa to lift the columella. Suspension sutures alone cannot remedy this situation.

## 7. Postoperative phase

Initially patients may worry that the tip of the nose has been lifted too much but if sensible exaggeration has been done, the nose takes up a pleasing position very quickly. (see Figures 10 through 1)

For the first four five days the nose looks over-corrected but rapidly changes as the swelling disappears and within a week the patient feels much more confident. By ten weeks. Weeks the nose has settled to very close to the final appearance.

The nose can be rather sensitive to minor trauma and even to kissing but that also settles quite soon. The patients may be aware of the suture for up to six months.

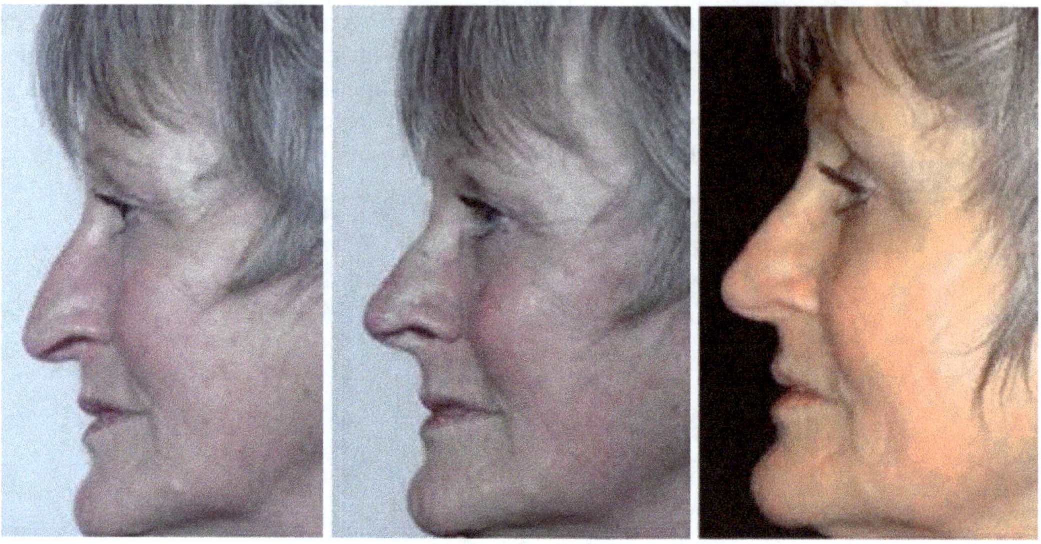

One realises quite quickly if the nose has not been over-corrected sufficiently. Patients should be warned that this is a possibility and that they might need a second minor procedure.

## 8. The advantages

This is a simple low cost procedure easily done in the office that does not disrupt the alar cartilages and yet shapes them easily. It is rapidly done with little morbidity and the patient can rapidly return to normal social activity. The worst luck is that the nose might need some modification with some extra sutures.

One of the greatest advantages for older people is the improvement in breathing through their nose when the tip has been lifted. Another major advantage for people who have had previous surgery is how easily their nose can be re-fashioned into the nose they hoped for.

## 9. Summary

A simple technique is always a benefit and this technique of lifting and compressing the nasal tip combines a very simple surgical procedure with rapid results and minimal discomfort. It can be used in old people whose nose tips have dropped and also in patients who have had a previous rhinoplasty. Its simplicity also makes it an inexpensive minimally invasive procedure that is also suitable for many minor nasal deformities.

## Author details

M. B. Des Fernandes
*The Renaissance Body Science Institute, Cape Town, South Africa.*
*Department of Plastic Surgery, Groote Schuur Hospital, University of Cape Town, Cape Town, South Africa*

3

# Chin Enhancement Using Serdev Suture: Five Case Reports

Meity Hidayani, Syarief Hidayat and Dali Amiruddin

Additional information is available at the end of the chapter

## 1. Introduction

The main goal of aesthetic facial cosmetic surgery is to achieve balance and harmony to the facial features. Chin augmentation and correction are the most important procedures to obtain overall facial beauty. Chin augmentation has been conducted since 100 years ago. Some synthetic implant alloplastic materials have been used including the observation of benefits, loss, and complication accompanied with it. The beauty of the chin is one of the important factors to enhance aesthetic facial features, where the chin is the lower most from 3 facial parts. Aesthetically, protrusion of the chin should be parallel to the line of facial profile. Protrusion of the chin gives character to the face. However imperfection and protrusion of the chin as a result of trauma, congenital or aging may hinder an individual's appearance. Inconsistency between the bone and soft tissue is a common cause of impaired aesthetic beauty. [1,2]

Aging causes the skin to wrinkle and an increase in subcutaneous tissue causes change in projection and facial contour. This is caused by the laxity of the skin and facial muscles that support the gravity force. The area of the face that creases due to age includes cheeks and chin, which causes face disproportion in some individuals. [1,3,4]

There are many techniques/methods used to correct and tighten sagging facial skin, one of them by employing Serdev suture. This method involves lifting part of the face to correct the volume and position of the soft tissue with fixation of the fascia/muscle percutaneous without conventional incision. This method is preferably chosen because it is relatively safe (with minimal side effects), easy, and quick with satisfactory results. This method was invented by Dr. Nikolay P. Serdev. Besides chin lift, the method can also be applied to lift other facial parts, buttocks and abdominal area. [2,5]

Serdev suture involves passing sutures by needle into the soft tissue under the skin and stitched according to the desired purpose. This action can be performed in an outpatient unit because it is relatively safe and complications are relatively mild, such as edema, hematoma, infection and scar (rare). Patients must be selected, amongst others, patients must not have a history of heart disease, hypertension, uncontrolled diabetes mellitus, blood clotting disorders, and not taking any anti-coagulant medications; also the surgery is suggested not to be performed to patients who are under 20 years old due tothe mandible bone has not yet fully grown. [2,3,5,6]

Five cases of chin enhancementis reported on women ages between 40-53 years old using Serdev suture and without any complication.

## 2. Case reports

### 2.1. First case

A 34-year old woman came to aesthetic clinic of Mintohardjo hospital for chin enhancement. From anamnesis, no chronic medical history is found like diabetes mellitus, hypertension, heart disease, or bleeding disturbances. In terms of physical examination, no abnormality to the chin is found. Routine laboratory blood test is within normal limits. With a clean medical

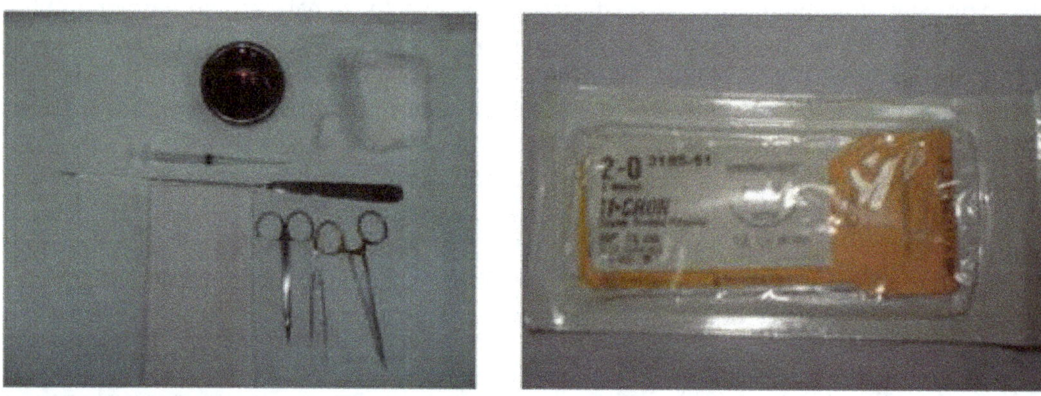

**Figure 1.** (A) and (B) Surgical instruments and materials prepared

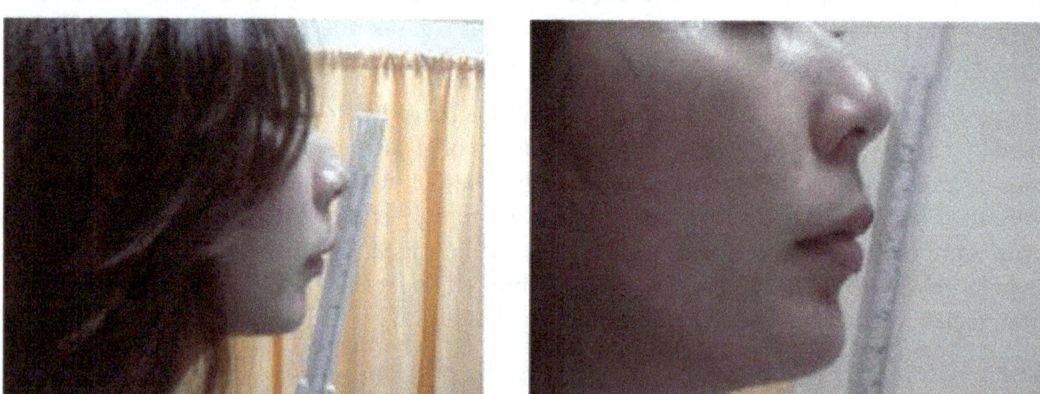

**Figure 2.** (A) Pre-Operation (B) Post-operation

record, chin lift can be performed using Serdev suture and after the patient read, understand, and agree to sign a medical consent.

SurgeryReport:

1. Document chin from different angle.
2. Chin position is measured by drawing a line between the lower lip and chin, then place a mark under the chin for needle insertion and exit point. .
3. The patient is laid on the operating bed.
4. Surgical instruments are disinfected using Betadine/povidone-iodine.
5. Sterile drapes are placed around the field to delineate sterile areas.
6. Local anesthesia is given by injecting 2% lidocaine on the lowermost of the chin, under inferior lip.
7. Chin skin that has been marked is punctured using a special needle by following the internal chin muscle until it penetrates the mark below inferior lip.
8. Serdev thread is inserted in the hole at the tip of the needle, and then pulled down, thus appearing under the chin.
9. Needle is inserted back to the lowermost chin following the outer chin muscle until it penetrates to the same mark below the inferior lip.
10. Thread is inserted to the needle tip then pulled again until the thread appears in the lowermost of the chin.
11. The tip of the thread is stitched to the first thread until reaching the desired chin lift.
12. The thread is cut just above the knot.
13. The skin around the knot is freed.
14. The wound is given betadine and covered with bandage as needed.
15. Document the results after operation is finished.

After the operation is completed, patient can perform activities as normal, however, the patient should take amioxcilin-clavulanic acid 3x500 mg for 5 days and administer mefenamic acid 3 times in one day if in pain.

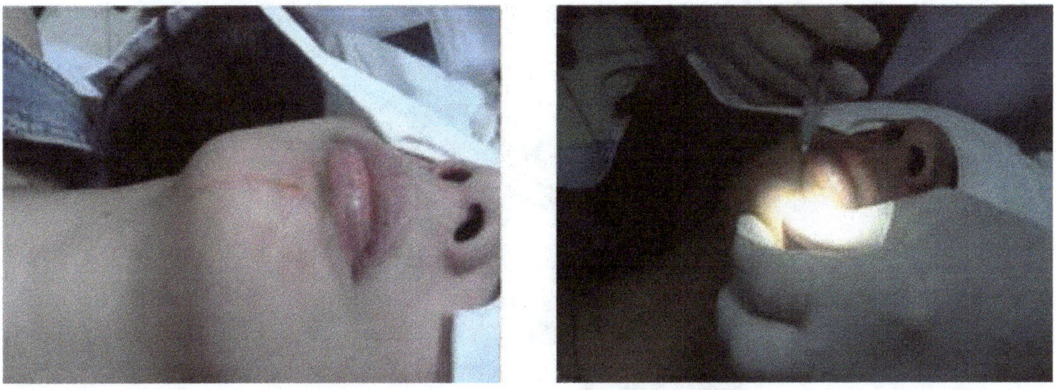

**Figure 3.** (A) marking for insertion and exit point (B) Anasthetic lidocaine 2%

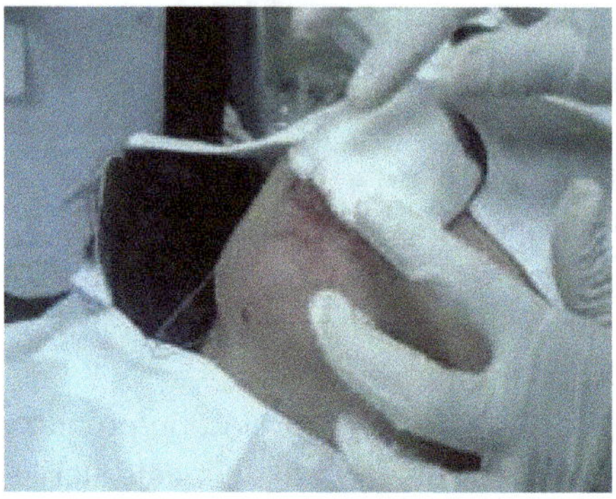

**Figure 4.** Thread is inserted to the tip of the needle and pulled until thread is seen in the lowermost of the chin.

## 2.2. Second case

A 42 year old woman came to aesthetic clinic of Mintohardjo Hospital to enhance the chin which she felt was slightly flabby. From anamnesis, no chronic medical history is found like diabetes mellitus, hypertension, heart disease, or bleeding disturbances. In terms of physical examination, no abnormality to the chin is found. Routine laboratory blood test is within normal limits. Thereby, chin lift can be performed using Serdev method after the patient read, understand, and agree to sign a medical consent.

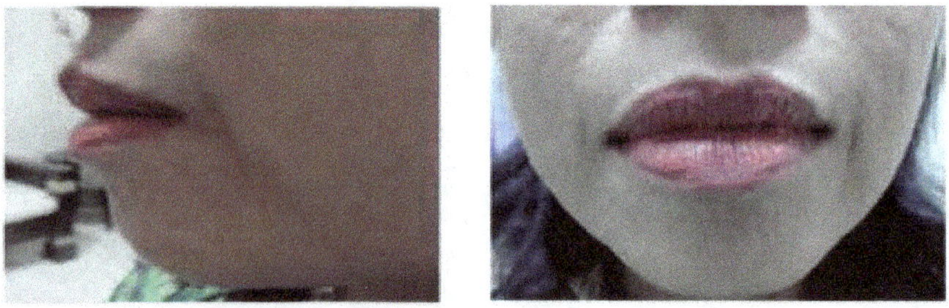

(A). Side view (B). Front view

**Figure 5.** Before procedure

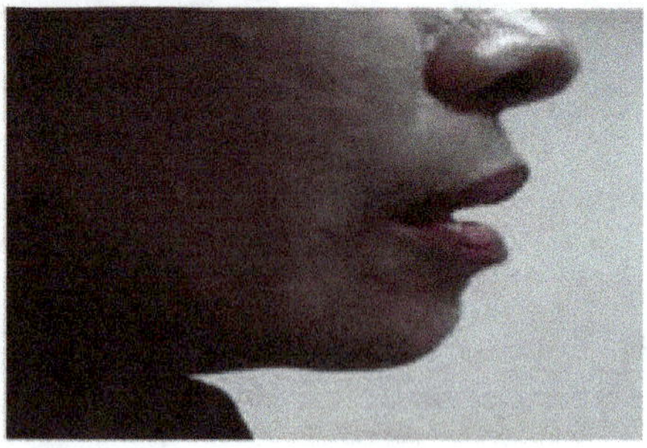

**Figure 6.** After procedure

Surgery report:

1. Document chin from different angle.
2. Chin position is measured by drawing a line between the lower lip and chin, then place a mark under the chin for needle insertion and exit point. .
3. The patient is laid on the operating bed.
4. Surgical instruments are disinfected using Betadine/povidone-iodine.
5. Sterile drapes are placed around the field to delineate sterile areas.
6. Local anesthesia is given by injecting 2% lidocaine on the lowermost of the chin, under inferior lip.
7. Chin skin that has been marked is punctured using a special needle by following the internal chin muscle until it penetrates the mark below inferior lip.
8. Serdev thread is inserted in the hole at the tip of the needle, and then pulled down, thus appearing under the chin.
9. Needle is inserted back to the lowermost chin following the outer chin muscle until it penetrates to the same mark below the inferior lip.
10. Thread is inserted to the needle tip then pulled again until the thread appears in the lowermost of the chin.
11. The tip of the thread is stitched to the first thread until reaching the desired chin lift.
12. The thread is cut just above the knot.
13. The skin around the knot is freed.
14. The wounds is given betadine and covered with bandage as needed.
15. Document the results after operation is finished.

After the operation is completed, patient can conduct activities as normal, however, the patient is advised to minimize the use of the lower jaw, like chewing hard foods. Patient is given amioxcilin-calvulanic acid 3x500 mg for 5 days and administer mefenamic acid 3 times in one day if in pain.

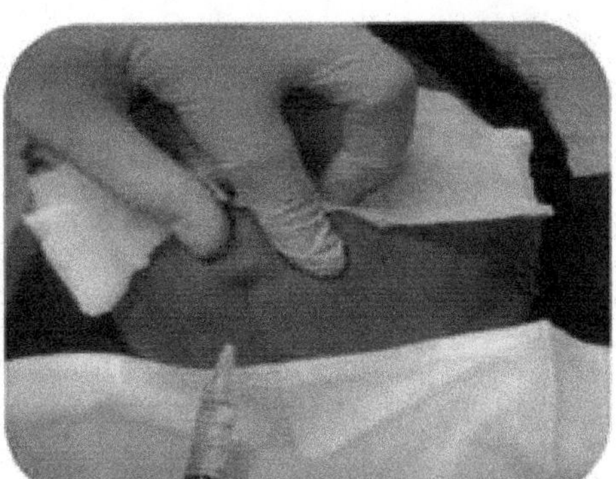

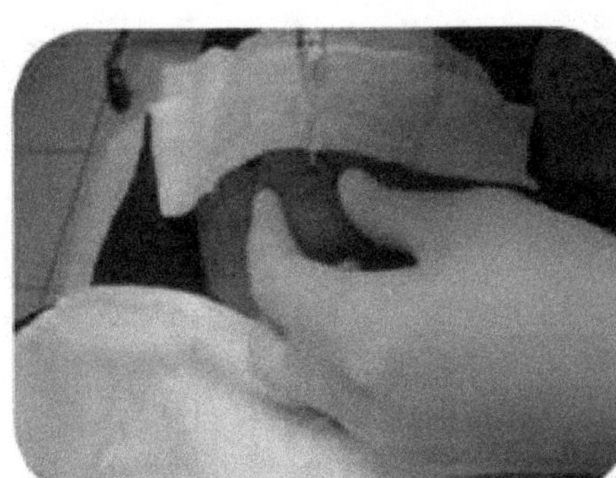

**Figure 7.** (A) and (B) Anesthetic lidocaine 2%

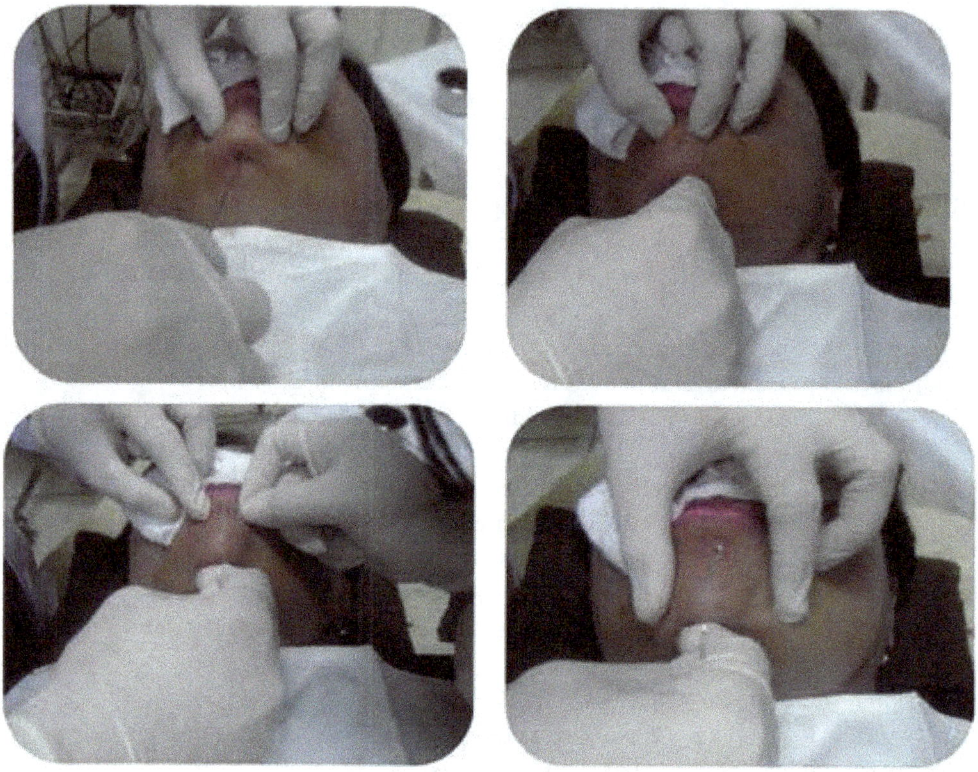

**Figure 8.** Thread is inserted to the tip of the needle and pulled until thread is seen in the lowermost of the chin.

## 2.3. Third case

A 30 year old woman came to Aesthetic Central RSAL Dr. Mintohardjo with the desire to perform chin lift because she feels her chin is lacking beauty and sagging.

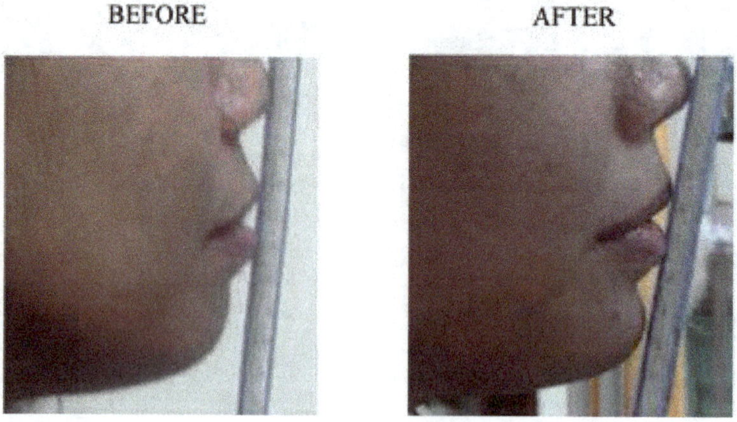


**Figure 9.**

From anamnesis, no chronic medical history is found like diabetes mellitus, hypertension, heart disease, or bleeding disturbances. In terms of physical examination, no abnormality to the chin is found. Routine laboratory blood test is within normal limits. Thereby, chin lift can be performed using Serdev method after the patient read, understand, and agree to sign a medical consent.

## 2.4. Fourth case

A 39 year old woman came to Aesthetic Center RSLA Dr. Mintohardjo with the desire to perform chin lift because she feels her chin is lacking beauty and sagging.

From anamnesis, no chronic medical history is found like diabetes mellitus, hypertension, heart disease, or bleeding disturbances. In terms of physical examination, no abnormality to the chin is found. Routine laboratory blood test is within normal limits. Thereby, chin lift can be performed using Serdev method after the patient read, understand, and agree to sign a medical consent.

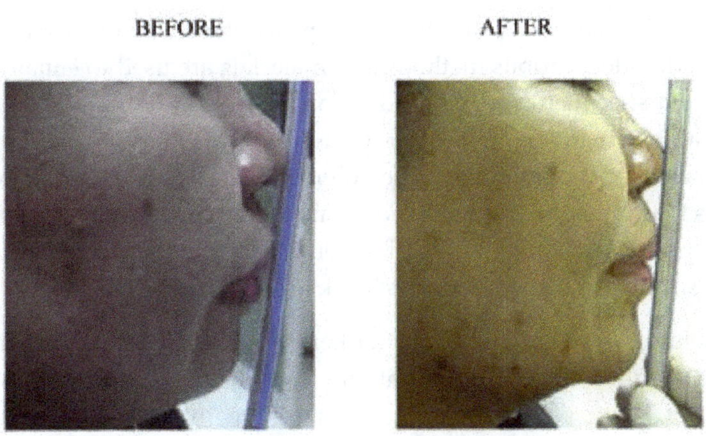


**Figure 10.**

## 2.5. Fifth case

A 45 year old woman came to Aesthetic Center RSAL Dr. Mintohardjo with the desire to perform chin lift because she feels her chin is lacking beauty and sagging.

From anamnesis, no chronic medical history is found like diabetes mellitus, hypertension, heart disease, or bleeding disturbances. In terms of physical examination, no abnormality to the chin is found. Routine laboratory blood test is within normal limits. Thereby, chin lift can be performed using Serdev method after the patient read, understand, and agree to sign a medical consent.

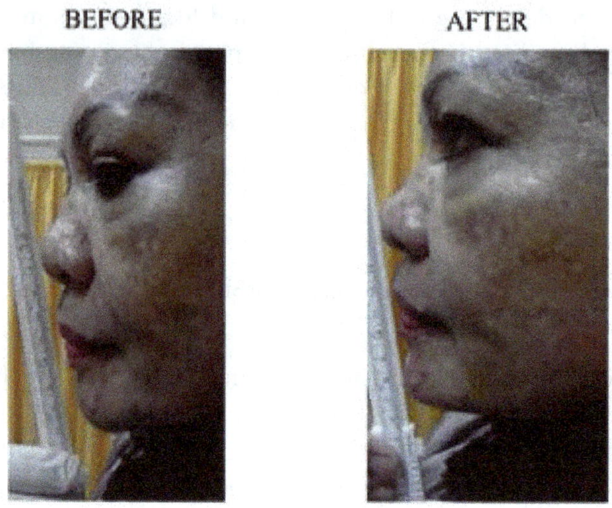


**Figure 11.**

## 3. Discussion

Chin enhancement is a surgical procedure to improve the shape or increase the size of the chin. For several decades, various methods and materials are used to enhance the chin. This includes implanted specimen from the body, transplantation of the bone and cartilage, fat, fascia, tendons and skin are the first materials used for this kind of procedure. A variety of alloplastic are then used to lift the chin. The polymer is used as a bone replacement. Sincethe 1950s, materials that can be used to enhance a small chin include silicon, collagen injection, expanded politetrafluoroetilan (e-PTFE), high density plyethylene (HDPE), polidimetiloksan (PDMS), proplast, and hyraxypatile porous block (PBHA) [1,2,7,8,9]

There are many injections available in the market over the last decade. But the materials are foreign for the body thus causing complications. Complications that occur include infection, position that is not fitting, parastesi, absorption, rejection, migration, implant, erosion of soft tissue, asymmetry, and indentation. [1]

There are no materials found that are perfect for the face, therefore a study is conducted to determine a method that is much more effective and less complicated. Surgery without implant is introduced by Dr. Nikolay P. Serdev, an aesthetic expert from Sofia, Bulgaria, which has become popularly known as Serdev method. This method is an operation without implant and only usesthread to pull/stitch soft tissue in the chin. This technique is done by changing the angle of the chin and keeping the chin align to the jaw line thus providing a better result. [1,10]

The advantages of Serdev method compared with other methods is that the result can be seen after the surgery, complications is minimal, more natural results, long-lasting, and can be applied to other areas of the face and body. [10,11]

Serdev thread is a woven polycapromide that is semi-synthetic, antimicrobial and non-absorbable. The result is more natural looking chin because an implant is not inserted and the operation only uses thread that is stitch to the soft tissue. The method can be used to correct flabby chin and does not cause scarring. [1,12]

Serdev method only requires a short amount of time and also requires only local anesthesia. The duration of the operation is dependent upon the area that is to be operated, the level of flabbiness, and the expertise of the doctor. Results can be seen immediately after the operation, but still accompanied with mild ederma. The pain will disappear by itself, and patients are recommended not to overly manipulate the chin. Serdev thread is not visible in the suface of the skin and the result can last 10-20 years. [1,12]

The report discusses cases for five women between the ages of 30 to 40 years old that complain sagging to the chin. From medical history record and check-up, there are no systematic diseases found or other contradiction, thus chin lift with Serdev method is chosen by patients.

Chin lift performed to the five patients are satisfactory with no complications after the operation. The patients are able to perform their usual daily activities after the operation. Although the patients are given antibiotic to prevent secondary infection and analgetic if in pain.

## Author details

Meity Hidayani and Dali Amiruddin
*Dermatovenereology Department Medical Faculty of Hasanuddin University Wahidin Sudirohusodo General HospitalMakassar, Indonesia*

Syarief Hidayat
*Dermatovenereology Department Mintohardjo Navy Hospital Jakarta, Indonesia*

## 4. References

[1] Serdev NP. Chin enhancement and form correcting using a suture of the soft tissue. *Intern Jof Cosmetic Surg*. 2002:11(1); 16-25

[2] Serdev NP. Chin enhancement using serdev suture. Available from www.google.com

[3] Serdev NP. Chin form correction and augmentation using simple suture. *Int J AesthCosm Beauty Surg*. 2001;3(1):42-66

[4] Pachigolla R, Calhoun K. Chin and malar augmentation. Available from www.google.com

[5] Serdev NP. Serdev Suture. Available from http://en.wikipedia.org/wiki/Serdev_suture

[6] Anonyme. Chin augmentation, nasal, and facial plastic cosmetic surgery institute and laser centre. Available from www.google.com

[7] Serdev NP. Principles of face beautification in liftings: aesthetic proportions, volume and angles. Available from www.what11.com

[8] Anonyme. Chin augmentation. Available from www.veri.google.com
[9] Berman M. Chin and cheek augmentation. Available from www.google.com
[10] Serdev N. Scarless suture liftings. Available from www.google.com
[11] Anonyme.Scarlessserdev suture miniinvasive suspension lift and volume technique suspension lift and volume techniques. Available from www.drserdev.com
[12] Anonyme. Facelift with minimally invasive threadlift enhancement. Available from www.parkwayaesthetics.com

# 4

# The Holistic Scarless Rejuvenation of the Face

M. B. Des Fernandes

## 1. Introduction

This chapter will concentrate on the holistic approach to harmonious facial rejuvenation by concentrating on the procedures that should accompany every face-lift procedure. In particular I will concentrate on facial rejuvenation in younger adults or those who do not need a full facelift with excision of skin. However, the principles of holistic rejuvenation of the face remain the same.

Rejuvenation of the face is commonly asked for yet, sadly, often not delivered. A Face-lift is not automatically facial rejuvenation. Surgeons who concentrate on surgery only fail to recognize that the very best surgery done without any attention to the skin will deliver only a semblance of rejuvenation and very often a disharmony between structure and surface appearance. For real rejuvenation, one needs to pay attention to the skin in particular and restore *naturally young,* and not just *smoother* skin. As aesthetic surgeons we have to be sure that our patients get the best advice for rejuvenation. This is my experience and when a patient comes for facial surgery I explain that there are three important steps that we should always attend to:

1. First of all we need to make sure that our patients use skin care that can actually rejuvenate skin. The only molecule so far described in the history of skin care that actually rejuvenates skin physiologically as well as in appearance is vitamin A. We do not need to use retinoic acid to get these effects because we can use the pre-cursors of retinoic acid e.g. like retinyl palmitate to get exactly the same end-result without the irritation normally encountered when using retinoic acid. However, there are very few products available that contain effective quantities of vitamin A. One way to ensure that you are recommending a product with sufficient vitamin A is to choose a product that presents vitamin A in gradually increasing doses till the maximum dose is reached. We have at the same time to remember that skin care alone cannot make photodamaged skin return to younger skin. This is where we need to add regeneration of youthful skin through skin needling.

2. The second step for the most convincing, scarless rejuvenation of the facial skin is Collagen Induction Therapy (CIT) by skin needling to generate platelet-derived growth factors and regenerate skin (P-CIT). [1] This is the only process yet described in the medical literature that causes regeneration of skin and the normal latticework matrix.
3. Finally, a simple face-lift without attention to the mid-face will not produce a convincingly younger face. The mid-face is the key to a youthful appearance because it not only addresses the naso-labial folds, but also rejuvenates the lower eyelids and lifts up the corner of the mouth. In fact the mid-face-lift addresses most of the concerns of many people seeking a face-lift. The ideal situation is where the intervention occurs at an earlier rather than a later time and the facial tissues can be lifted by sutures or threads and repositioned in their youthful position. [2]

## 2. Restoring the skin surface through scientific skin care

Vitamin A is a normal component found in our skin and is absolutely essential for healthy skin. [3] However, vitamin A is rapidly destroyed by exposure to light because it is in fact a natural sunscreen and absorbs UVA and UVB rays [4]. As a result our skin develops a chronic, progressive and unrelenting deficiency of vitamin A that manifests as pigmented blotches, wrinkles, thin skin, and pre-cancerous lesions that eventually develop into skin cancer. This is exactly the sort of person who may present to you for a face-lift. Fortunately, by restoring normal levels of vitamin A we can reverse these effects and create healthier skin. The earlier the patient starts to use Vitamin A topically, the better. Do not waste time thinking about Alpha hydroxyacids except to enhance the effects of vitamin A products. Only vitamin A has this power to rejuvenate the skin cells and restore more normal function.

While sunscreens can give protection, the safety of the skin depends to a large extent on the quantity of vitamin A and other antioxidants in the skin. Keep the skin rich in Retinyl palmitate (RP) because it is the major form of cellular vitamin A. RP is relatively non-irritating and is converted into every possible metabolite of vitamin A. As a result, when used topically at adequate dosage, it affords us the most acceptable method of vitamin A replacement. Research shows us that Retinyl palmitate plays a role in preventing skin cancer [5] and squamous skin cancer cells have an impaired ability to esterify retinol [6]

Doctors generally think retinoic acid is the only effective vitamin A but retinyl palmitate, as described above, is the major form of vitamin A in the human body and skin [3]. Retinyl esters are de-esterified to retinol, which is then oxidised by alcohol dehydrogenases to retinal and finally retinoic acid [7]. There seems to be a feedback mechanism whereby retinoic acid production is controlled by increasing or decreasing the esterification of retinol to retinyl palmitate. [8] The ratio is tightly controlled with the retinyl esters being 91% and retinol, retinal and retinoic acid each at 3%. By increasing the RP one automatically increases the quantity of retinoic acid that is the molecule that interacts with the DNA.

Guide your patients to healthier, lovelier skin by using products containing vitamin A, especially RP. [9] [10] [11]. Make sure that the creams are adequately supported by antioxidant vitamins at the same time. Pay particular attention that they contain vitamin C (preferable in its ester form and particularly ascorbyl tetra-isopalmitate. Vitamin C and E are the dominant antioxidant vitamins of the skin [12].

Figure 1 shows the degree of photo-damage often seen in "sun-worshipping" people who may come to you for surgery and Figure 2 shows the changes that can be expected from using topical vitamin A as retinyl palmitate in doses that I recommend. The skin is clearly healthier.

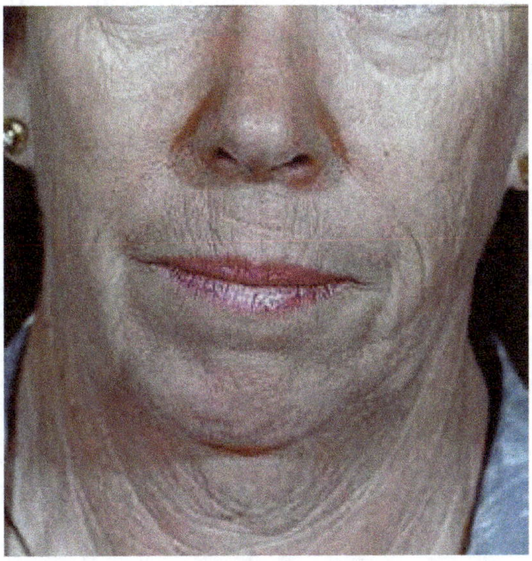

**Figure 1.** Before using vitamin A, C and antioxidant skin care.

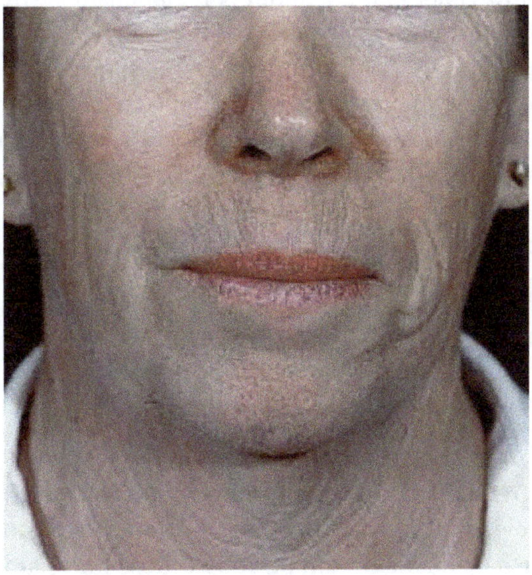

**Figure 2.** Six months after using vitamin A, C and antioxidant skin care.

**Clinical effects of topical retinyl palmitate**

- It affects the genes of the stem cells so that the keratinocytes grow and look more normal. It increases the growth of the basal layer (growth layer) of skin cells that causes thickening of the epidermis. Not only does the skin get thicker; it also heals faster because the cells are growing faster.
- Vitamin A improves the horny layer, so it makes the skin more resistant to environmental pollution. [13]
- Melanin in keratinocytes becomes more evenly distributed. [14]
- The production of melanin by melanocytes is generally reduced to the normal constitutional colour of the skin.
- The production of sebum is decreased in oily skin. [15]
- Vitamin A supports and potentiates the Langerhans cells of the skin. [16]
- It affects the fibroblast cells, the most important cell in the dermis, particularly the genes for the production of collagen. Healthier collagen is formed and unhealthy collagen is removed by enzyme activity. [17]
- It increases the secretion of natural moisturising factors by the fibroblast cells of the dermis into the space between the cells, allowing the skin to retain more water with some puffing out of the wrinkles. These natural moisturising factors filter up into the epidermis between the cells. Glycosaminoglycans are some of the chemicals created by the fibroblast to help retain moisture. [18]
- The blood supply to the deeper layers of the skin is improved, which means that nutrition of the skin is improved. The skin also assumes a healthier colour.

Vitamin A should be used twice daily and if used during daylight hours it should be accompanied with anti oxidant vitamins like vitamin C, E and beta carotene, so that it is better protected from ultra violet light. Vitamin A metabolism is strongly tied to vitamin C, and vitamin C is essential for the proper function of vitamin E. The concept of the balanced use of these vitamins as the main way of maintaining skin health is becoming more and more certain with current research work. Our skin is constantly exposed to light and light destroys certain essential chemicals in our skin. We can never escape this fact. A reliable UVA and UVB sunscreen with sun protection factor SPF 15 – 20 should be used at the same time in preference to high SPF products over 30. Vitamin A should also be replaced every evening as a topical application to the skin to try and address the loss of vitamin A from being in light. Because we cannot prevent the damage to the vitamin A in the skin, it is essential to replace the vitamin A each day so that we minimise the signs of photoaging that are really also the signs of accumulative vitamin A and antioxidant deficiency of the skin.

**Recommended skin care regime:**

Select a skin care regime that offers vitamin A as retinyl palmitate especially, or retinyl acetate, retinol or even retinaldehyde. I prefer a heavy bias towards retinyl palmitate and the vitamin A should be offered in a series of creams that increase from low levels right up to 50,000 i.u. per g., which is the maximum permitted dose for vitamin A in cosmetics in the European Union. You cannot start at high doses because that would induce a retinoid reaction that would dissuade the patient from using the product. Start on the lowest and even that levels will still give excellent changes [19]. Then for maximum results gradually build up to the strongest permitted concentration. The simultaneous use of stable versions of vitamin C and other antioxidants is essential. Peptides such as Matrixyl are particularly valuable in giving tighter smoother skin. The patient ideally should start this skin care regime before surgery and continue forever afterwards to maintain the best, healthiest skin.

The effects of topical vitamin A and C and antioxidants and even peptides can be enhanced by using a device that punctures only the stratum corneum[1] Even greater tightening of the skin may be obtained as witnessed by Figures 3 and 4 which show skin before being treated with vitamin A and antioxidants[2] and the Skin-Roller and then the appearance after one year. This demonstrates tightening that is normally only achieved after heavy peels or intensive treatments with fractional laser or radio-heating devices. However, this was done by the patient herself with a simple device that caused absolutely no pain or discomfort.

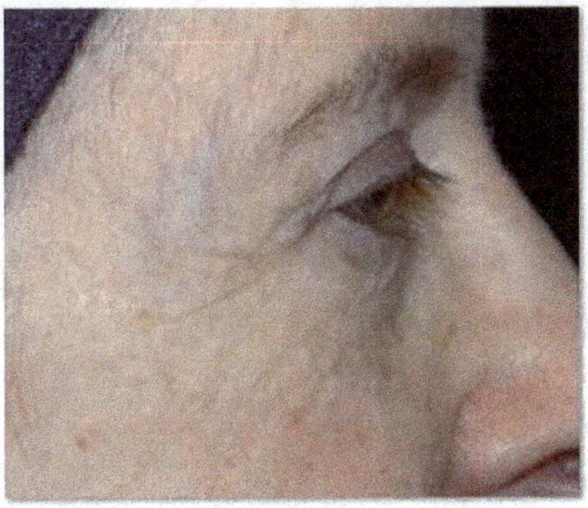

**Figure 3.** photo-damaged skin before starting vitamins A, C and antioxidants.

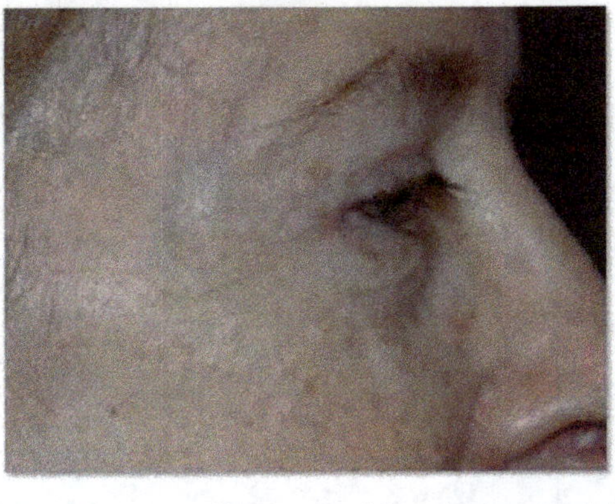

**Figure 4.** One year later with no surgery peeling or anything else except daily skin care enhanced by using the Cosmetic Skin Roller

[1] The Environ Cosmetic Skin-Roller

[2] Environ Skin Care

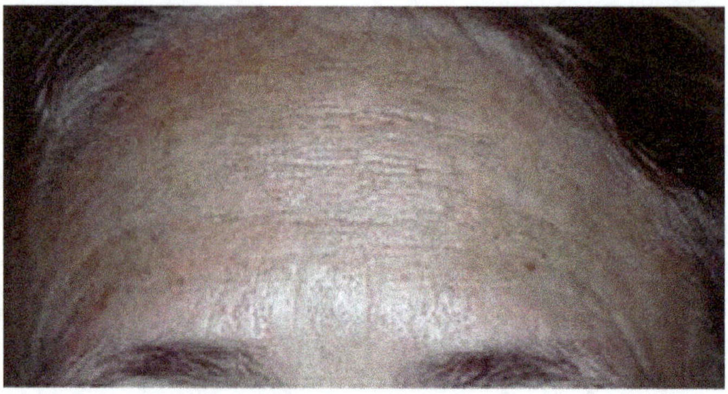

**Figure 5.** Lower face before needling with 3 mm Roll-CIT

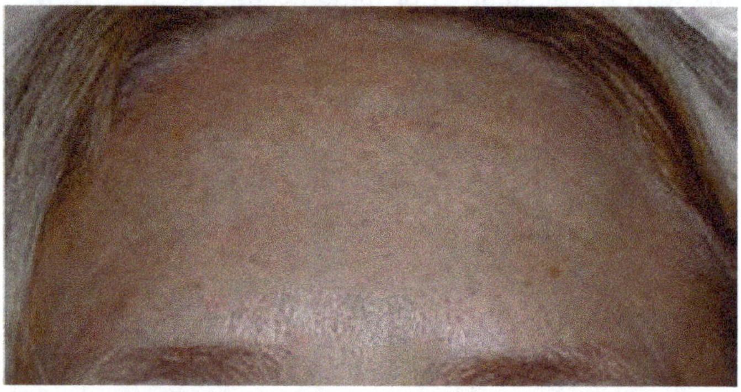

**Figure 6.** After Roll-CIT and skin care.

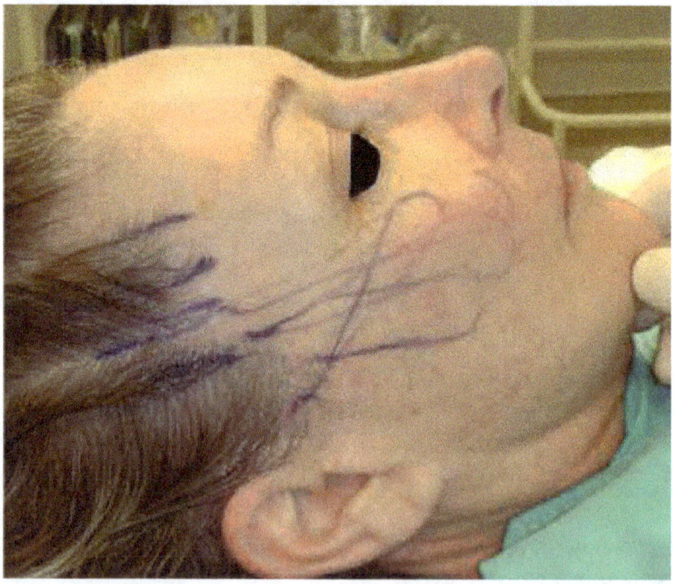

**Figure 7.** Markings for suture loops of the cheeks. In this case a number of loops have been marked in case they will be needed to get full tightening of the facial tissues. Generally by adding the Silhouette sutures, one can avoid adding extra loops.

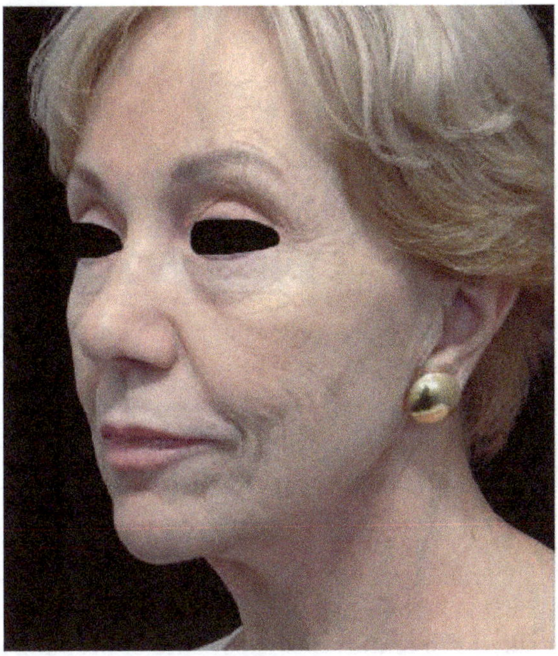

**Figure 8.** This patient has had a face-lift but was not given a mid-face-lift and is unhappy with the result. One can understand this because the corners of her mouth turn down and she still has a heavy naso-labial fold.

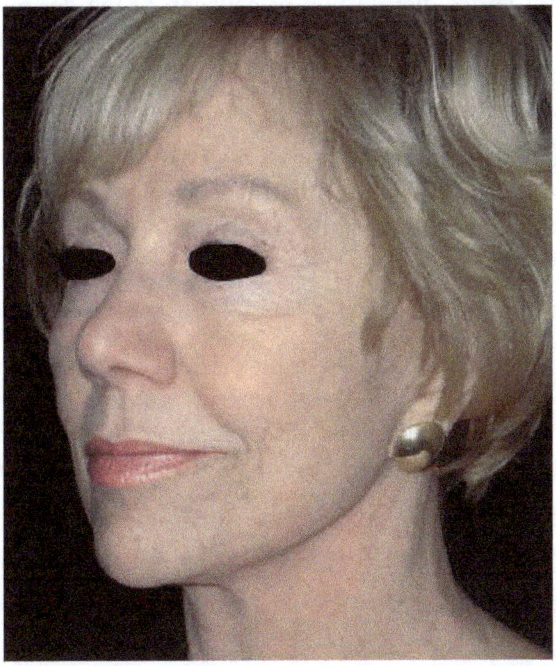

**Figure 9.** One year after a scarless suture suspension mid-facelift only and skin care with vitamins A, C and antioxidants enhanced by the use of the Cosmetic Skin Roller.

**Summary of Skin Care**

Vitamin A, particularly as retinyl palmitate, is probably the safest way to protect skin from solar irradiation and may also be used for protracted periods to rejuvenate skin. The ideal treatment would be to apply topical vitamin A to the skin starting at an early age, soon after our first exposure to light, and continuing the daily replenishment of vitamin A into old age. Not only would this maintain healthy young looking skin, but most likely would also protect against cancer.

While skin care can make a big difference and when used under ideal conditions, may hold back the clock of photoaging, most patients present to us with well established damage and skin care needs to be supplemented with a more radical and new technique that actually regenerates younger skin.

## 3. Regenerating skin through percutaneous Collagen Induction Therapy (p-CIT)

Needling skin is rapidly becoming an established method to rejuvenate skin and refine scars that is competing with ablative and minimally ablative procedures. [1] While the technique may seem new, we actually have centuries of experience of needling skin because tattooing has been practiced in both "civilized" and "primitive" cultures all around the world. Needling stands above all other currently used treatments because it has been shown to be the first method described, as far as we can determine, that conclusively regenerates tissue and restores the natural lattice-distribution of collagen of the dermis. Neither fractionated laser or any other treatments induce regeneration of tissue. To date it is the only described skin treatment that regenerates elastin [20]. It has a wide list of indications and can be used on all ages and all different coloured skins with safety.

To achieve results one has to cause bleeding of the skin because it is the release of platelets that stimulates the regeneration of tissue, and the degree of improvement is directly related to the amount of bleeding. Since I first started needling in 1994 I have been searching how to get the best out of needling.

**Here are my guidelines:**

I always insist that the patient should use topical vitamin A and C and antioxidants for at least three weeks before the procedure. I persuade my patients to use a device with needles protruding only 0.2 mm as a "rolling massage" system so that only the stratum corneum is punctured and this allows better action of the applied vitamin A etc. See figure 3 and 4

I first started experimenting with needling of the skin in the early 1990"s and by 1996 started the micro-needling of skin in the way that we now do it.

I called the process Collagen Induction Therapy and that term is used around the world and usually abbreviated to CIT. [21] [22]

Then I recommend **The Medical Roll-CIT** that has needles that protrude 1.0 – 1.5 mm so that the needles will penetrate right down into the dermis and rupture the tiny arcade capillaries in the dermal papillae (rete pegs). Bleeding releases platelets and the platelets in turn release growth factors and particularly TGF-Beta-1, 2 and 3. TGF-beta-1 and 2 soon disappear after needling in direct contrast to the levels seen after a surgical incision. TGF-beta-3 disappears within 24 hours after a surgical incision whereas with needling it is raised for more than two weeks and that seems to be responsible for regeneration [23] of tissue and natural lattice arranged collagen fibres and elastin.

Generally I recommend that the patient should have six sessions of needling done once a week under topical anaesthesia, or if they prefer, then they could have one intensive session done with nerve block and local anaesthetic infiltration. The difference is that with the lighter sessions under topical anaesthesia, they can return to work the very next day whereas after an intensive needling, they will be swollen and bruised for about four days.

I use a unique cream-form of low concentration TCA cream[3] that I apply for 20 minutes before and then for only four minutes after the needling session. I believe this gives me better results. I do this to clean the skin and reduce the chance of an infection in people with acne spots. The second reason for doing this is that I deduce that lower pH levels induce the release of growth factors from the keratinocytes.

The technique for needling is simple and has been well described. [21] Basically one keeps rolling until one has made as many holes as one can either physically or when topical anaesthesia is used, until the patient finds it uncomfortable.

By doing skin care and then skin needling I can offer my patients a safe way to get smooth clear healthy younger-looking skin without any risks. The results, according to many observers, outrank the results achieved with fractionated lasers and radio-frequency devices etc.

I have used iontophoresis and sonophoresis of vitamin A and C immediately after the needling treatment to maximize the induction of healthy collagen. Iontophoresis also tends to reduce the swelling of the skin and I also recommend it after all facial surgery. Low Frequency Sonophoresis can be used to enhance penetration of peptides to induce more collagen and elastin production.

**In summary, Skin needling**

1. Tightens skin laxity and restores normal skin tension in the early stages of ageing. Some patients who are worried about face-lift surgery may be satisfied with simple Percutaneous CIT. The arms, hands, abdomen, thighs, and buttocks can also be treated to give total rejuvenation. In fact this has become the only "anti-ageing full body treatment that we have.
2. Treats fine wrinkles. The interesting feature about skin needling is that it sets up a metabolic mechanism that replaces photo-damaged fibres and re-invigorates cells to regenerate skin. As one would expect, this cannot happen overnight, so it is not

[3] Environ Acid Cream Mask

surprising that the regeneration phase is prolonged and there is continual improvement over many months. I believe the best time to judge the final result is about one year after the needling sessions. Our photographs show that the three-month picture is not as good as the six-month picture and the photograph at the end of the year is the best. This is quite different from the commonly used soft lasers etc. where the best time to take the post-intervention picture is within three months after the treatment otherwise the results become more difficult to see.

3. Reduces Acne scarring and it is gratifying to see that previously scarred skin is slowly replaced by normal looking skin. Interestingly enough, histology shows reduction of scarring and restoration of the normal architecture of the skin.
4. Stretch marks respond well to skin needling even when they have become "silvery" after a long time. This however, is not a problem with facial work except in rare cases where there are stretch marks on the neck.
5. Scars are always improved - even if they are white, old scars they can become more skin coloured.
6. Burn scars – both flat and hypertrophic scars can be treated with success and de-pigmented areas are restored to even normal coloured skin.

**Advantages of PCI**

1. PCI does not damage the skin. The epidermis remains intact. Histology done at 24 hours, a week, and several months after needling fail to show any signs of damage.
2. Any part of the body may be treated. It is excellent for rejuvenating hands so that younger looking hands can accompany facial rejuvenation.
3. Skin becomes thicker as has been repeatedly demonstrated in histological studies. The epidermis is thickened by vitamin A and antioxidant creams but the restoration of a healthy lattice of collagen and elastin results from skin needling. We have never seen excessive deposition of collagen or any sign of scar collagen after skin needling.
4. The healing phase is short. With milder needling under topical anaesthesia, the patients can normally return to work the next day. Most patients select this form of needling but some people choose intensive needling because of time constraints and even do needling at the same time as the scarless minimally invasive face-lift. That way their healing period from needling over-laps with the healing of the facial lifting.
5. Not as expensive as laser resurfacing.
6. The skin does not become sun sensitive so this can be done any time of the year.
7. Can be done on people who have previously had laser resurfacing, or those with very thin skin. The skin always thickens up so the ugly complication of translucent skin following CO2 laser re-surfacing can be treated. I like these patients to use topical vitamin A for a minimum of three months prior to needling.
8. I have never seen hyper-pigmentation in patients with darker skins e.g. African, Indian, Malaysian, Chinese and Mediterranean skins.
9. Telangiectasia may disappear totally. I think the explanation for this may lie in the fact that the tiny vessels are repeatedly fractured and cannot be easily re-constituted.

10. Does not really have to be done by a doctor but should be done under their supervision. In my office the skin-care therapists and nurses, do the needling and that makes it more affordable for the patient.
11. The technique of Medical Roll-CIT is easy to master and is easily taught by a demo DVD. Medical Focus-CIT is also useful for smaller areas and makes the treatment more affordable.
12. Can even be done with topical anaesthesia.

**Disadvantages of PCI:**

1. Exposure to blood. If the procedure is done properly there will be exposure to blood so the proper precautions have to followed
2. While we cannot achieve as intense a deposition of collagen as in laser resurfacing, we can repeat the treatment and get even better results that will last even longer. The scar collagen following laser resurfacing is dense and often reflects white through the skin. These scar collagen fibres, as with any other scar, are resorbed over time. It seems that the normal collagen latticework is not affected in the same way and is only damaged by light.
3. Local anaesthetics limit the area that may be treated and in some cases a general anaesthetic is required e.g. when extensive areas or virtually the whole body is needled.

This is a simple technique and with the right tool it is easy and fast to puncture any skin thoroughly. While one treatment may not give the smoothening seen with ablative laser re-surfacing, the epidermis is normalised and if the result is not sufficiently improved it can safely be repeated as often as necessary. The technique can be used on areas that are not suitable for peeling or laser re-surfacing.

**Some Pitfalls to avoid.**

1. Never use retinoic acid after needling. It irritates the skin and the patient is also less likely to use it properly.
2. Never use Ascorbic acid preparations immediately after needling. Experience has shown me that the ascorbic acid can cause a deep, destructive peel.
3. Never use any strong peeling agents immediately after a peel. The peel will be very much deeper than expected and may cause scars.
4. Needling is painful for about 20 minutes after the operation so, if the procedure has been done with general anaesthesia and without local anaesthetic infiltration, do make sure that the patient is given adequate analgesia before waking up.

Skin Needling induces collagen and elastin induction by employing the body's natural mechanisms that for the first time, as far as we know, produces regeneration of the skin and it's matrix. There is no scar formation and the procedure can safely be repeated until the desired effect is achieved. This can be repeated as often as necessary after face-lift surgery.

## 4. Lifting the most important component of the face with the scarless Mid-face-lift

Younger patients in their thirties and early forties are presenting to the plastic surgeon because they want to

- Reduce the early tear-trough shadows that run obliquely across their cheeks, and
- Early naso-labial grooves that make them looked tired and jaded. This results from the medio-inferior descent of malar fat and Sub Orbicularis Oculi Fat. There is a loss of the "ogee" curve of the face and in order to restore a youthful appearance to the face the surgeon has to reposition these two essential "padding" structures. However, this is not achieved even with the standard full face-lift, which tends to address the lower face and hardly deals with the mid-face. Improvement of the sagging mid-face can only be achieved by re-positioning of the malar and SOOF pads. We cannot approach this area without causing noticeable scars and because we are aesthetic surgeons we have to try and do this with virtually no scars.

I believe the solution is to anchor the tissues of the cheek with loops of non-absorbable sutures, to the temporal fascia on the side of the head and avoid making visible scars. I call this "Suture Suspension Loops" which I started doing in 1994. Alternatively, or in combination one can use specially designed anchoring threads to lift the midface tissues. After using various types of these threads I prefer Silhouette threads [24] either alone or in combination with suture suspension loops.

**Suture suspension Loops**

By using a number of 4/0 non-absorbable suspensory suture-loops, positioned in the malar fat pads with a spinal needle, one can easily lift the malar and sub-orbicularis oculi fat to create a youthful lower eyelid and ogee curve to the face. The principle is surprisingly simple and will be described in more detail [2]. However, there are many small tips and I found a rather steep "learning curve" in developing this procedure.

These threads are anchored by using 4-6 stab-incisions in a special pattern behind the temporal and side-burn hairline. Then I define the tissues of the malar fat pads and one easily can see that traction on these tissues will eliminate the jowls and improve the corner of the mouth. This creates the classical "ogee" cheek contour [25]. One of the major advantages of this procedure is that the anchoring area can be marked with silicon or even metallic rings and then at a later date, when the tissues start to sag again, they can be tightened up with a small operation in the temporal area without any signs of surgical intervention in the face. This is a unique feature of the technique and stands out as an important difference from virtually all other facelift operations. This novel idea is derived from the anchoring system for the Silhouette suture-lift.

In some cases it is useful to use the described suture loop to lift heavier tissues of the cheek, but in other cases with very little malar fat, I prefer to use "Silhouette" threads with absorbable cones to lift the cheek. These threads are also anchored onto the same anchoring system as the suture loops. I often use both sutures and threads.

**Markings**

You must mark the patient in the upright position and draw the guidelines that will give you the most appropriate lift. Some people only need moderate lifting of the actual mid-face whereas many require lifting of the tissues pushing down the corners of the mouth. In these people an extra loop is required.

The first loop should be designed (see figure 7) about 1.5 cms from the naso-labial groove at about the level of the nostril curving on its upper line over the malar arch, infero-laterally to the orbital margin, towards the temple about 2 cms behind the hairline. This point on the temple will be the anchor point. Mark the area where this line reaches the hairline. We will need to make a small stab incision at this point. The inferior part of the loop curves sufficiently to catch a good volume of malar fat and then goes straight up to the temple anchor point. Plan to anchor the Silhouette threads, if they will be used, in the same place.

If there is heaviness of the lower midface, then a similar loop is designed catching tissue more inferiorly but anchored to the same temporal area. If necessary other loops can be added. I prefer often to add another loop in a different horizontal vector just below the lateral canthus as shown in figure 7.

## 5. Methods and instruments

The following instruments and materials are required:

1. 11 or 15 blade scalpel
2. A 22 (yellow) gauge spinal needle.
3. Sharp pointed fine scissors
4. Fine dissector
5. Toothed "Adson's" forceps.
6. Fine needle-holder to tie the knot.
7. Skin hook to free the skin from the buried thread
8. 4/0 non-absorbable suture. I use a "Provein" polypropylene suture but this could be an elasticised suture as described by Serdev.
9. A Mayo style thick curved suture needle

**Surgical technique.**

The reason why this technique is called a scarless mid-face-lift is because no incisions or scars are made on the face at all. Only a needle prick is necessary on the facial skin. A stab incision is made on the hairline where the guidelines transect on their way to the temporal anchoring point as shown in figure 7. A slightly larger incision is made at the anchor point so that an anchoring silicon ring marker can be inserted into the depths. These incisions are carefully dissected away from the surrounding tissue so that the skin is totally free.

Push the needle into the skin in the cheek on the most medial part of the upper loop. The needle should be directed perpendicularly into the substance of the cheek fat, then upward towards the orbital margin to catch the greatest volume of cheek fat and finally directed to the upper incision at the hairline. The needle tip is "fished" out with the `Adson's forceps and then the non-absorbable suture is passed through the barrel of the needle till it emerges from the hub. Then the needle and the contained suture are withdrawn until the needle reaches the starting point in the depths of the cheek tissue. The needle is then re-directed in the opposite direction and then towards the lower incision at the temporal hairline. The needle is once again "fished" out and the thread inside the needle is pulled out. The needle can be totally withdrawn and the loop of the suture remains and can be checked to make sure that it pulls the tissues upwards without any retraction of skin. If necessary the suture should be replaced if it is not perfect.

WE now have a suture loop that can be anchored on the temporal fascia by taking each end respectively and then threading it through the mayo needle which is passed from the stab incision through the temporal fascia to the anchoring incision. The loop is tightened carefully with only mild over-correction and knotted. Once it has been knotted a silicon ring is used to mark the knot and the loop is tied onto the ring. I use six throws at least. At a later date if the face tissues become a little loose, one can open the incision again, find the silicon ring and tug it further backwards to restore the tightness.

Any other loops are similarly made and connected to the silicon ring.

I believe that it is necessary to change the vector of pull and introduce horizontal traction at the level of the lower orbital margin. For that reason I place a horizontal loop as shown in figure 7 after the malar lift. This restores a natural curve to the malar area.

Then if necessary, the upper silhouette threads are positioned and tied and also attached to the silicon ring. One needs to bury the silicon ring carefully and without any tension. If necessary I use a deep suture to close the skin as well as a skin suture. The stab wounds do not need to be sutured.

Once you have finished the one side you can easily see the difference between the tightened and the untreated side. I have learned to be sure not to have any traction areas or bumps because I have found that small irregularities do not always disappear. Often these irregularities can be pulled out with the skin hook.

I use this easy and safe procedure for younger patients as well as when I do a full face-lift with skin excision. The recovery can be rapid but some people swell rather more than one expects.

This can be a rather painful operation for about 50% cases in the initial 24 hours. The pain does not seem to be related to the tension of the loops. I tend to prescribe a special program of two unrelated analgesics to be taken alternately at 4-hour intervals. I usually use oral diclofenac as the one and a standard analgesic for moderate to severe pain as the other. That keeps the total daily dose down to minimal levels of each of these agents and also gives great pain relief.

PRE-OPERATIVE CARE – notes I give to the patient

1. To reduce bruising, avoid products that contain ASPIRIN, high doses of Vitamin E, high level Omega Oils and Evening Primrose oil for a period of 4 weeks before surgery. Avoid strong alcoholic drinks prior to surgery. I recommend that you use Vitamin C

1000 mg daily prior to surgery to reduce bruising and facilitate healing. You may use antioxidants, as usual. The use of bovine colostrum is also recommended.

2. It is also my impression that iontophoresis treatment with vitamin A and C by your beauty therapist may promote rapid healing if it is done a day or two before your operation. This may promote lymphatic drainage.
3. Do not smoke before or for a few days after surgery. Smoking interferes with the circulation of your skin. For people who cannot stop smoking, I will still operate because there is no threat of skin necrosis.
4. Wash your hair the night or the morning before surgery. We supply a medicated shampoo.
5. If you develop any signs of infection, pustules or boils on the face or body before surgery, please notify my office. We will be able to stop the infection rapidly.
6. Do not wear any make-up to surgery: this includes mascara and nail polish. If you tint, dye or bleach your hair then this should be done about one week prior to surgery.
7. Wear comfortable loose clothes that you don't have to pull over your head.
8. I always recommend a skin care with vitamin A and C and antioxidants for as long as possible before the operation and then continue post-operatively indefinitely to keep your skin as healthy and young-looking as possible.
9. I recommend Medical Roll-CIT skin needling to maximise the rejuvenation of your skin. Generally a course of six treatments should be done prior to surgery but can be done after surgery and repeated as often as necessary to achieve eradication of fine wrinkles.
10. I have designed a special pillow to remove the distorting pressure on your face that is partially responsible for the aged appearance and the development of the naso-labial grooves and upper lip lines. This pillow will also be essential to help you sleep comfortably after the operation.

POST-OPERATIVELY

1. It is important to remember that even though this delicate, extensive operation has been done under local anaesthetic, you must treat yourself as if it had been done under a general anaesthetic. Do not laugh, talk much, or run about. You have had a very large operation and you must rest properly. The fine suturing of the deep muscle layer and the re-positioning of the facial fat must be protected from rupturing in the first 2 weeks. Failure to take care may compromise the long-term result.
2. If you have had an intensive medical Roll-CIT at the same time then apply your topical skin products as normal.
3. Blood may stain the bandages. You may remove the bandages the morning after surgery. Do not remove any facial support that I have placed on the skin. You can have a shampoo one day after surgery.
4. You will be given a special mask to use post-operatively that will prevent distortion of your facial tissues no matter what pillow you chose to use. This also allows you to sleep on your side immediately after the operation. As soon as I have removed the support tapes, then you should use the "facial support mask" to protect the repair.

5. Do not turn your head from side to side but turn your body as a unit. Keep your chin in an elevated position and your head above shoulder level at all times. I prefer that you do not sleep flat. The head of the bed should be elevated with bricks if necessary so that you may sleep comfortably and still have your head elevated.
6. Use the special Pillow to support the face without placing stress on the repair while sleeping.
7. If eyelid surgery has been done at the same time as your face-lift, apply cold eye pads as frequently as possible for the first 48 hours.
8. Swelling and discoloration, and uneven swelling (more on one side than the other) are expected. Bruising and discoloration may rarely persist for 2-3 weeks after surgery. There might also be some lumpiness of the neck or cheeks and this may persist for 6-8 weeks, but it will disappear. In unusual cases it may be necessary to anaesthetise areas and tug on the skin.
9. Swelling may be improved by having Lymphatic drainage by a qualified skin-care therapist. A Facial treatment involving pulsed iontophoresis and low-frequency-sonophoresis is recommended a few days after surgery to reduce swelling and promote a tighter skin.
10. Avoid strenuous activity, getting overheated and sunbathing for 2-3 weeks.
11. Excessive swelling or pain should be reported as soon as it is noted.
12. If you have pets then please be particularly careful not to allow them close to you during the early stages of healing. Their hairs etc. can contaminate your scars and cause an infection.
13. Generally you may use topical vitamin A and C products again within a day or two of the operation.
14. You will have had a major operation so please remember to be gentle with yourself. Many people laugh in the initial phases after the operation and are euphoric but then become depressed as they realize the gravity of the operation, and the local anaesthetic. You should not be surprised to feel a little depressed about a week after the operation. Slowly, as the swelling in your eyes disappears, you will regain your confidence, and feel much happier.
15. You may drive as soon as you feel comfortable and safe to do so.
16. Usually, after a scarless facelift with or without intensive Roll-CIT needling, the patients feel comfortable to be out socially by about 5-7 days.
17. If the forehead has been lifted, you may have bruised eyes for 10-14 days.

## 6. Conclusion

It is easier to achieve impressive results when one ensures that the patient who wants a face-lift for rejuvenation, first treats their skin with vitamin A and C to get the youngest skin possible and reverse as much of their photoaging as possible. By adding six sessions of Roll-CIT done with topical anaesthesia one can make the skin actively more vital and convincingly younger. Finally, one can do a scarless mid-face-lift or total scarless face-lift with or without upper blepharoplasty or forehead lift and achieve a holistic and truly scarless rejuvenation of the face.

## Author details

M. B. Des Fernandes
*Renaissance Surgical Clinic, Cape Town, The Renaissance Body Science Institute, South Africa*
*Department of Plastic Surgery, Groote Schuur Hospital, University of Cape Town, Cape Town, South Africa*

## 7. References

[1] Fernandes, D., Percutaneous collagen induction: an alternative to laser resurfacing. Aesthet Surg J, 2002. 22(3): p. 307-9.
[2] Hudson, D.A. and D.B. Fernandes, Caveats for the use of suspension sutures. Aesthetic plastic surgery, 2004. 28(3): p. 170-3.
[3] Randolph, R.K. and M. Simon, All-trans-retinoic acid regulates retinol and 3,4-didehydroretinol metabolism in cultured human epidermal keratinocytes. J Invest Dermatol, 1996. 106(1): p. 168-75.
[4] Antille, C., et al., Vitamin A exerts a photoprotective action in skin by absorbing ultraviolet B radiation. J Invest Dermatol, 2003. 121(5): p. 1163-7.
[5] Moon, T.E., et al., Effect of retinol in preventing squamous cell skin cancer in moderate-risk subjects: a randomized, double-blind, controlled trial. Southwest Skin Cancer Prevention Study Group. Cancer Epidemiology, Biomarkers and Prevention, 1997. 6(11): p. 949-56.
[6] Guo, X. and L.J. Gudas, Metabolism of all-trans-retinol in normal human cell strains and squamous cell carcinoma (SCC) lines from the oral cavity and skin: reduced esterification of retinol in SCC lines. Cancer Res, 1998. 58(1): p. 166-76.
[7] Bailly, J., et al., In vitro metabolism by human skin and fibroblasts of retinol, retinal and retinoic acid. Exp Dermatol, 1998. 7(1): p. 27-34.
[8] Kurlandsky, S.B., et al., Auto-regulation of retinoic acid biosynthesis through regulation of retinol esterification in human keratinocytes. J Biol Chem, 1996. 271(26): p. 15346-52.
[9] Idson, B., Vitamins in cosmetics, an update: 1. Overview and vitamin A. Drug Cos Ind, 1990. May, 1990.
[10] Counts, D.F., F. Skreko, and J. McBee, The effect of retinyl palmitate on skin composition and morphometry J Soc Cosmet Chem, 1988. 39(44): p. 235-240.
[11] Hill, D.L. and C.J. Grubbs, Retinoids and cancer prevention. Annu Rev Nutr, 1992. 12: p. 161-81.
[12] Lin, J.Y., et al., UV photoprotection by combination topical antioxidants vitamin C and vitamin E. J Am Acad Dermatol, 2003. 48(6): p. 866-74.
[13] Goffin, V., et al., Topical retinol and the stratum corneum response to an environmental threat. Skin Pharmacol, 1997. 10(2): p. 85-9.
[14] Ortonne, J.P., Retinoid therapy of pigmentary disorders. Dermatol Ther, 2006. 19(5): p. 280-8.
[15] Shalita, A., The integral role of topical and oral retinoids in the early treatment of acne. J Eur Acad Dermatol Venereol, 2001. 15 Suppl 3: p. 43-9.

[16] Murphy, G.F., S. Katz, and A.M. Kligman, Topical tretinoin replenishes CD1a-positive epidermal Langerhans cells in chronically photodamaged human skin. J Cutan Pathol, 1998. 25(1): p. 30-4.

[17] Varani, J., et al., Vitamin A antagonizes decreased cell growth and elevated collagen-degrading matrix metalloproteinases and stimulates collagen accumulation in naturally aged human skin. J Invest Dermatol, 2000. 114(3): p. 480-6.

[18] Edward, M., Effects of retinoids on glycosaminoglycan synthesis by human skin fibroblasts grown as monolayers and within contracted collagen lattices. Br J Dermatol, 1995. 133(2): p. 223-30.

[19] Watson, R.E., et al., Repair of photoaged dermal matrix by topical application of a cosmetic 'antiageing' product. Br J Dermatol, 2008. 158(3): p. 472-7.

[20] Aust, M.C., et al., Percutaneous collagen induction-Regeneration in place of cicatrisation? J Plast Reconstr Aesthet Surg.

[21] Fernandes, D., Minimally invasive percutaneous collagen induction. Oral Maxillofac Surg Clin North Am, 2005. 17(1): p. 51-63.

[22] Fernandes, D. and M. Signorini, Combating photoaging with percutaneous collagen induction. Clin Dermatol, 2008. 26(2): p. 192-9.

[23] Aust, M.C., et al., Percutaneous collagen induction-regeneration in place of cicatrisation? J Plast Reconstr Aesthet Surg, 2010.

[24] de Benito, J., et al., Facial rejuvenation and improvement of malar projection using sutures with absorbable cones: surgical technique and case series. Aesthetic plastic surgery, 2011. 35(2): p. 248-53.

[25] Little, J.W., Volumetric perceptions in midfacial aging with altered priorities for rejuvenation. Plastic and reconstructive surgery, 2000. 105(1): p. 252-66; discussion 286-9.

# 5

# Serdev Sutures® in Upper Face: Brow and Temporal Lift; Glabella Muscle Ligation

Nikolay Serdev

## 1. Introduction

Closed approach transcutaneous Serdev Suture® lifts encompass the principale concept of stable suturing and fixation of mobile fascias to immobile periosteum, tendons and fascias, resulting in suture suspension and/or volume augmentation and/or repositioning.

21 techniques and individual modifications are used on face and in body areas, even where open surgical techniques cannot be directly applied. Serdev Sutures® are scarless and uncomplicated in the post-operative period. These techniques use curved semi-blunt semi-elastic needles and smooth surgical sutures to elevate and fixate mobile fascial tissue. Polycon surgical sutures are preferred for these techniques. They are characterized by short elasticity to prevent mobilized tissue from rupture and are characterized by delayed resorption (in 2-3 years, after the fibrosis is finalized). This enables stable fibrotic fixation before suture degradation.

Fixed mobile facial tissue using Serdev Sutures® is SMAS in all face areas: upper facial SMAS (galea aponeurotica), zygomatic SMAS extension, cheek SMAS, platysma and others. It is fixed by suture to stable, immobile tissues, such as periosteum, temporal fascia, zygoma, coli fascia, mastoid, occipital bone etc.

In addition to the possibility of lifting, Serdev Sutures® follow aesthetic principles of beautification: adaptation of aesthetic proportions, volumes and angles. In art and theatre, face masks called "mask of tragedy" and "mask of comedy" are well known and used to express age, status and emotions. The concept of scarless suture lift in face is to convert the "mask of tragedy" into a "mask of comedy", i.e. to uplift the subcutaneous facial mask – the SMAS. As soft tissue and skin are attached to the SMAS by a trabecular system, an intrinsic consequence of SMAS lifting is reflected in the lifting of the face and its most important elements in the same direction.

The structuring and positioning of different face elements is not limited to facial ptosis and elderly cases. Unaesthetic face angles, volumes and proportions are responsible for lack of beauty in young patients as well. Beautification is most important in youth and rejuvenation incl. beautification in elderly. Changing SMAS position by sutures can restore aesthetic angles, shape, volume and proportions as a basis for beautification and rejuvenation, imparting a happy, youthful appearance and a smiling expression.

## 1.1. History

Scarless closed approach Serdev Suture® lifts present skeletal fixation using skin punctures, without incisions and excisions, as a first alternative to classic excision lifts. Sutures are the same as in open surgery, but with much more variations and even in areas not reachable in open surgery. The anatomy study, instrument creation and surgical suture selection commenced in 1990 and the entire understanding of local topographic anatomy, instrumentarium and technique of this new method was ready in 1993. Needle preparation and selection of surgical sutures was experimental. For sutures stretch, elasticity and cut through tests were performed. The long term absorption of the sutures is crucial in the author's method. In 1994, at the Second annual meeting of the National Bulgarian Society of Aesthetic Surgery and Aesthetic Medicine, most of the scarless suture techniques for correction of early ptosis and flabbiness in areas of face and body were presented, as well as the initial results with 54 patients, operated during the period from 1993 to 1994. The author's contribution is that the transcutaneous closed approach suture techniques lift the SMAS and the facial skin attached to it, without traditional incisions. Operations were ambulatory with excellent results, reported by the patients. The trauma is minimal and the follow-up period is no longer than 3 days with fast and mostly immediate return to work and social life. There are no visible scars and the needle perforations on the skin are no longer visible after days.

## 1.2. Technique and anatomical fixations

Operations are ambulatory, without hospital stay. Trauma is minimal. The techniques consist of passing closed sutures, by needle perforations only, to lift mobile fascias supporting the skin and fix them to immobile skeletal structures (such as periosteum) in several facial and body areas.

The author has invented and performs the following scarless transcutaneous closed approach **suture lifts**:

1. **In face areas**: **Temporal lift** (upper SMAS to upper temporal line and temporal fascia) and **supra-temporal lifting** (upper SMAS to upper temporal line), **Brow lift** (orbito-cutaneous brow fascia, discovered by the author, to upper temporal line periosteum 1.5 cm above the upper orbital rim or at the hair line), **Lateral canthus lift** (to orbital rim or to upper temporal line and temporal fascia), **Mid-face lift** (SMAS zygomatic extension to temporo-parietal tendon and to upper temporal line periosteum), **Cheekbone lift** (fascial tube of Bichat fat pad, SMAS and zygomatic SMAS extension to zygoma

periosteum, to upper temporal line and temporal fascia, to temporo-parietal tendon etc.) **as well as Augmentation** using patient's own tissue, **Smiling dimple formation, Lower SMAS-platysma face and neck lift** (platysma fixation to mastoid), **Chin enhancement, form and position correction** with or without fixation to the menton periosteum, **Chin dimple formation**, **Sutures in rhinoplasty** for **tip rotation** (medial crura of greater alar cartilages to nasal bone periosteum), **tip refinement** (suturing together all 4 crura of both greater alar cartilages at the dom), **alar base narrowing** (suturing the alar base incl. accessory alar cartilages), **Otoplasty** (perihondrium suture to obtain the antihelix fold) etc.

2. **In body areas: Breast lift** (fixation of breast fascia and upper glandular tissue to clavicle and/or to pectoralis major tendon), **suture technique for Simmastia, or implant position correction, Buttocks lift** (fixation of the fibrous soft tissue to the sacro-cutaneous fascia, found by the author), **Abdominal flaccidity tightening** (linea alba shortening, superficial fascia to costal line, spina iliaca superior anterior), **Inner thigh lift** etc.

## 1.3. Results

The suture methods became possible after creating specific curved, semi-elastic, semi-blunt needles. Best results were obtained with the Bulgarian polycaproamide sutures Polycon, which ensure semi-elastic fixation of mobile to immobile tissue (unlike other available non elastic and non-absorbable surgical sutures). The author has experimentally evaluated that they do not cut through the tissues.

Preferred **surgical suture** qualities are – short elasticity, absorbable within two-three years - after final fibrosis formation, and anti-microbial action. The author's tests have shown that only Polycon surgical sutures ensure these qualities. - http://medicaldevices-bg.com/MDI/Threads.html.

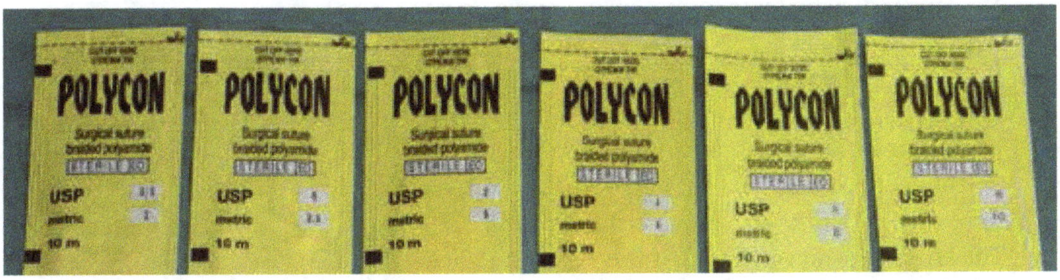


**Figure 1.** Polycon surgical sutures (3/0, 0, 2, 4, 6, 8) are semi-elastic (short elasticity), braided polycaproamide sutures of different thickness and have anti-microbial qualities.

USP depends on application. **6 different USPs** are suitable for different procedures and body areas:

- **USP 3/0** - for ear and nose: tip & base
- **USP 0** - for chin & brow lift
- **USP 2** - for facial, inner thigh, abdomen lifts

- **USP 4** - for temporal, mid-face lifts, buttocks & breast lifts
- **USP 6** - for bigger buttocks & large breast lifts
- **USP 8** - for bigger buttocks lifts (mostly used in Latin America)

Polycon surgical sutures are absorbed in the human body within 2-3 years, i.e. after the final fibrosis. According to the author, these are the best surgical sutures for lifting methods, because they permit semi-elastic movement of the sutured tissues.

## 1.4. Contributions

Serdev Suture® lifts, suspensions and volumizing present the first lifting method to replace scarring classic excision lifts as a complete method for scarless transcutaneous closed approach in total face and body lifts, where mobile fascias (holding skin by trabecular system) can be lifted and fixed to immobile periosteum, tendons and fascias.

### *1.4.1. Author suture techniques present*

- A new method for closed approach face and body liftings – a new alternative to classic excision lifts;
- Scarless lifting, using skin punctures only (no incisions or excisions);
- Mini-invasive, no downtime procedures;
- Beautification and rejuvenation methods;
- Volumizing method without implants and transplants. When needed, tissue augmentation is performed using patient's own tissue – a new alternative without implants;
- Can be used in cosmetic, aesthetic and plastic-reconstructive surgery;
- Downtime is shortened from weeks into some days;
- No danger of hematoma formation, no nerve damage, no scars.

**Serdev® Needles** are specially designed and developed for best use and have the following qualities:

- Elastic curve (the curve cannot be deformed when applying pressure in patients tissue);
- Smooth surface (does not cut periosteum);
- Conical semi-blunt tip (trauma is minimized);
- Thickness depends on length (from 50 mm to 250 mm) and application - http://medicaldevices-bg.com/MDI/Serdev_Needles.html.

**11 different needle lengths** were developed specifically for one or more face & body lifting techniques:

- Mini Mini 50 - for ear and nose: tip and alar base
- Mini Mini 50 (bended) - for fine chin subperiosteal fixations
- Mini 60 - for brow, chin, temporal, mid-face, cheekbone etc. lifts
- Mini 60 (bended) - for fine mid-face subperiosteal fixations

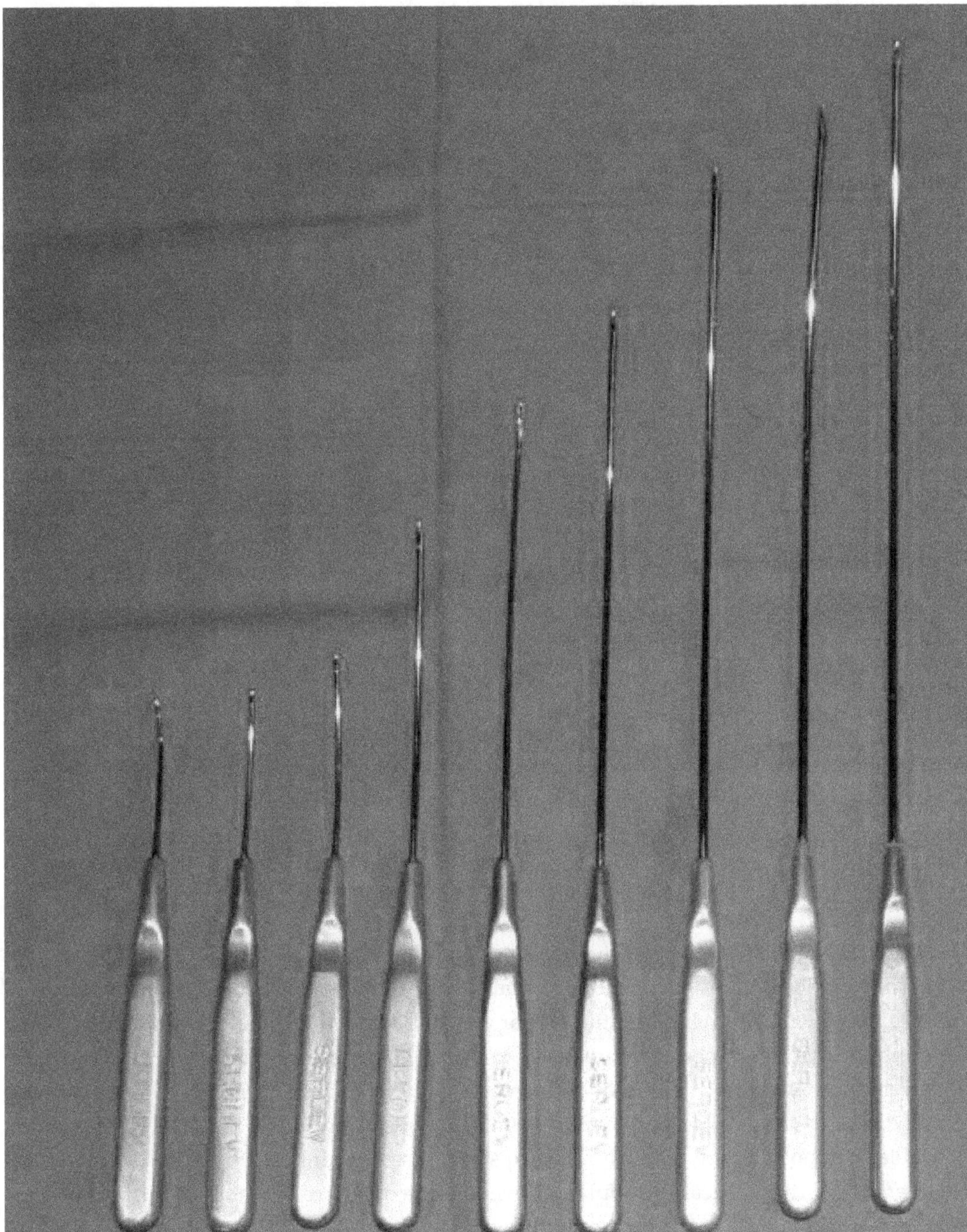

**Figure 2.** Serdev® needles (from left to right): Mini Mini 50 mm (bended), Mini Mini 50 mm, Mini 60 mm, Small 100 mm, Medium 140 mm, Long 170 mm, Super Long 210 & 230, and Super Super Long 250 mm (mostly used in Latin America).

- Small 80 - for neck lifts
- Small 100 - for facial, inner thigh, abdomen lifts
- Medium 140 - for mid-face, breast, abdomen lifts
- Long 170 - for buttock and breast lifts
- Super Long 210 - for buttock lifts *
- Super Long 230 - for buttock lifts *
- Super Super Long 250 - for buttock lifts *

*The choice of length depends on patient's physical characteristics

The needles are similar in shape to the currently used surgical needles with a handle to ease manipulation, with an eye at the needle tip (example Reverdin needles). However, Serdev® Needles are different in surface, elasticity, shape, size, thickness and have a curved elastic section (that retains structural curve memory regardless of the applied pressure). The elasticity and smooth polished surface allows the needles to safeguard bone-periosteal structures against cutting, regardless of the length and change of direction of the moving needle. The semi-blunt tip and elastic needle characteristics combine to avoid tissue trauma. The needle curve is specifically designed to provide ease of skin ingress, fluid movement through different soft tissue levels and periosteum, and the capture of fascial tissue. The semi-blunt tip exhibits variable penetrative qualities adapting to the application of the respective methods. The handle is flat and has a concavity mark for secure handling and display of needle tip position in the tissue.

## 1.5. Discussion

Scarless Serdev Suture® liftings use closed approach fixation of specific mobile fascial tissue to immobile skeleton periosteum without incisions. In Brazil they are known as "fio elastico" or "fio bulgaro". The Serdev Suture® techniques are used to correct early ptosis and flaccidity in areas of face and body, without traditional incisions. They are used also for tissue augmentation.

Observing Dr. Serdev's videos without proper training and understanding of anatomy led to "modified" techniques using non-original or straight needles, performing superficial barbed threads that are neither sutured, nor fixed, free floating in subdermal fat tissue or fixed only superiorly. Superficial threads and sutures fixed solely to the trabecular system in the subdermal fat cannot guarantee outcome longevity. Using straight needles is an over simplification that fails to secure deep fixation of mobile to immobile tissues that is essential for stable fixation. These are easy procedures for non-surgeons and this is the reason that this oversimplification became popular. However, outcomes are insecure. As little as a 1 or 2 mm change is enough to miss the topography of the important anatomical fixations such as bony rim, level of fascias and tendons. Therefore it is essential that doctors have a critical perception about the differences between suture lifts of mobile to immobile stable tissues and superficial thread lifts in subdermal fat.

## 2. Brow lift

Multiple invasive techniques have been described for fixation of the scalp and upper face. However, these methods do not allow the direct positioning of the brow as in the suture method described by the author. Within the past decade the demand for minimally invasive surgery, fast recovery and immediate beautification outcomes have revised the trend toward extensive surgical procedures and radically changed surgery in face-forehead beautification and rejuvenation. Even minimal incision approaches to brow lifting, using endoscopic methods or excisions of supra-brow skin, are associated with longer down time and have become undesirable options for beautification in younger patients. Improved understanding of eyebrow anatomy, pathophysiology of the aging face and advances in small - and non-incision surgery, have contributed to the new approach in correction of the eyebrow position for beautification and rejuvenation. The Serdev Suture® method with needle skin perforations between the eyebrow hairs has been reported and introduced internationally since 1994. The concept is to capture mobile but stable tissue (the orbito-supercilliar fascia, discovered by the author) and attach it to firm, immobile upper temporal line bone and periosteum.

The eye-eyebrow is the most influential region in determining facial expressions. There is only a narrow range of eyebrow positions that are perceived as attractive. Artistic location of the eyebrow is a guide line for eyebrow repositioning. The author has reviewed the young position of the eyebrow in models and also the artistic experience and aesthetic criteria for ideal female eyebrow height and shape in both international fashion models and movie stars. The preferred distance from the upper orbital rim to the eyebrow tail is on average 1.5 cm. Eyebrow shape should have a lateral apex slant. In male patients a lesser rise of the eyebrow tail has to be considered. The importance of aesthetic anatomy, aesthetic assessment and treatment planning in evaluation of the face must take into account considerations of patient selection, indications, and contraindications.

The author performs brow lift by suture in cases of ptosis, asymmetry, or in patients who desire a non-scarring and non-invasive procedure. Indications are beautification, rejuvenation, correction of proportions and angles.

### 2.1. Procedure

The brow lift suture is done by needle punctures only between the eyebrow hairs to prevent scaring. It presents a stable fixation of the orbito-supercilliar fascia to the periosteum of the rim of the upper temporal line, 1.5 cm above the orbital rim or at the hair line. The subperiosteal bite line (1.5 cm above the orbital rim) defines the eybrow design. An important instrument that facilitates performing this technique is the curved, semielastic, semiblunt mini-mini Serdev® needle with length of 50 mm that can be turned down and up in order to enter through the skin, capture periosteum or fascias and exit through another skin perforation point (Fig. 5). It is most important that we have at our disposal the 0 polycaproamide surgical sutures with marked elasticity that are biodegradable in the longer term (in 2-3 years), antimicrobial and braided (Fig. 1, 4). The semielastic, braided, USP 0 suture permits movements of face and muscles, fixation under elastic tension and does not traumatise or cut the sutured tissue. The extended period of resorption quality allows time for a stable fibrosis formation and does not leave foreign bodies in the tissue after the fibrotic fixation formation process and suture absorption is complete.

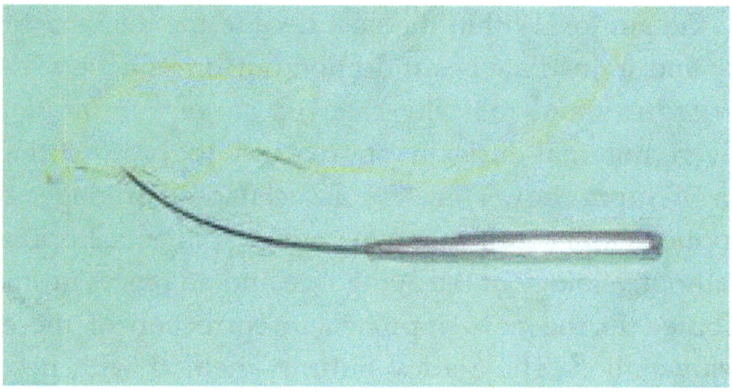

**Figure 3.** Curved, elastic, semi-blunt 50 mm or 60 mm Serdev® needle.

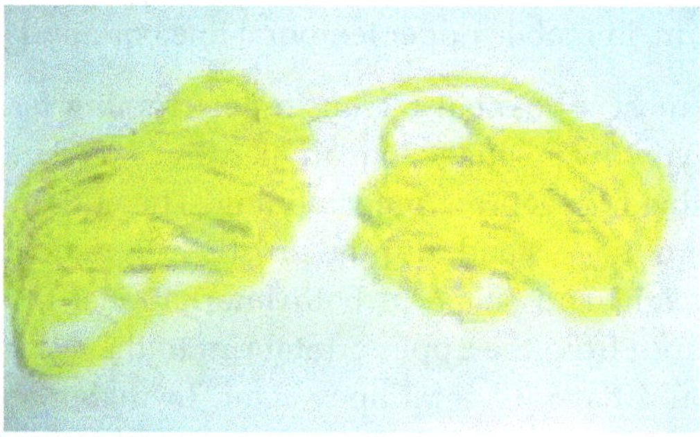

**Figure 4.** Semi-elastic, absorbable, braided, anti-microbial, polycaprocamide surgical sutures USP 0 are preferable and give best results.

## 2.2. Method for scarless brow lift by suture

### 1. Fixation of the orbito-supercilliar fascia to the periosteum of the upper temporal line, 1.5 cm above the orbital rim

To perform and accomplish the brow lift suture, the author uses 2 perforation points between the hairs of the brow, using the tip of a No. 11 scalpel blade. The perforation points are located on both sides of the intersection of the lateral canthus line and the eyebrow (Fig. 5A, B). The lateral canthus line is very important as the upper temporal line rim is located along this line, above the upper orbital rim. To position the eyebrow for artistic fixation, the forehead skin is pulled with a thumb placed 1 cm higher than the eyebrow, at the lateral canthus line. The maximum pull positions the eyebrow tail at the desired level of 1.5 cm over the upper orbital rim, without exeption. **NB!** Do not pull the eyebrow itself, which is looser and more mobile - it will result in a wrong brow tail position. After local anesthesia, while holding the eyebrow lifted, a 50 mm Serdev® needle is introduced through the lateral skin perforation point A with the tip pointing down, slides down on the rough surface of the upper temporal line rim, taking its periosteum, and becomes fixed. **NB!** If the needle is not

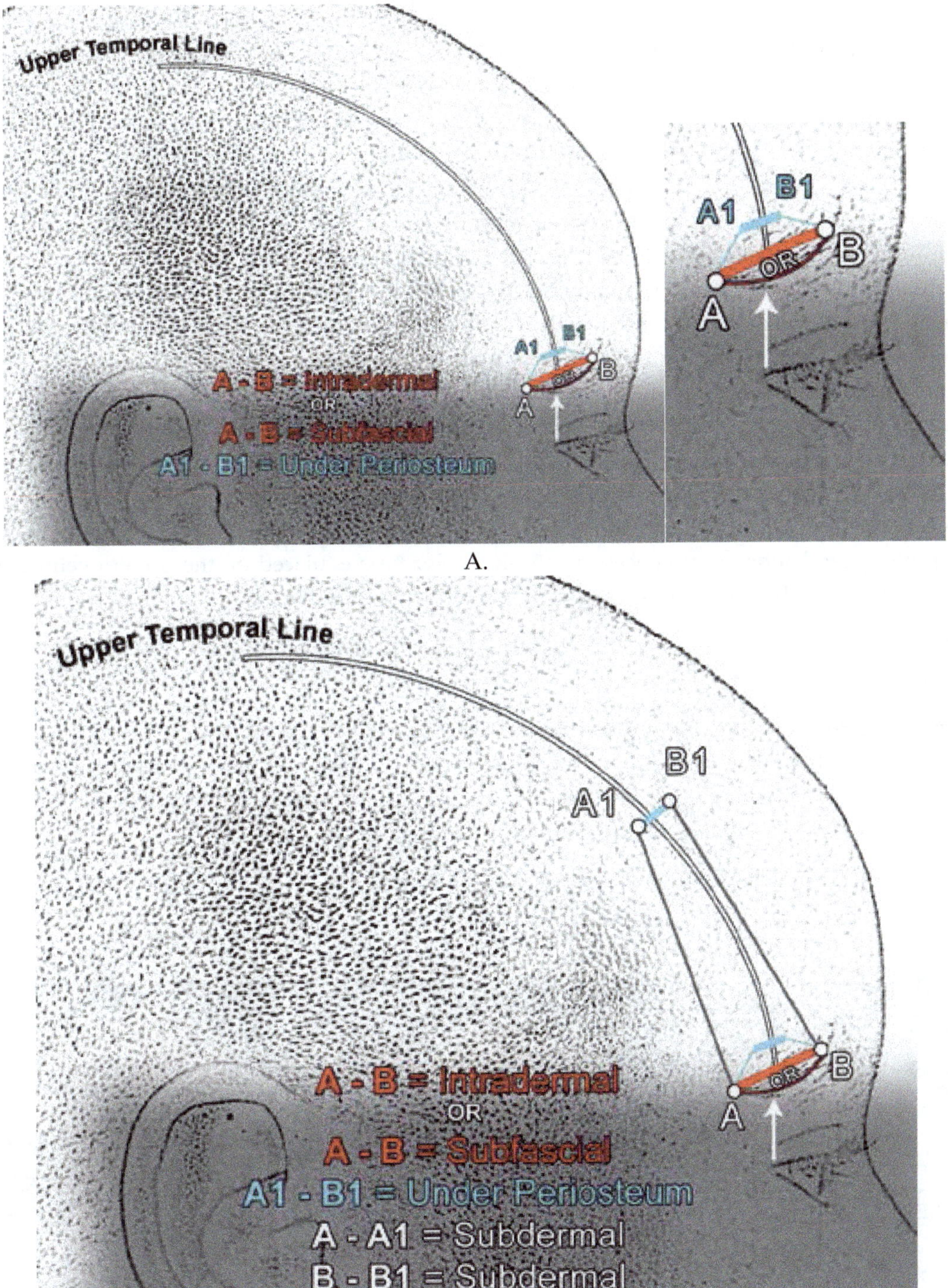


A.



B.

**Figure 5. A.** Eyebrow lifting by suture to the upper temporal line, 1.5 cm above the superior orbital rim. **B.** Eyebrow lifting by suture to the upper temporal line at the hair line.

fixed and can be moved lateraly, it is wrongly located in a superficial tissue plane and its position should be changed deeper subperiosteal. Turning the tip up, the needle exits through the medial skin perforation - point B. **NB!** Prevent dermis fixation. The needle should not feel any resistance when passing through the skin perforation points. This could be facilitated twisting the needle gently forward and backward. Do not push or pull. After threading the needle eye, the surgical suture is introduced and positioned through the first needle pass – stable immobile subperiosteal fixation. The second needle pass is done through the lower dermis layer between the points A and B at the lower eyebrow line. After exiting through point B and re-threading the needle, the second end of the surgical suture is pulled out through the second needle pass that presents fixation of the mobile orbito-supercilliar fascia, found by the author to hold the eyebrow to the upper orbital rim. The knot of the suture is done under medium elastic tension. A symmetry check follows. Equal lift of the skin on both sides gives us symmetry in all cases. If even a slight asymmetry is noted, an additional suture is performed to solve it. Then, pressure is used to flatten the brow over the suture and stop any bleeding. Still using pressure, skin at perforation points A and B is pulled away from the suture with a mosquito clamp, in order to remove any dimpling. No bandages are necessary. A skin color tape is placed on the upper eyelid that stays on overnight to reduce (suck) swelling by the hypertensive quality of the glue.

Additionally, through a 3-mm medial brow incision, glabellar muscles can be excised or ligated.

**Post-op care**: Next day, tapes are removed from upper lids. Face washing is obligatory to remove residual blood. Swelling in the suture area and the upper lid is nearly invisible for observers. No bruising appears in 99% of the cases. Patients can return to social life. Wound disinfection should be performed several times in the next 2-3 days.

**Video** http://www.youtube.com/watch?v=cLUf6-OrMPg

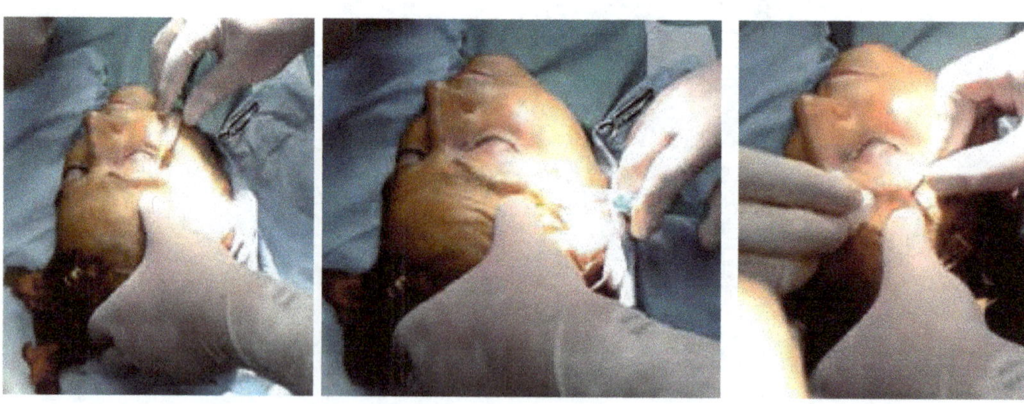

A. B. C.

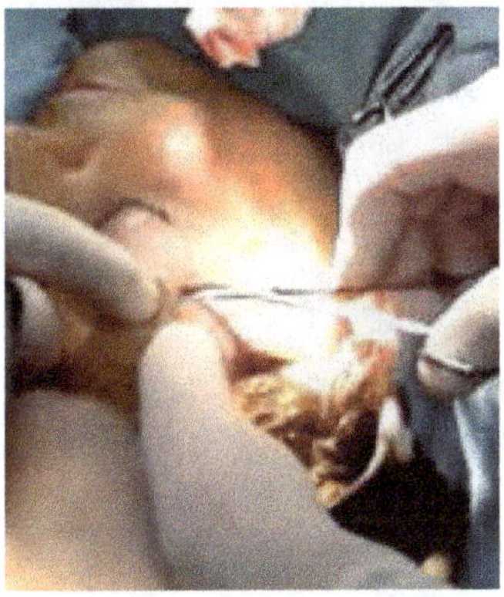
D.

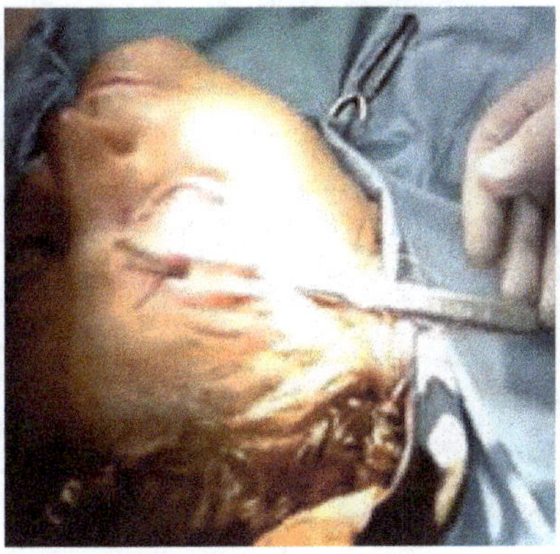
E.

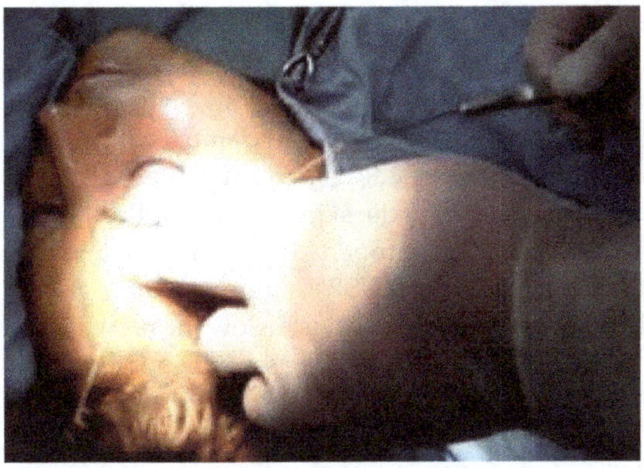
F.

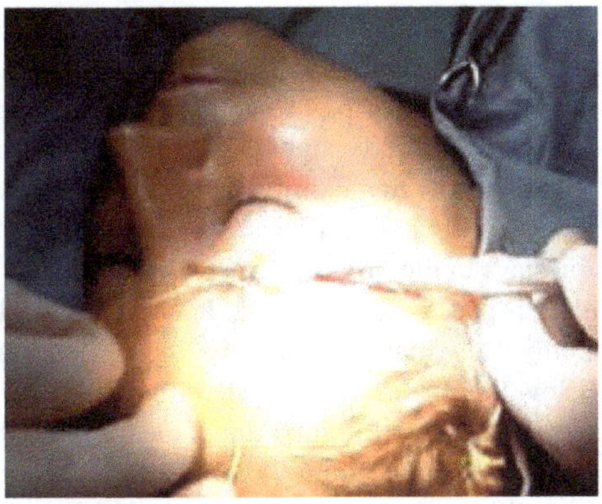
G.

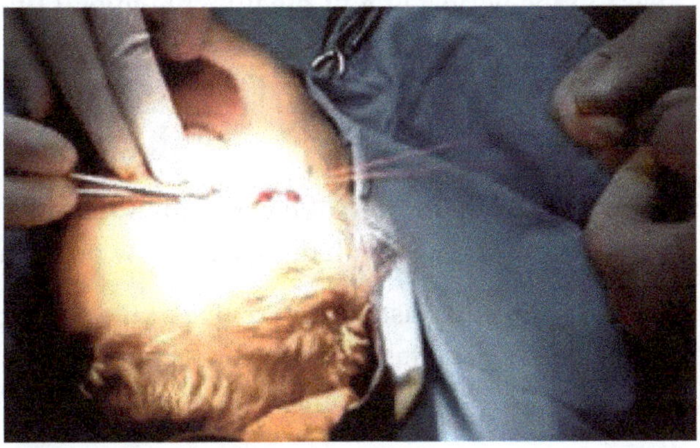
H.

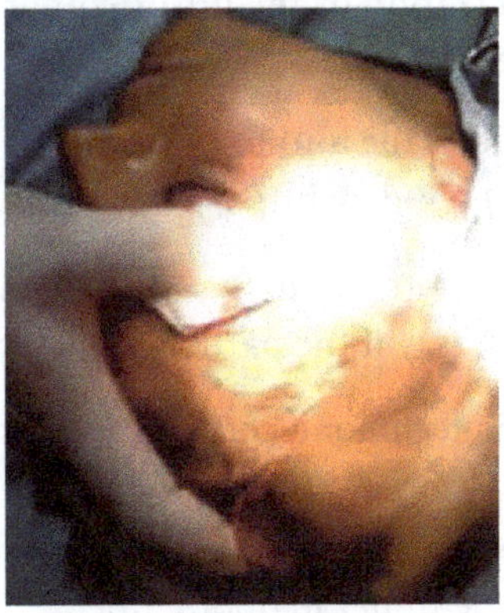
I.

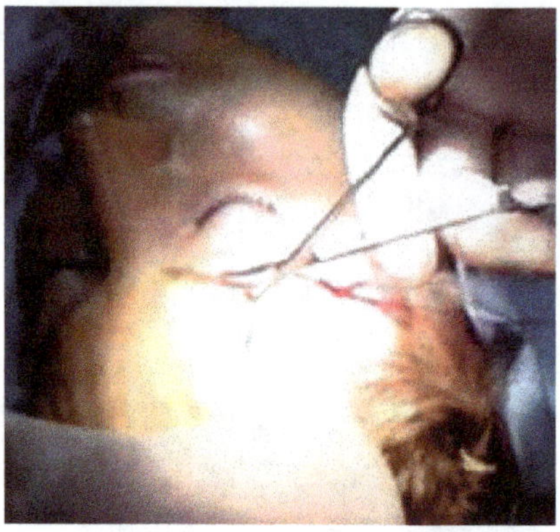

J.

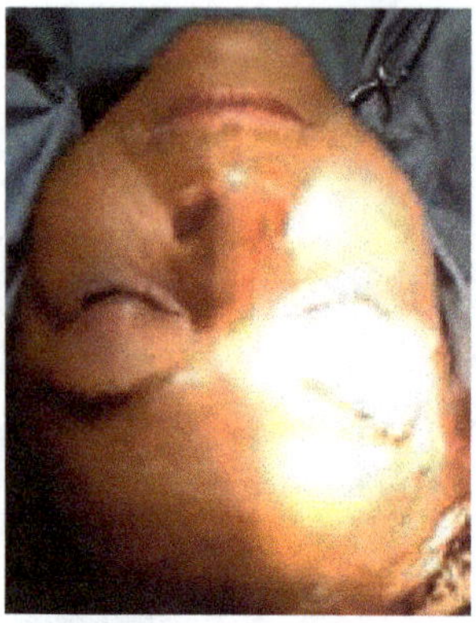

K.

**Figure 6. Steps of eyebrow lift by suture. A.** The needle shows where the lateral canthus line is crossing the brow. Skin perforation points A and B are located on both sides of this intersection point. Higher, on the lateral canthus line, the upper temporal line (rim) can be palpated with the thumb. Locate your thumb on the rim, 1 cm higher than the eyebrow; **B.** Lift the eyebrow with the thumb maximally and hold the brow in this position. Infiltrate point A and B, then the periosteum between, and also intradermally. Use a small amount of local anesthesia, injecting a few drops per line, to prevent swelling; **C.** Still holding the thumb in the same position, perforate points A and B with a No. 11 blade; **D.** Perforate the subdermal fascia at points A and B with the tip of a thin mosquito clamp; **E.** Still holding the brow in maximum lifted position, introduce the Serdev® needle 50mm subperiosteally between A and B. To test for proper placement, release your hand from the skin and the needle. If the needle stays in the proper subperiosteal position without moving, it is properly fixed. If needle moves, repeat this pass subperiosteally; **F.** Load the needle tip and introduce the USP 0 surgical suture subperiosteally in the line B-A; **G.** Second A-B needle pass is just subdermal, just below the brow line i.e. below the Serdev orbito-supercilliar fascia. Load the needle and introduce the second end of the surgical suture into the subcutaneous line B-A; **H.** The suture circle is finalized; **I.** Press for a minute and a half to stop any bleeding; **J.** Remove dimples at points A or B; **K.** The brow lift result is immediate. Perform the same steps the other side, holding the skin maximally lifted at the upper temporal line (rim), 1 cm higher that the brow. If the traction with the thumb is equal on both sides, the eyebrows will be lifted equally. Flex the head to check for equality.

### 2. Fixation of the orbito-supercilliar fascia to the periosteum of the upper temporal line at the hairline

Rarely, the author performs eyebrow fixation to the upper temporal line at the hair line (Fig .5B) – Video: http://www.youtube.com/watch?v=71n9oveGapc.

It is more traumatic and the author uses it only if higher lifting of the eyebrows is requested and only if the particular face permits aesthetic proportions with higher eyebrow position.

This technique consists on: Subdermal suture pass A-B (just below the line of the eyebrow), in order to attach the mobile Serdev orbito-superciliar fascia; two Connecting subdermal passes – A-A1 and B-B1; and Subperiosteal pass A1-B1: immobile subperiosteal attachment to the upper temporal line

## 2.3. Clinical cases

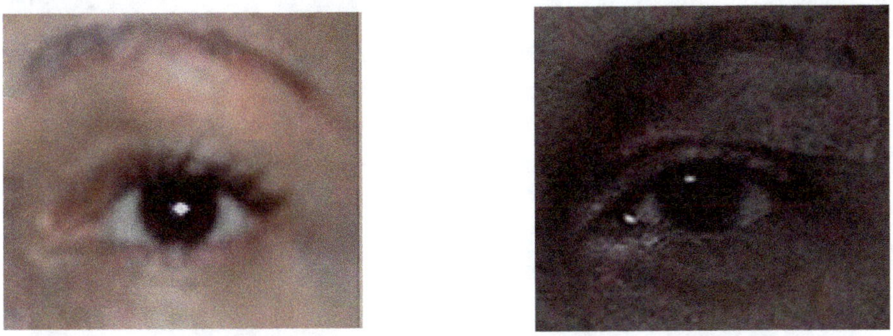

A. B.

**Figure 7. A., B.** Before and after brow lift by suture. A skin color tape is placed on the upper lid below the eyebrow to reduce swelling.

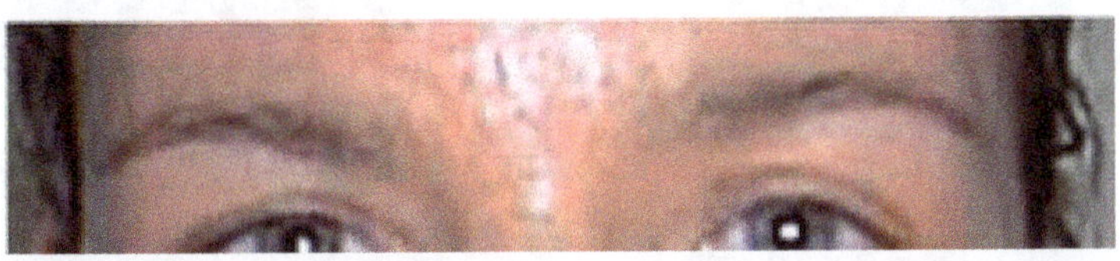

A.

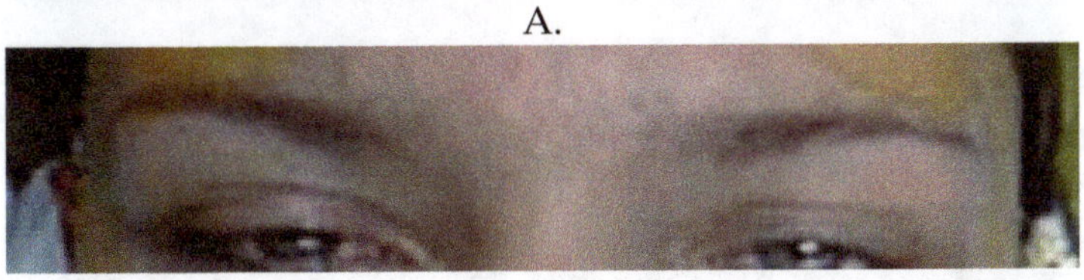

B.

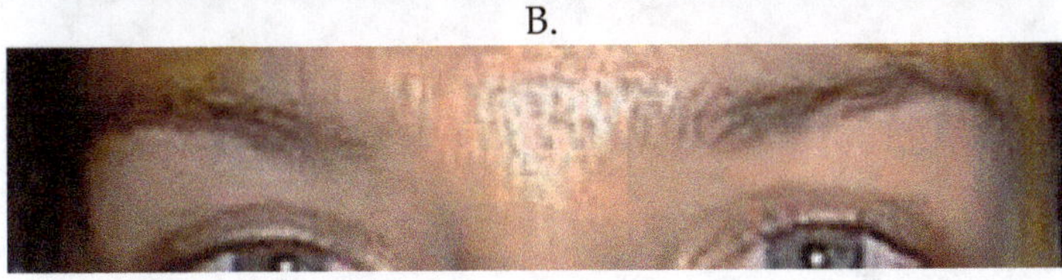

C.

**Figure 8. A.** Before, **B.** Intraop: right eyebrow is lifted without visible scars. Visible lift of the lateral canthus of the right eye, **C.** After: both eyebrows are lifted at the end of the operation. No visible scars. No operated-on appearance. No down time.

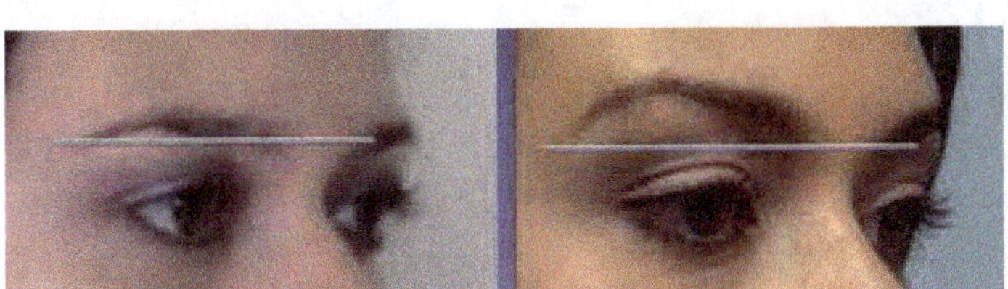

A. B.

**Figure 9. A.** Before and after Brow lift by Serdev Suture®. Artistic lifting and positioning of the eyebrow in a young lady.

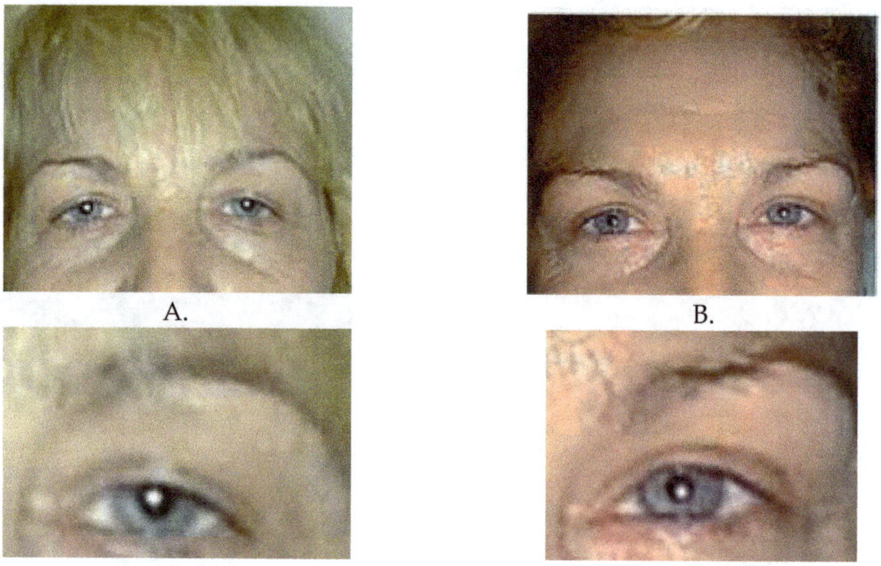

A. B.

C. D.

**Figure 10.** **A., C.** Before and **B., D.** 3 years after brow lift by suture. Visible lift of the eyebrow and lateral eye canthus.

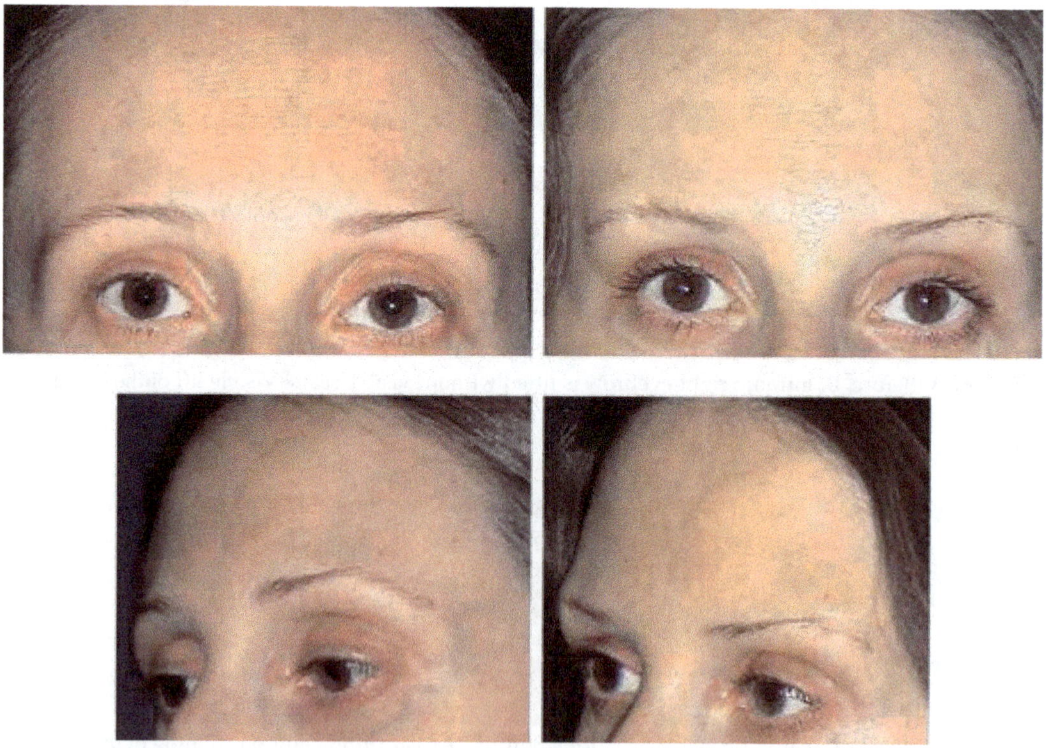

**Figure 11.** Eyebrow lift enhances appearance of the eyes.

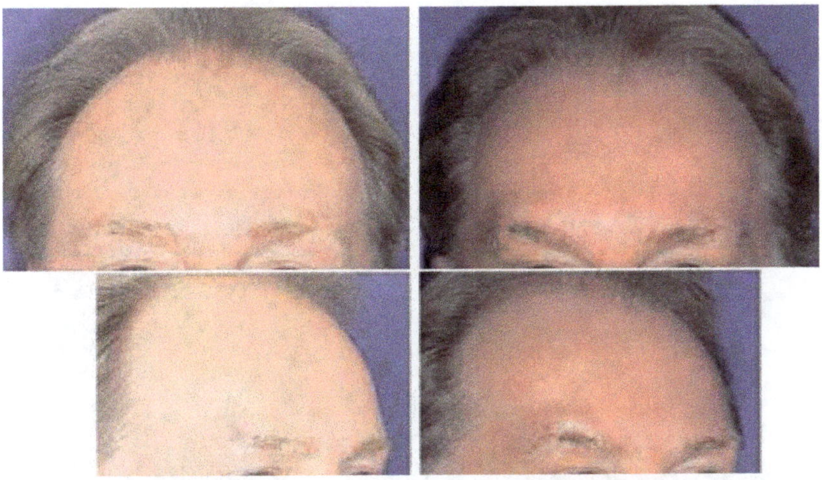

**Figure 12.** Lifted eyebrows solve the problem with proportions in high fronts and baldness.

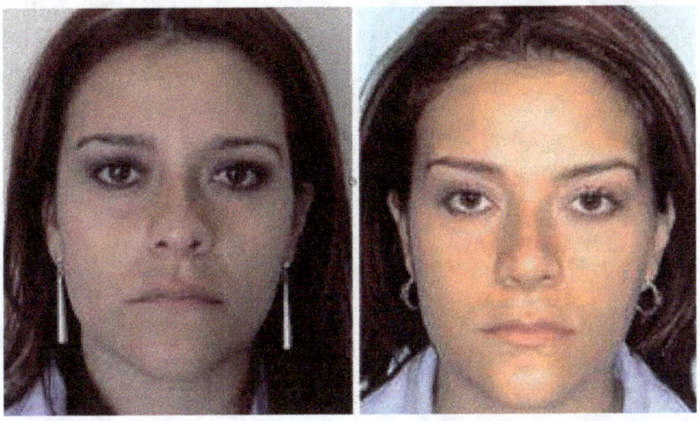

**Figure 13.** Total face beautification in the above 22 years young female obtained by a combination of operations: Brow lift + Nasal tip and allar base narrowing by suture + Chin enhancement + Cheekbone lift – all done by sutures + nasal hump removal. Result 4 days after surgery.

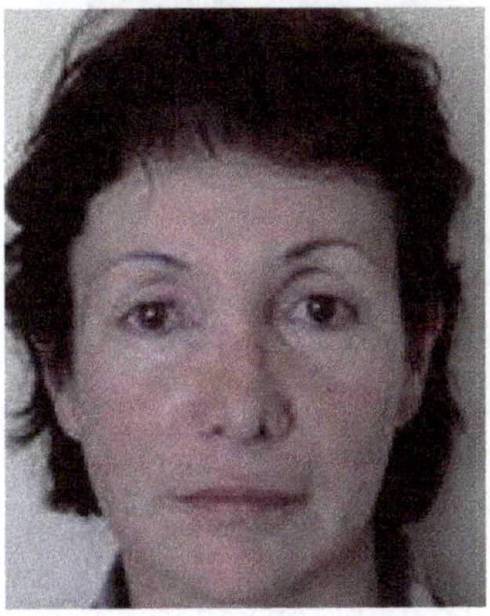

A.

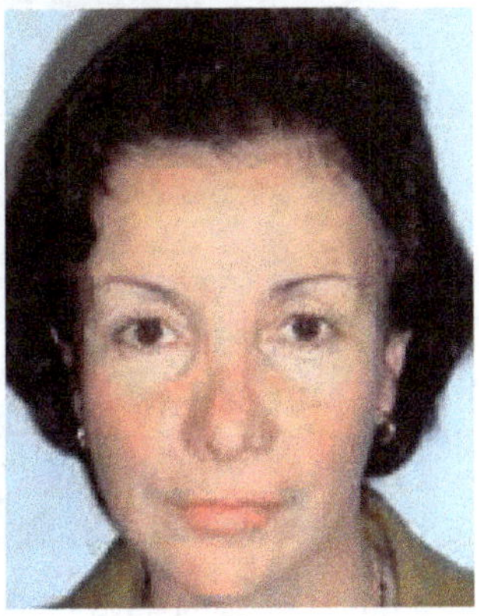

B.

**Figure 14. A.** Before and **B.** After Brow lift and Temporal SMAS lift by suture

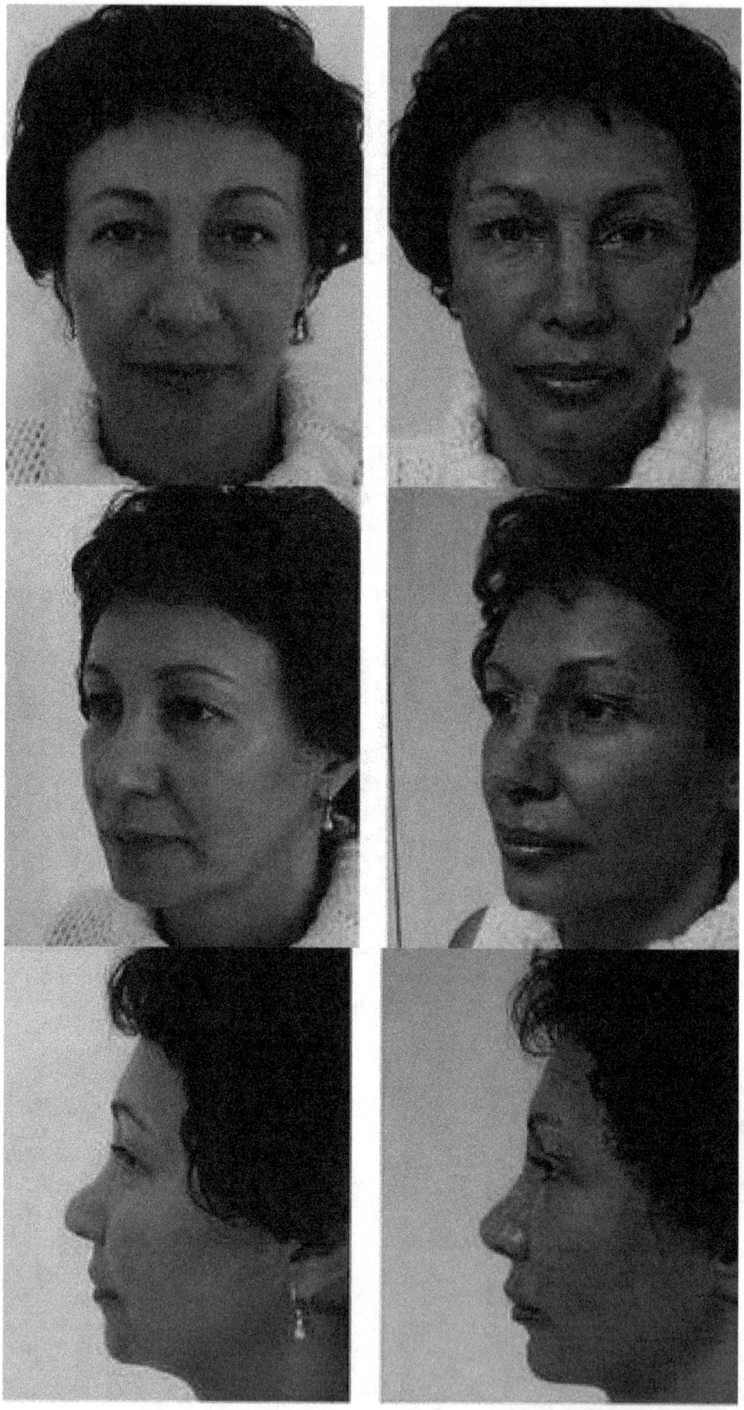

**Figure 15.** Beautification is mostly obtained by a combination of multiple operations – in this case: Brow lift + Chin enhancement + Chin dimple – all done by suture +secondary Rhinoplasty + Lip wy-plasty augmentation – immediate result

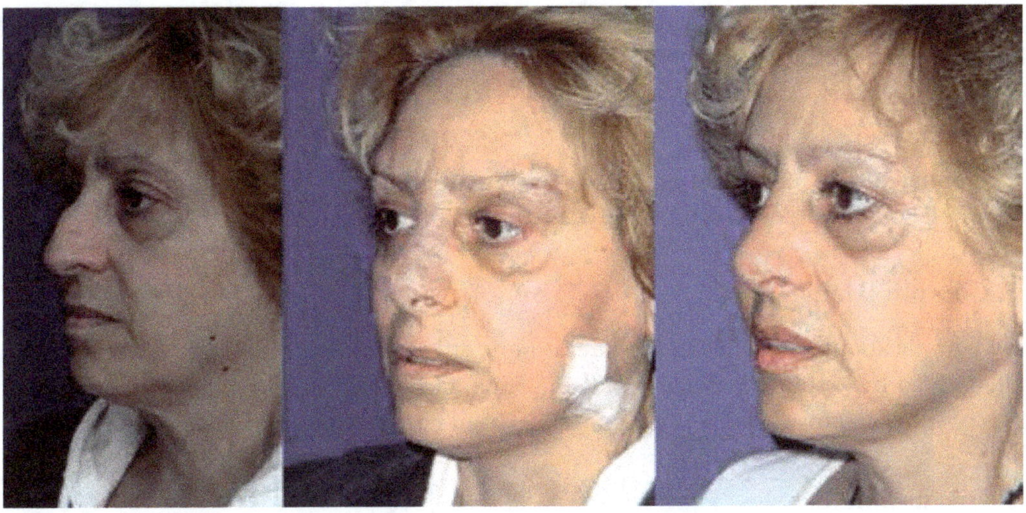

**Figure 16.** Beautification and rejuvenation obtained by a combination of operations: Brow + Temporal + Lower SMAS lifts by sutures + Rhinoplasty – Immediate and late result.

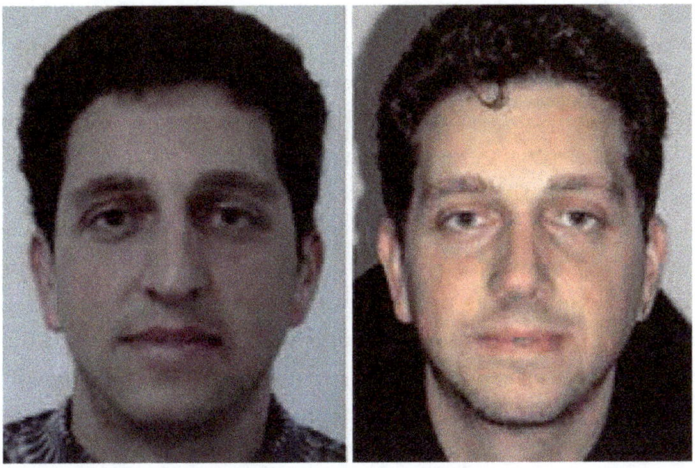

**Figure 17.** Total face beautification in a young male: Brow lift + Chin enhancement by sutures + Rhinoplasty. Brow lift in male patients has to be a bit lower than in female patients.

## 2.4. Results

During the period from 1994 to 2012, brow elevations using sutures were carried out in 982 patients. The follow up period varies from one month to 15 years. 96% of the patients reported excellent results, while 4% experienced good results. 68 % of the patients were followed during the first 5 years after surgery with very good rates of satisfaction. Only one 59 years old patient experienced aesthetic lack of satisfaction due to differences in appreciation of aesthetic proportions and angles in her age group. Complications were minimal – only 2 cases of infection in the lateral skin punctures which were treated by wound cleaning and disinfection for 2-3 days.

There were no instances of scarring, skin problems, or hair loss. The post operative period is characterized by a small percentage of swelling, no bleeding or bruising, no nerve injury, no scars, near to zero complications, immediate return to social life, preservation of facial expressive function.

In the patients with more than one year of follow up, the author has observed stable results and no ptosis was discovered with the years during follow up.

## 2.5. Complications

Two complications, infection in the lateral perforation point, 2 and 3 weeks after surgery, were treated by wound cleaning and disinfection and healed in 2 to 3 days. There were no cases of suture removal. No nerve damage has been noted in any patient.

## 2.6. Discussion

The purpose of this section is to present new trends in brow lifting philosophy and techniques.

There are a lot of procedures for brow lift that can have some negative effects for patients in modern society life: scars on the face that are only partially acceptable or non acceptable, asymmetries, increased tension across the healing wound, tension-related trophic skin changes, alopecia, paresis, ptosis etc. We can devide the proposed methods into invasive and mini-invasive surgeries. This chapter aims to describe an innovation in scarless brow lifting without any incision, without undermining but through suturing in situ the brow subdermal fibrous tissue and the orbito-supercilliar fascia higher to stable periosteum, using special needles and skin punctures only between the hairs of the brow. The method was introduced in 1994, with protocol description and was presented around the world as a part of author's "fashion art" face beautification in young patients and for correction of ptotic eyebrow and rejuvenation. In his hands it has the following advantages compared to incision and excision metods: short intervention time (about 5 minutes per side), no visible scars, minimal trauma, immediate result, a short and easy post-operative period with immediate return to social life. The suture absorbs over the longer term – in 2-3 years, so that it remains until the fibrosis is finally completed in 6 to 18 month after surgery and disappears later. The results are long lasting and pleasing.

The brow lift by suture without scars is an effective and safe technique for beautification of the eye region and rejuvenation of the upper face, producing a natural result with minimal complications and high level of longevity. It is a beautification method, ambulatory, under local anesthesia and i.v. sedation, with immediate results and near to 0 complications. It is done without visible scars, preserves the expression, the movement of the brow, and also preserves the natural look. A combination of local anesthesia and intravenous sedation provides excellent patient tolerance and comfort, both intraoperatively and postoperatively. Postoperative recovery is uneventful. Complications are very rarely encountered.

The eye-eyebrow region is the center for facial expression. The position of the eyebrows expresses emotion and even a minor change in brow position can be important for the understanding and contact between individuals. Lifting the eyebrows can change the expression into a more pleasant, young and natural one. We believe that this technique provides a more permanent and stable result. This brow lift method can be one of the most beneficial surgical procedures in cosmetic surgery. This very simple procedure allows lifting in any degree and elevation of any brow point. It supports the upper lid with lateral face improvement. It may be utilized for eyebrow ptosis alone or for fashion beauty, whether unilateral or bilateral; in conjunction with other suture techniques for equalizing asymmetrical eyebrows and for further support of markedly ptotic upper lids. It has been used by the author in instances of facial paresis or paralysis in conjunction with other procedures in the face to accomplish better symmetry. The stable duration of results with this procedure depends on the tissue quality and healing, the non-traumatic surgical technique, care given to the area during healing by the patient, amount of frowning and vigorous facial muscle use by the patient, and aging. It is a useful adjunct, especially when used with temporal SMAS lift, other suture methods on the face, beautification rhinoplasty etc. to adjust proportions, volumes and angles for beautification and rejuvenation of the individual's face.

The author's experience indicates that this specific method of scarless brow lift by suture adds a great deal to appearance and satisfaction. The procedure has taken its place as an integral part of facial beautification and rejuvenation.

## 3. Temporal SMAS lift

Since Mitz and Peyronie described the superficial muscle-aponeurotic system, or SMAS, in 1976, the SMAS facelift has become common and has risen into an operation to which others are compared. The author's concept to lift the whole SMAS in temporal direction is realised using the scarless Serdev Suture® method for changing the "mask of tragedy" into the "mask of comedy" in cases of beautification, soft tissue laxity, early facial ptosis and revision facelifts.

The temporal SMAS lift by suture was started in 1990 using traditional surgical instrumentarium. The author's needles and semi-elastic surgical sutures were introduced in 1993. In 1994 the author firstly reported his concept of a scarless ambulatory temporal SMAS lift by sutures, as lifting of the suprazygomatic SMAS with effect on the infrazygomatic SMAS, i.e. the whole SMAS. It became a routine ambulatory procedure for beautification and rejuvenation, presented and demonstrated around the world.

Since soft tissue and skin are attached to the SMAS in the temporal region, the lifting of the SMAS in temporal direction reflects in lifting of the face and its most important elements in the same direction (Fig. 18). It affects the lower face as well.

Anatomic landmarks for this method are: 1. The upper temporal line; and 2. The crosspoint (intersection) of the upper temporal line and the coronal line.

The aim of this method is to obtain beautification in patients of any age and rejuvenation in elderly, using minimally invasive cosmetic surgery procedures. It is performed in the ambulatory setting under local anesthesia with i.v. sedation. It is scarless with immediate results and near to 0% complications.

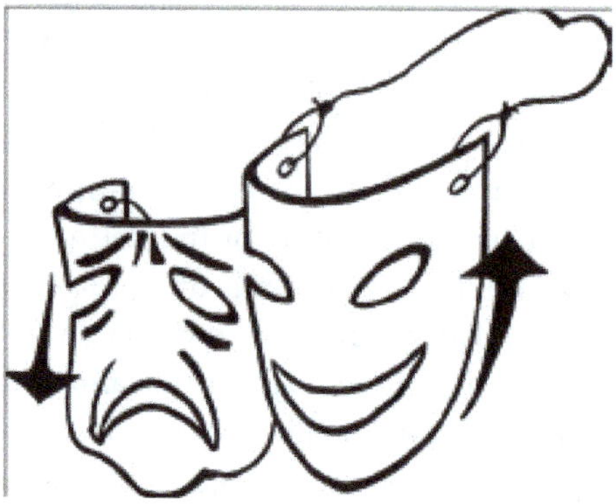

**Figure 18.** Mechanism of temporal SMAS lift – lifting of facial fascial mask (upper SMAS). Effect on facial structures. Transforming the old appearance into a young one. In ancient theater these masks are known as "Mask of tragedy" and "Mask of comedy".

Same idea of a temporal lift is easily created in any lady's mind, beautiful or not (Fig.19).

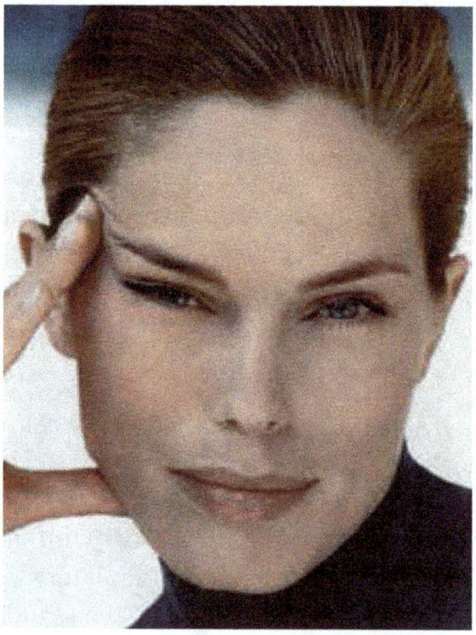

**Figure 19.** Ladies with no exception are thinking about temporal lift of the face.

With age, cranium volume shrinks and ptosis is reflected in the SMAS, which we can name Loose SMAS, and skin laxity changes expression into a sad and tired one. On the other hand, re-positioning of face elements could be used without restriction in face ptosis of the elderly. Aesthetically wrong face angles make young people look sad. Fixing the SMAS in a higher position allows repositioning of other soft tissue facial structures, fixed to SMAS. In young patients, the aim of the temporal SMAS lift is beautification, based on facial aesthetics.

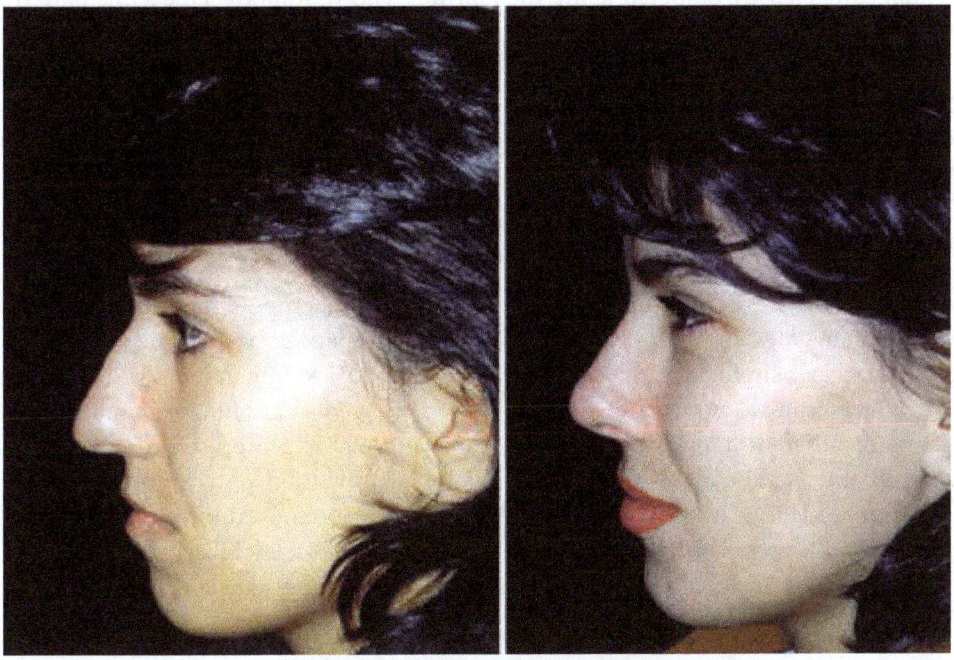

**Figure 20.** Before and after surgery. Temporal SMAS lift changes hanging eyebrow tail, lateral canthus angle of the eye and oral commissure. After: Better expression of cheek-bone prominence, due to the lifting of the skin and the fat pad. Additional rhinoplasty is made to correct the "golden section rule" of facial proportions in 3 equal parts; Lip augmentation to equalize lip and eye volume; Chin augmentation to obtain the "beauty triangle" and the straight line of the profile. Embellishment of the face is obtained and "smiling" expression is present ("mask of comedy" = fresh and young look).

### 3.1. Anatomic description of the temporal area and the SMAS

The SMAS is spread from the vertex to the platysma. It lies superficially to facial nerves. The SMAS acts as a suspension for the overlying facial skin and distributes forces of facial expression.

The Galea aponeurotica, as the upper part of the SMAS, is a muscle-aponeurotic tissue and extends from the vertex to the brow and the zygoma. It is named "superficial temporal fascia" as well, but it does not cover the temporal area solely. The temporal region, or "temporal pocket", is located over the temporal muscle, bordered by the superior temporal line above, by the lateral orbital rim in front, and by the zygomatic arch below. The layer, covering the temporalis muscle, is a bright and thick aponeurosis, the Temporalis Fascia, named also (wrongly) "deep temporal fascia". Both galea and temporal fascia are described with different names that causes confusion. At the level of the superior orbital rim, the temporal fascia (or "deep temporal fascia") splits in two layers: Superficial and Deep layer of the temporalis fascia (or /wrongly/ "deep temporal fascia"). These two fascial layers:

Superficial and Deep layer of the temporalis fascia enclose intermediate fat, including nerve and vessels. An important landmark in the temporal region is the superficial temporal artery that can be easily palpated along the hairline. The vein follows the same pattern. The frontal branch of the facial nerve, which innervates the frontalis muscle, the orbicularis oculi and corrugator supercilii lies in the intermediate fat interposed between the deep and the superficial layer of the temporalis fascia (or /wrongly/ "deep temporalis fascia"). It is considered to travel along a line connecting the base of the tragus to a point 1.5cm above the eyebrow.

### 3.2. The procedure

The concept of the scarless closed approach transcutaneous temporal face lift by sutures is to lift loose mobile galea and to fix it to stable immobile upper temporalis line periosteum and temporalis fascia. Skin fixed to the galea follows this repositioning in temporal direction that reflects in face lifting. To obtain such lifting, special curved semi-blunt, semi-elastic Serdev® needles with different lengths of 50 mm, 60 mm and 100 mm are used to introduce long-term absorbable, semi-elastic, braided, antimicrobial Bulgarian polycaproamide (Polycon) surgical sutures USP 2 or 4. Other surgical sutures could be used, but the short elasticity quallity of the Bulgarian suture reduces trauma to the fixated mobilised tissues. Rigid thin USP 2/0 threads work as a scalpels to mobile tissue, when under tension.

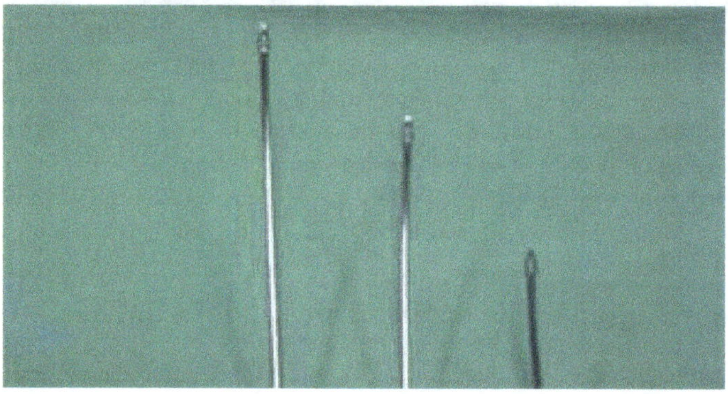

**Figure 21.** Curved semi-blunt and semi-elastic needles 50 mm, 60 mm and 100 mm

### 3.3. Surgical method

**Video:** http://www.youtube.com/watch?v=qFF3lr9jHqs

**1. Using needle perforation only - without skin incisions**

**1a. First Temporal SMAS Lift Suture**

Two lines A-B and A1-B1 are marked as parts of a rhombus inside the temporal area (Fig. 22 A). Line A-B represents the subperiosteal (upper temporal line) and subtemporal pass of the suture. Point A is located above the intersection point of the upper temporal line and the coronal line and point B is marked about 3-4 cm below at the coronal line. Starting from A, a line A-A1 is marked in 45 degrees angle to the line A-B in direction to the eyebrow tail. Point A1 is located at the end of that line in a distance from A, depending on the laxity, usually at 3-5 cm away from A. Line A1-B1 is the line of supragaleal fixation of SMAS. Lines A-A1 and B-B1 are subgaleal passes of the suture, connecting the two fixation lines. They mark the direction of movement of the galea to temporalis fascia. In cases of a very loose SMAS, mostly in elderly, it is advisable to perform a second suture, lower than the first one, to lift the medial and lower facial SMAS and soft tissue.

The wide spread temporal fixation (to temporal fascia) is not advisable, because temporalis fascia fibers are perpendicular and cannot hold a suture fixation with tension in distal direction. The suture will slide down and the lift will lose on longevity (Fig. 23).

**1b. Second (Lower) Suture for Temporal Lift**

A second line of galea fixation A2-B2 (below A1-B1) is marked (Fig. 22B) and a second suture is performed. in cases when laxity in the lower face is still presented after the first suture, mostly in elderly. The needle and surgical suture are introduced as follows: A-B – subperiosteally/subtemporally at the upper temporal line; A2-B2 – supragaleally; A-A2 and B-B2 – subgaleally.

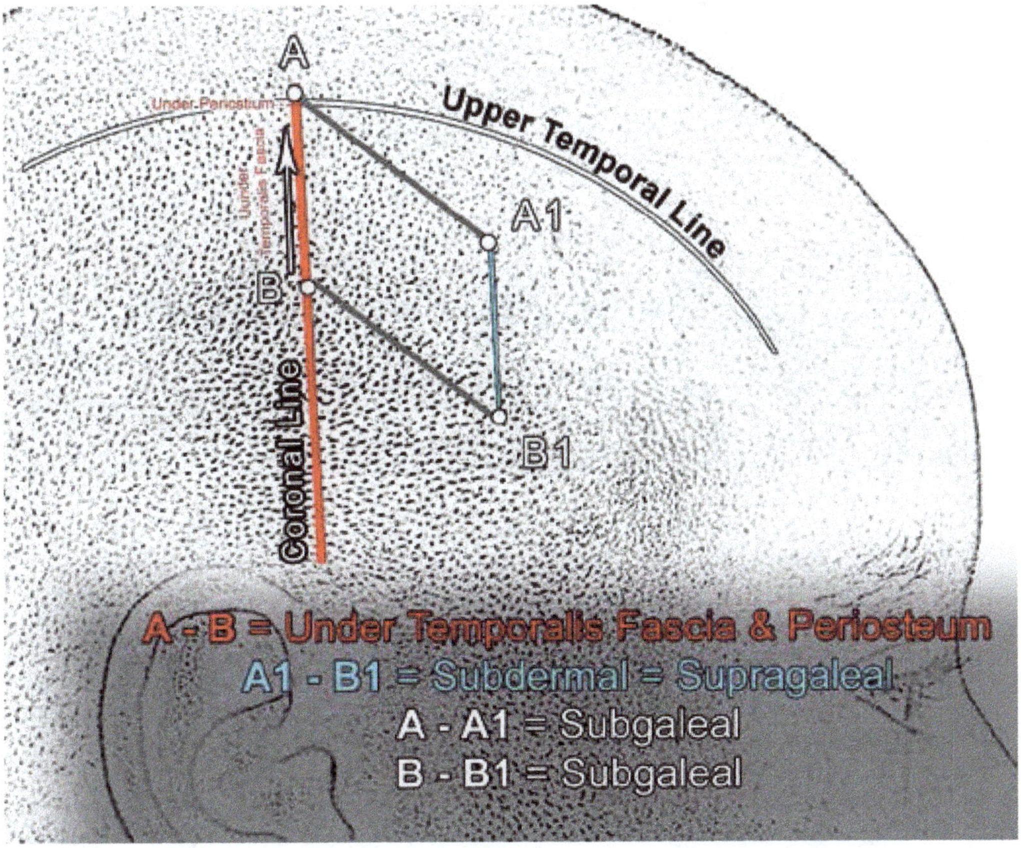


A.

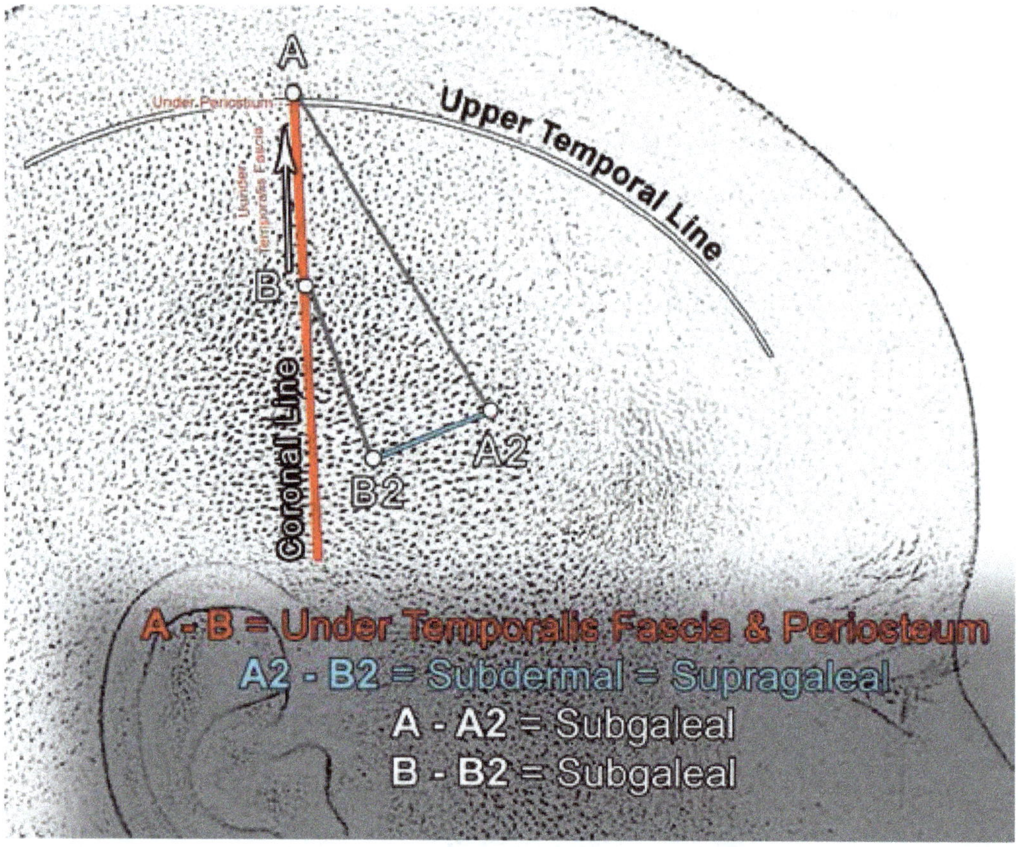


B.

**Figure 22.** **A.** Upper temporal line and coronal line are marked. The upper immobile fixation - subperiosteal (upper temporal line) and subtemporal pass of the suture (3-5 cm in the coronal line) is marked in red color. Line A1-B1 of supragaleal SMAS fixation will be lifted and fixed to A-B line of subperiosteal and subtemporal fixation. **B.** Same with the second lower suture in elderly: line A2-B2 of supragaleal fixation will be lifted and fixed by the suture to A-B line of subperiosteal and subtemporal fixation. Line A-A1 in direction to eyebrow and line B-B1 in direction to the cheekbone are subgaleal passes only. Lines A-A2 and B-B2 in direction to the lower face are subgaleal passes as well.

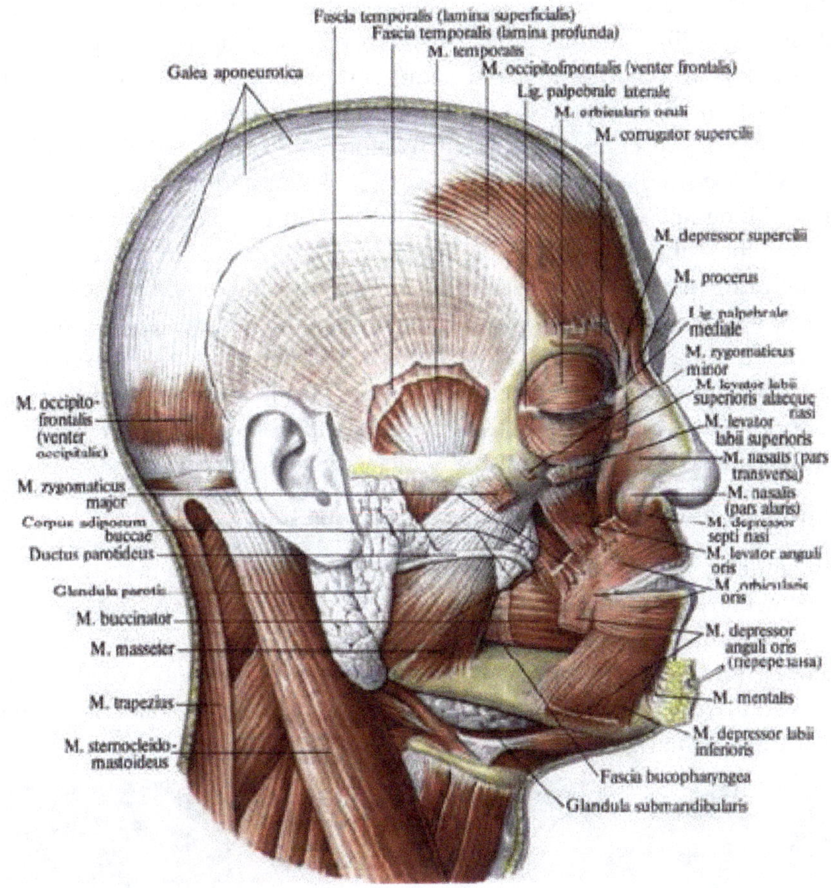


**Figure 23.** Temporal fascia fibers* are in distal direction and cannot hold the suture if the fixation is not attached to upper temporal line bone and periosteum. ***Anatomy figures from Sinelnikov - Atlas Of Human Anatomy, GIML, Moscow, 1963**

After local anesthesia, a No. 11 scalpel blade is used to make skin perforations at points A, B, A1 and B1. The order of needle entries should be convenient to right or left handed surgeons and could be as follows: the needle is introduced supragaleally in line A1-B1, just under the skin (between skin and galea, where a thin layer of subdermal fat allows to pass without any resistance). After threading the needle, the surgical suture is introduced in the A1-B1 supragaleal plane. The next subgaleal passes are directed from A to A1 and from B to B1 to take the suture ends. The final A-B pass is through the bone of the upper temporal line, subperiosteally and subtemporally. So, we have 3 levels of needle passes i.e. 3 levels of positioning of the surgical suture in the tissue: A1-B1 is supragaleal/subdermal (mobile fixation), A-A1 and B-B1 are subgaleal, and A-B – subperiosteal and subtemporal (immobile fixation). The location of the needle in each level has its characteristics. In the subdermal plane, the needle is not fixed by stable tissue – it is movable laterally and is covered only by a thin layer of skin. In the subgaleal plane, the needle is introduced deeper (in the tunnel of the lifted skin and galea, fixed together), and is mobile laterally again (Galea is mobile), and is covered by a thicker layer that includes skin, subdermal fat and galea. As galea is fixed to skin in that region, pulling of skin like a tunnel pulls galea as well and subgaleal entry in that tunnel is made easy. In this plane, one has to avoid taking temporalis fascia that is located below the needle. If temporalis fascia is captured with the needle, movement of the needle is impossible without movement of the entire head. Such fixation is incorrect and the needle has to be repositioned. **NB!** The needle should pass through all 4 skin perforations, in and out (or vice versa), without biting any dermal tissue, so as to prevent dimpling. The suture should not invert hair into the subdermal plane, in order to prevent foreign body reaction. When tightening, the suture dives in the subdermal tissue. Skin should not be engaged in the suture. When the circle of the suture is finished, a knot is made under medium elastic tension. The idea is to prevent trauma of the tissue. After the knot is tightened, a mosquito clamp is used to pull the skin perforations away from the suture, in order to free the skin and reduce dimpling at the perforation points. Some bulging effect (due to suture and edema) will disappear in a month, but is not visible in the temporal area, which is covered by hair.

**2. Using a minimal, hidden skin incision in the coronal line:**

In the very beginning, the author was using a 3 cm temporal incision in the coronal line A-B, which, working under visual control, is more comfortable for beginners to perform the subperiosteal and subtemporal fixation. In this technique we start with anesthesia and make a 2-3 cm long A-B incision along the coronal line. The skin and subdermal fat are opened and the red vascularised galea below becomes visible. After the galea is opened with a mosquito instrument, the white shiny temporal fascia is presented (Fig. 24).

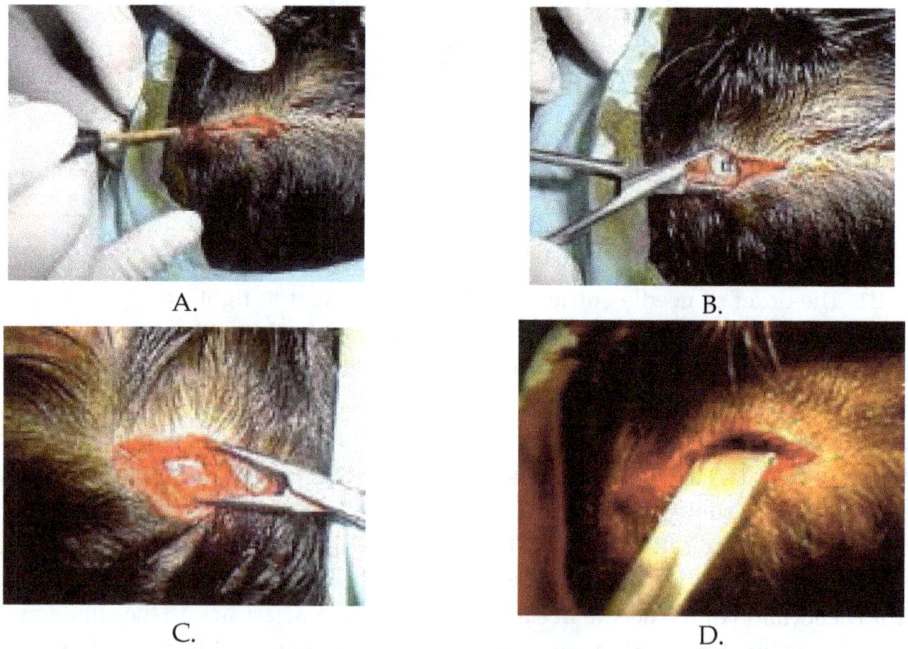

A. B. C. D.

**Figure 24. A.** Skin incision, **B., C.** blunt opening of skin and red galea; then white, shiny temporal fascia is visible, **D.** Blunt dissection between galea and temporal fascia.

A blunt subgaleal dissection follows till the hairline. It should be very easy because there is no stable fixation between these two fascias – galea and temporal fascia. Further, the same surgical technique is done as described above. Lines A-A1 and B-B1 are subgaleal passes of the suture, done under visual control, A1-B1 is a supragaleal i.e. subdermal pass, and A-B is a subperiosteal and subtemporal pass under visual control as well. A very important part of the technique is prevention of hair insertion with the suture loop into the subdermal plane that will lead to granuloma formation and local infection. Deep biting of the temporal muscle instead of a subfascial pass should be avoided to prevent pain, which is described by patients as headache. The galea, presenting the SMAS, is pulled up and fixed higher to the upper temporal line with one or two sutures on each side, under elastic tension. Thus, the whole SMAS is pulled up in temporo-occipital direction. Following this, the skin is closed with single stitches and no dressing is necessary. A hair wash is recommended on the next day to remove any residual blood. Wound stitches are removed after 7 days.

## 3.4. Clinical cases

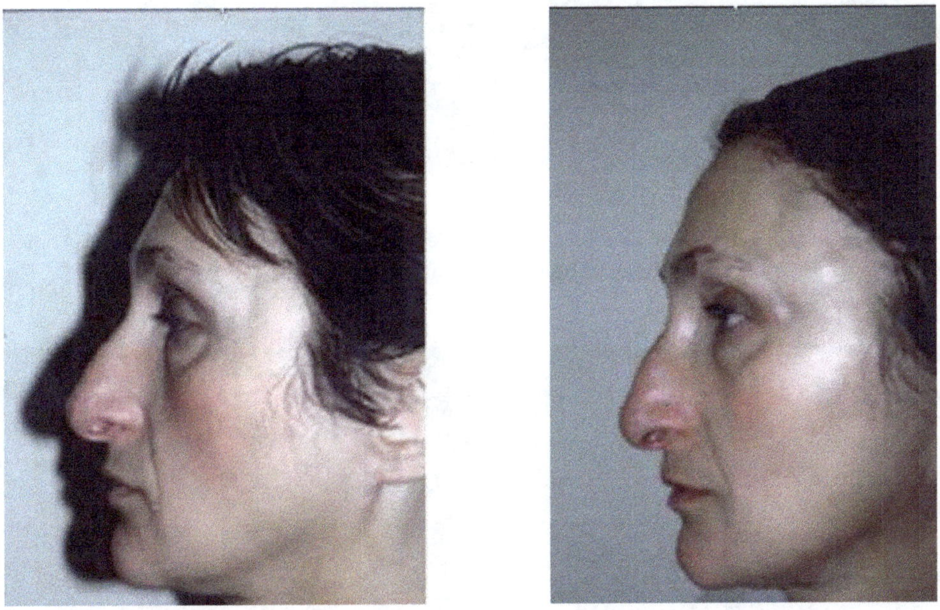

A. B.

**Figure 25. A, B.** Before and after a temporal SMAS lift. Visible elevation of the eyebrow tail and the lateral canthus of the eye, reduction of the crows-feet wrinkles, elevation of the cheeks' fat pad into a better cheekbone prominence; tightening, better texture and beautification of the skin.

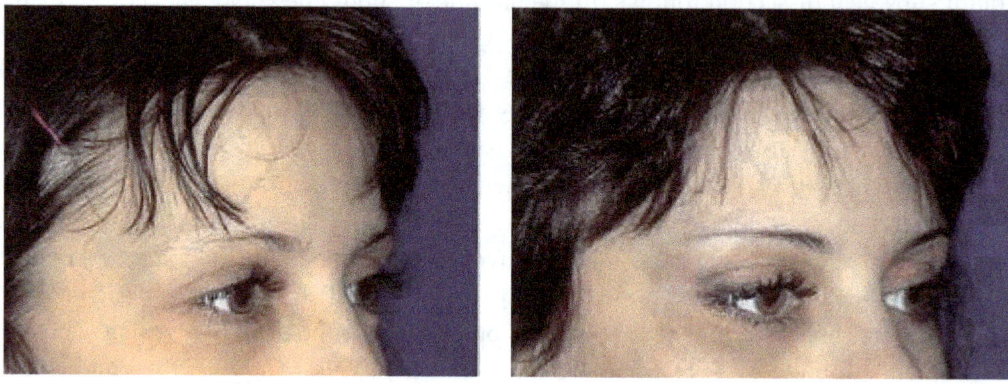

A. B.

**Figure 26.** **A.** before, **B.** after a temporal face lift in a young patient using Serdev Suture®. Angles of the eyes and eyebrows are changed, resulting in beautification.

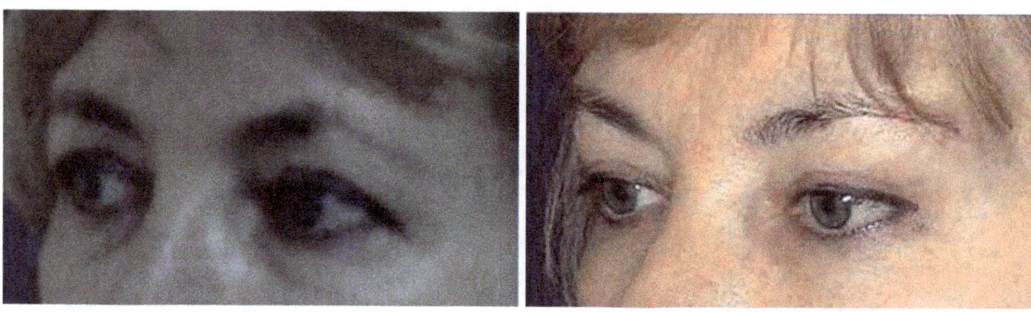

A. B.

**Figure 27.** **A**. before, **B.** after a temporal face lift using Serdev Suture® in an elderly patient. Angles of the eyes and eyebrows are changed resulting in rejuvenation and beautification.

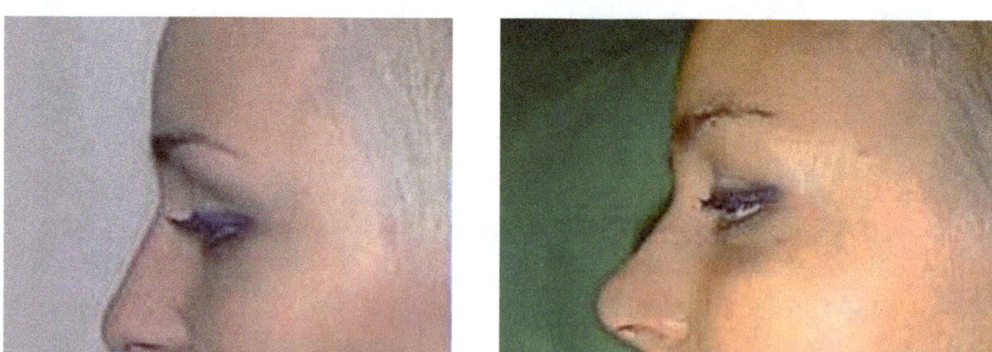

A. B.

**Figure 28.** **A, B.** Before and immediately after a temporal SMAS lift and tip rotation rhinoplasty. The absence of visible signs of operation permits immediate return to social life. Rhinoplasty in the author's technique does not need tampons and plaster fixation. No bruising when tip rotation only.

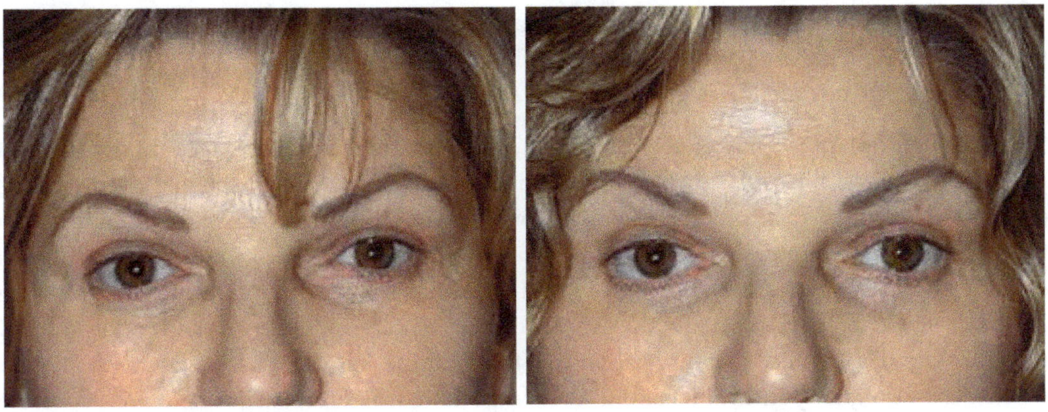

A. B.

**Figure 29.** **A.** Before. Asymmetric ptosis of the face with aging, **B.** After a temporal face lift using Serdev Suture®. The whole face is lifted resulting in beautification and rejuvenation, solving the different flabbiness on both sides. The face symmetry is equalized.

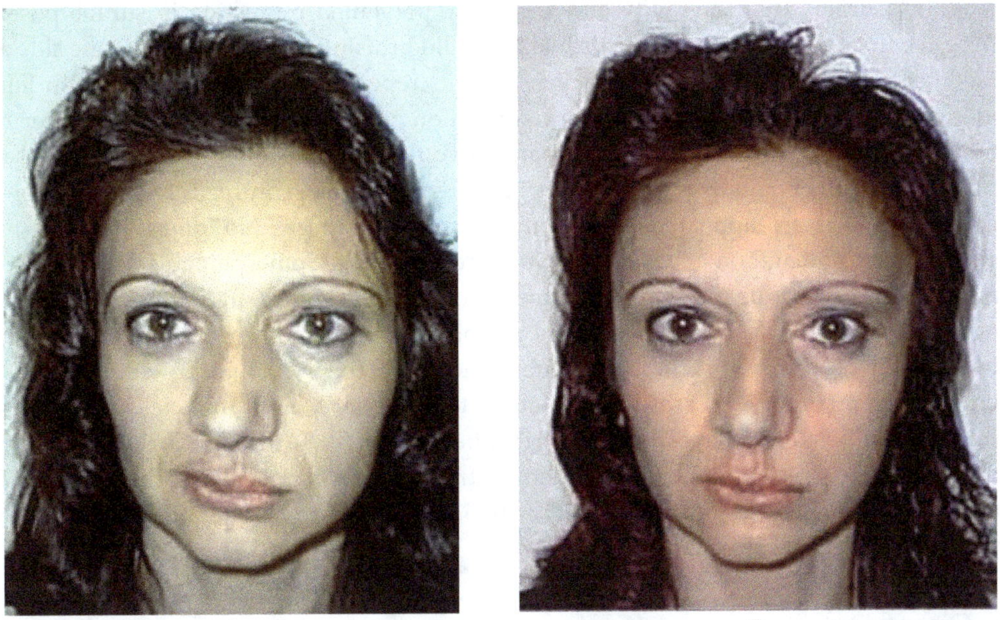

A. B.

**Figure 30.** **A, B.** Before and after unilateral temporal SMAS lift in facial paralysis. A 4-years result. The whole left side is elevated and the nose is repositioned in the middle by the temporal SMAS lift. Further equalization is possible using mid-face and cheekbone lifts, as well as chin movement to the left (see mid face and lower face chapters).

## 3.5. Results

1427 patients were followed up for more than 3 years, operated from 1993 to 2001, using the Temporal lift suture method, firstly with a minimal incision in the coronal line and later with needle perforations only. Patients' age ranges from 19 to 68 years. The operation was performed in ambulatory settings. After washing and styling the hair, patients could return to their social life next day, if necessary on the same day.

The temporal SMAS lift has effects on the suprazygomatic area: it reduces the lateral and forehead wrinkles; raises the eyebrow tails and the lateral canthus of the eyes; reduces the crows-foot wrinkles, raises the cheekbone prominence and tightens the skin. The effects on the lower face are collateral. The SMAS elevates the lateral canthus of the eyes, and the oral commissure. It improves the skin texture, reducing cheek flaccidity; gives a clearer outline of the jaw. Generally, the method gives excellent results in younger and middle aged patients whose lower face flacidity is minimal to medium. The facial tissues are repositioned to the desired higher youthful location. The temporal hair is preserved. There are no visible scars, no signs of operative intervention, and no "operated-on" appearance. A moderate feeling of tension in the face could be present for hours or days. The feeling is mostly pleasing. Only 7 patients described the tension as uncomfortable for one or two days. During the first week 12 patients reported headache. Lower eyelid swelling could appear on day 3 after surgery due to gravity and should be prevented by resting in supine position during the first two days. Five patients had lower lid bruising on the 3rd day on one side and four other patients – on both sides. Seven patients reported a crust formation with liquid under the crust. The reason was subdermal position of hair by the suture sling. After hair removal, the wounds healed in approximately two to four days. One patient had the same problem in another country and the surgeon removed the suture. Due to the fibrosis formation, no ptosis appeared after removal of the suture. No other infections, no hematomas or damage on the facial nerve were observed. Some palpable bulging in the temporal area could be present for some weeks. Most important in face lifting is its longevity. Numerous factors act against face stability, such as gravity and facial movements. The longevity of the result is improved due to the SMAS fixation to periosteum. This is best seen years after surgery in cases of a unilateral temporal SMAS lift in facial paralysis, post traumatic and postoperative canthal abnormalities etc. (Fig. 30). Two patients could not see the difference, despite the photograph demonstrations, contesting the aesthetic result. The effect of lifting angles was not satisfactory with 5 patients. With 3 of them the operation was repeated after 3 to 5 years.

### 3.6. Discussion

Currently, there are plenty of techniques used for face-lifts: conventional rhytidectomy, composite face-lifting, deep layer rhytidectomy, sub-SMAS, extended face-lifting, subcutaneous temporofacial lift combined with SMAS suspension, medial SMAS lift with aggressive temporal skin removal, temporal lift via blepharoplasty approach. Stretching the skin solely is obsolete. New techniques were proposed, such as endoscopic, subperiosteal, extended face lifts etc. There is no general agreement and no definitive answer as to which operative technique is most effective or preferable for each specific case. This is due to the subjective nature of aesthetics, aspirations and to the variability of skills and anatomy.

In the last years, an increasing number of patients ask for non-invasive or minimally invasive surgery for beautification or rejuvenation with minimal trauma and short recovery downtime, corresponding to the modern lifestyle. The suture method for temporal SMAS lift is the most preferred option by author's patients as an optimal solution for upper (and total) face beautification and rejuvenation, which preserves the natural look.

The temporal SMAS lift is a nice, weekend ambulatory procedure that gives a pleasing rejuvenation and beautification of the skin, eyes, brows, cheekbones, and most importantly - changes the expression. Complications rate is very low and the methods to solve the complications are easily performed. In young ladies, only one suture per side is usually enough to lift the lateral canthus of the eye, the eyebrow and to pull the ptotic malar fat into place, which restores and forms a nice malar eminence. It is also possible to combine the temporal lift by suture with other suture procedures: the author uses additional suture methods for brow, mid-face, cheekbone, and lower SMAS lift, simultaneous rhinoplasty, chin and lip augmentation, fat reduction and/or augmentation, skin resurfacing or blepharoplasty to obtain facial beautification and or rejuvenation. The closed approach Serdev Suture® method for temporal SMAS lift provides a safe and effective beautification, as well as rejuvenation in early laxity and face ptosis, and in some revision facelifts.

## 4. Supra-temporal lift

Supra-temporal lift presents fixation of the mobile galea aponeurotica at the hairline to the upper temporal line periosteum.

## 5. Glabella muscle ligation for permanent glabella relaxation

**Video:** http://www.youtube.com/watch?v=F7r-W7-kK20

### 5.1. Directions

**1.** Mark the glabella muscles: 1. Corrugator supercillii muscle; 2. Procerus muscle; 3. Depressor supercillii muscle. The glabella muscles are V-shaped. Select and mark A , B and C skin perforation points to tie and ligate that muscles in 3 lines: A-B line to ligate the Procerus muscle and Depressor supercillii muscle, A-C and B-C lines to ligate the Corrugator and Depressor supercillii muscles (Fig. 31).

**2.** Local anesthesia in points A, B and C intradermal and in direction A-B, A-C and B-C at periosteum and subdermally. Note: Inject local anesthesia sparingly, drop by drop as necessary, to prevent from visible swelling.

**3.** Perforate points A, B and C using a No. 11 scalpel blade. Using a mosquito clamp, perforate bluntly the subdermal fascia in the points A, B and C. **NB!** If not previously perforated, superficial fascias will be engaged in the suture, forming a dimpling effect on the skin surface.

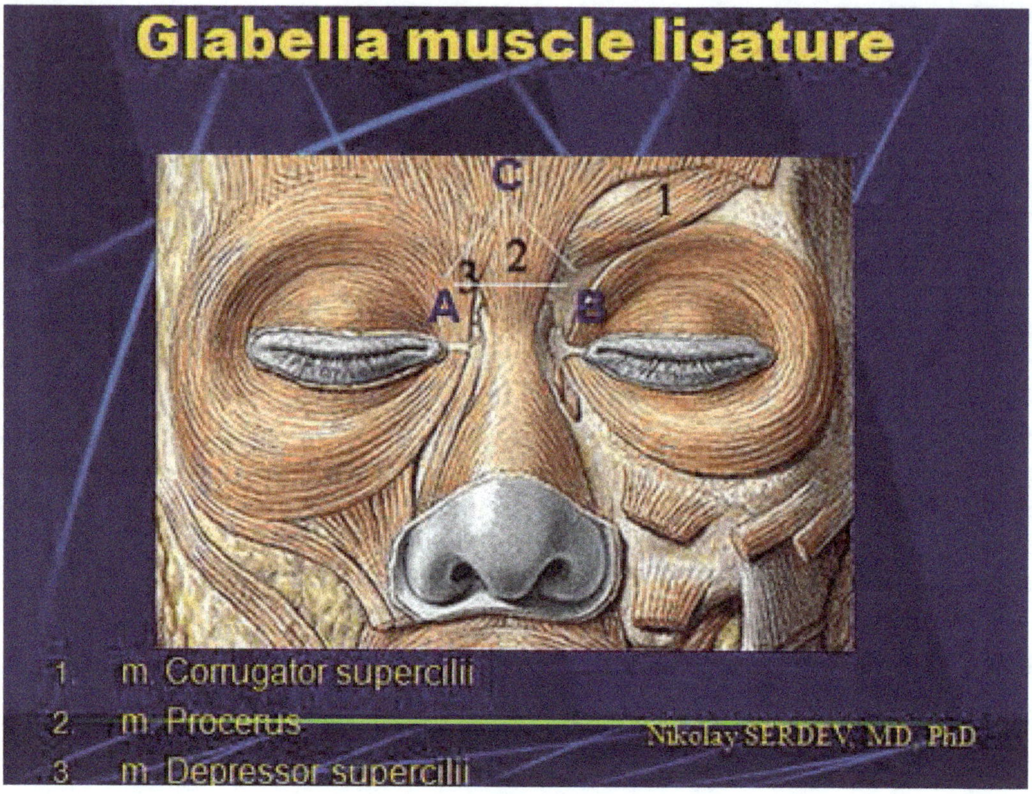


**Figure 31.** Suture lines A-B, B-C and A-C to ligate glabella muscles

### 5.2. A-B Suture - procerus & depressor supercilii muscle ligation

**A.** Introduce an unloaded "mini mini" Serdev® 50 mm needle from point A to point B, below the Procerus muscle, touching the periosteum. Load the needle with a surgical suture USP 3/0 and introduce it on the way of the needle pass A-B. **NB!** In skin perforation points, pass the needle perpendicularly to the skin surface, without resistance in front (to prevent engagement of dermal and fibrotic tissue), by smoothly twisting the needle. Do not push to bite dermis as this will result in a dimple. Do not push, do not pull – twist the needle smoothly forward and backward.

**B.** Introduce the unloaded needle from point A to point B subdermally, above the muscles. Feed the second suture end into the Serdev® needle at point B and introduce it toward A to finalize the circle of the suture. **NB!** The needle tip is always in direction to the suture end - to reach and load it.

**C.** Tie strongly at point A to ligate the muscles and obtain muscle necrosis at that place. After securing the knot, release any dimpling with a hemostat at point A and B.
**NB!** Serdev Sutures® should not engage skin.

### 5.3. A-C suture - corrugator supercilii & depressor supercilii muscle ligation

**A.** Introduce an unloaded "mini mini" Serdev® needle from point C to A, below the muscles Corrugator supercillii and Depressor supercillii, touching periosteum. Load the needle with suture USP 3/0 and introduce it on the way of the needle pass A-C.
**B.** Introduce the unloaded Serdev® needle from point C to A subdermally, above the muscles. Feed the second suture end into the Serdev® needle at point A and introduce it from A to C to finalize the circle of the suture.
**C.** Tie strongly at point C to ligate the muscles and to obtain muscle necrosis at that place. After securing the knot, release any dimpling with a hemostat at point A and C.

### 5.4. B-C suture - corrugator supercilii & depressor supercilii muscle ligation

**A.** Introduce an unloaded "mini mini" Serdev® needle from point B to C, below the muscles Corrugator supercillii and Depressor supercillii, touching periosteum. Load the needle with surgical suture USP 3/0 and introduce it on the way of the needle pass C-B.
**B.** Introduce the unloaded Serdev® needle from point B to C subdermally, above the muscles. Feed the second suture end into the Serdev® needle at point C and introduce it at B to finalize the circle of the suture.
**C.** Tie strongly at point B to ligate the muscles and to obtain muscle necrosis at that place. After securing the knot, release any dimpling with a hemostat at point B and C.

### 5.5. Results

20 patients were followed up to 3 years after operation with the suture ligation method to block glabella muscles. 3 years results show 80-95% relaxation of the glabella muscle function that is permanent.

Serdev Sutures® glabella muscle ligation provides a minimally invasive, scarless glabella muscle ligation, necrosis and relaxation with no downtime and near to zero complications. Longevity is very satisfactory. Aesthetic results often exceed patient expectations.

## 6. Lateral canthus lifting

There are 2 methods for lateral canthus lifting:

**1. Fixation to the lateral orbital rim.** Using 2 skin perforation points, the needle passes once below the lateral canthus and perforates orbital rim periosteum, and second time it passes above the orbital rim, subcutaneously. The suture fixes the lateral canthus to the lateral orbital rim periosteum.

**2. Fixation to the upper temporal rim and temporal fascia.**

**First pass:** Two skin perforation points are necessary on both sides of the lateral canthus to pass below or through the lateral canthus (using the 50 mm "mini mini" Serdev® needle), and introduce the surgical suture through that sub- or trans-canthal line.

**Second pass:** Then, a small (100 mm) or medium (140 mm) Serdev® needle is introduced through a third skin perforation point in the temporal line area to perforate the periosteum of the upper temporal line and the temporal fascia, take one of the suture ends and introduce it subtemporally and subperiosteally.

**Third pass:** This pass is subdermal, in order to take the second end of the suture, pull it through subdermally and fulfill the suture.

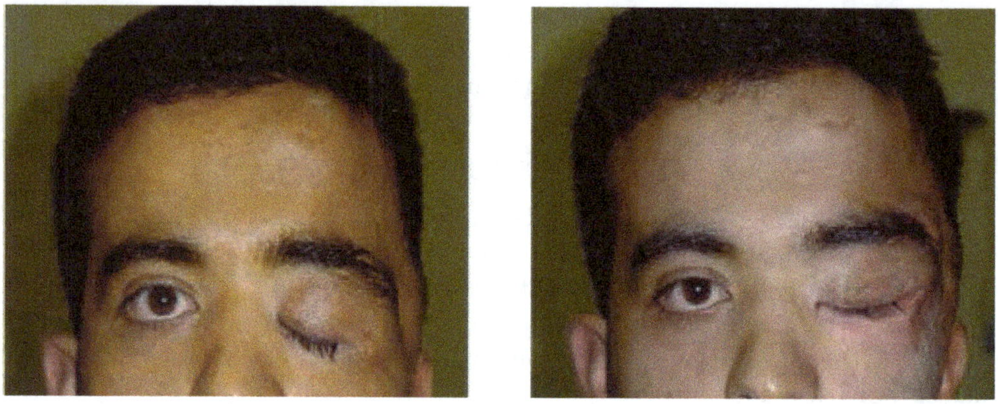

A. B.

**Figure 32. A.** After eye tumor enucleation, **B**. After lateral canthus fixation to upper temporal line and temporal fascia.

Lateral canthus repositioning is performed mostly in reconstructive surgery. Serdev Suture® lift permits beautification as well. Another possibility for lateral canthus lifting is the Serdev Suture® brow lift, which also reflects in a lateral canthus lifting.

## Author details

Nikolay Serdev
*New Bulgarian University, Sofia, Bulgaria*

## 7. References

[1] Serdev, N.P. Year 1994, Suture Suspensions For Lifting Or Volume Augmentation In Face And Body (English version), presented at the 2nd Annual Meeing of the National Bulgarian Society for Aesthetic Surgery and Aesthetic Medicine, Sofia, 18 March 1994, Int J Aesth Cosm, 2001,1:1, 2561-2568

[2] Serdev, N.P. Eyebrow lifting by suture (from "Serdev Sutures. Scarless face and body liftings"), Int J Aesth Cosm, 2011,11:3, 1-2

[3] Serdev, N.P. Brow lifting to the upper temporal line 1.5 cm, Int J Aesth Cosm, 2012,12:1, 1-62

[4] Serdev, N.P. Brow lifting with fixation to the upper temporal line at the hairline, Int J Aesth Cosm, 2012,12:1, 3-6

[5] Paul MD. The evolution in aesthetic cosmetic surgery. Plast Reconstr Surg 2001 Oct;108(5):1409-24
[6] Wang TD. Rhytidectomy for treatment of the aging face. Mayo Clin Proc 1989 Jul;64(7):780-90
[7] Cook TA, Musgrave-Zwetsch J. Adjuncts to face lifting procedures. Otolaryngol Clin North Am 1980 May;13(2):321-35
[8] Forrest CR, Phillips JH, Bell TA, Gruss JS. The biomechanical effects of deep tissue support as related to brow and facelift procedures. Plast Reconstr Surg 1991 Sep;88(3):427-32
[9] Rafaty FM. Elimination of glabellar frown lines. Arch Otolaryngol 1981 Jul;107(7):428-30
[10] Liebman EP, Webster RC, Berger AS, DellaVecchia M. The frontalis nerve in the temporal brow lift. Arch Otolaryngol 1982 Apr;108(4):232-5
[11] Webster RC, Gaunt JM, Hamdan US, Fuleihan NS, Giandello PR, Smith RC. Supraorbital and supratrochlear notches and foramina: anatomical variations and surgical relevance. Laryngoscope 1986 Mar;96(3):311-5
[12] Whitaker LA, Bartlett SP.Skeletal alterations as a basis for facial rejuvenation. Clin Plast Surg 1991 Jan;18(1):197-203
[13] Fogli A. Orbicularis oculi muscle and crow's feet. Pathogenesis and surgical approach Ann Chir Plast Esthet 1992 Oct;37(5):510-8
[14] Yeatts RP. Current concepts in brow lift surgery. Curr Opin Ophthalmol 1997 Oct;8(5):46-50
[15] Bruck JC, Baker TJ, Gordon H. Facial mimics and the coronal brow lift. Aesthetic Plast Surg 1987;11(4):199-201
[16] Bruck JC, Baker TJ, Gordon H. Facial mimics and the coronal brow lift. Aesthetic Plast Surg 1987;11(4):199-201
[17] Freund RM, Nolan WB 3rd. Correlation between brow lift outcomes and aesthetic ideals for eyebrow height and shape in females. Plast Reconstr Surg 1996 Jun;97(7):1343-8
[18] Arteaga DM, Taylor CO. Esthetic evaluation and treatment of the upper one third of the face. J Oral Maxillofac Surg 1991 Jan;49(1):27-32/
[19] Quantitative analysis of facial motion components: anatomic and nonanatomic motion in normal persons and in patients with complete facial paralysis. Plast Reconstr Surg 1997 Jun;99(7):1894-902; discussion 1903-4/
[20] Elkwood A, Matarasso A, Rankin M, Elkowitz M, Godek CP.National plastic surgery survey: brow lifting techniques and complications. Plast Reconstr Surg 2001 Dec;108(7):2143-50; discussion 2151-2
[21] Matarasso A, Elkwood A, Rankin M, Elkowitz M. National plastic surgery survey: face lift techniques and complications. Plast Reconstr Surg 2000 Oct;106(5):1185-95; discussion 1196
[22] Forrest CR, Phillips JH, Bell TA, Gruss JS. The biomechanical effects of deep tissue support as related to brow and facelift procedures. Plast Reconstr Surg 1991 Sep;88(3):427-32

[23] Webster RC, Fanous N, Smith RC. Blepharoplasty: when to combine it with brow, temple, or coronal lift. J Otolaryngol 1979 Aug;8(4):339-43
[24] Adamson PA, Cormier R, McGraw BL. The coronal forehead lift -modifications and results. J Otolaryngol 1992 Feb;21(1):25-9
[25] McKinney P, Mossie RD, Zukowski ML. Criteria for the forehead lift. Aesthetic Plast Surg 1991 Spring;15(2):141-7
[26] Rafaty FM, Goode RL, Fee WE Jr. The brow-lift operation. Arch Otolaryngol. 1975 Aug;101(8):467-8.
[27] Ortiz-Monasterio F, Barrera G, Olmedo A. The coronal incision in rhytidectomy--the brow lift. Clin Plast Surg. 1978 Jan;5(1):167-79.
[28] Ellenbogen R. Transcoronal eyebrow lift with concomitant upper blepharoplasty. Plast Reconstr Surg. 1983 Apr;71(4):490-9.
[29] Fett DR, Sutcliffe RT, Baylis HI. The coronal brow lift. Am J Ophthalmol 1983 Dec;96(6):751-4
[30] Riefkohl R. The forehead-brow lift. Ann Plast Surg 1982 Jan;8(1):55-63
[31] Nassif PS, Kokoska MS, Homan S, Cooper MH, Thomas JR.Comparison of subperiosteal vs subgaleal elevation techniques used in forehead lifts. Arch Otolaryngol Head Neck Surg 1998 Nov;124(11):1209-15
[32] Troilius C. A comparison between subgaleal and subperiosteal brow lifts. Plast Reconstr Surg 1999 Sep;104(4):1079-90; discussion 1091-2
[33] Dempsey PD, Oneal RM, Izenberg PH. Subperiosteal brow and midface lifts. Aesthetic Plast Surg 1995 Jan-Feb;19(1):59-68
[34] Riefkohl R, Kosanin R, Georgiade GS. Complications of the forehead-brow lift. Aesthetic Plast Surg 1983;7(3):135-8
[35] Gasperoni C, Salgarello M, Bajaj-Luthra A, Mueller T, Johnson PC. Karabulut AB, Tumerdem B. Forehead lift: a combined approach using subperiosteal and subgaleal dissection planes. Aesthetic Plast Surg 2001 Sep-Oct;25(5):378-81
[36] Camirand A, Doucet J. A comparison between parallel hairline incisions and perpendicular incisions when performing a face lift. Plast Reconstr Surg 1997 Jan;99(1):10-5
[37] Holcomb JD, McCollough EG. Trichophytic incisional approaches to upper facial rejuvenation. Arch Facial Plast Surg 2001 Jan-Mar;3(1):48-53
[38] Johnson CM Jr, Waldman SR. Midforehead lift. Arch Otolaryngol 1983 Mar;109(3):155-9
[39] Johnson CM Jr, Anderson JR, Katz RB. The brow-lift 1978. Arch Otolaryngol 1979 Mar;105(3):124-6 The We discuss the surgical technique in detail.
[40] Lewis JR Jr. A method of direct eyebrow lift. Ann Plast Surg 1983 Feb;10(2):115-9
[41] Byrd HS, Andochick SE. The deep temporal lift: a multiplanar, lateral brow, temporal, and upper face lift. Plast Reconstr Surg 1996 Apr;97(5):928-37
[42] Miller TA, Rudkin G, Honig M, Elahi M, Adams J.Lateral subcutaneous brow lift and interbrow muscle resection: clinical experience and anatomic studies. Plast Reconstr Surg 2000 Mar;105(3):1120-7; discussion 1128
[43] Gasperoni C, Salgarello M, Gargani G. Subperiosteal lateral browlift and its relationship to upper blepharoplasty. Aesthetic Plast Surg 1993 Summer;17(3):243-6

[44] Gargani G. Subperiosteal lateral browlift and its relationship to upper blepharoplasty. Aesthetic Plast Surg 1993 Summer;17(3):243-6
[45] Ramirez OM. Transblepharoplasty forehead lift and upper face rejuvenation. Ann Plast Surg 1996 Dec;37(6):577-84
[46] Ramirez OM. Endoscopically assisted biplanar forehead lift. Plast Reconstr Surg 1995 Aug;96(2):323-33
[47] Dayan SH, Perkins SW, Vartanian AJ, Wiesman IM. The forehead lift: endoscopic versus coronal approaches. Aesthetic Plast Surg 2001 Jan-Feb;25(1):35-9
[48] Pakkanen M, Salisbury AV, Ersek RA. Biodegradable positive fixation for the endoscopic brow lift. Plast Reconstr Surg 1996 Nov;98(6):1087-91
[49] McKinney P, Celetti S, Sweis I. An accurate technique for fixation in endoscopic brow lift. Plast Reconstr Surg 1996 Apr;97(4):824-7
[50] Namazie AR, Keller GS. Current practices in endoscopic brow and temporal lifting. Facial Plast Surg Clin North Am 2001 Aug;9(3):439-51
[51] Byrd HS. The extended browlift. Clin Plast Surg 1997 Apr;24(2):233-46
[52] Putterman AM. Intraoperatively controlled small-incision forehead and brow lift. Plast Reconstr Surg 1997 Jul;100(1):262-6
[53] Kikkawa DO, Miller SR, Batra MK, Lee AC. Small incision nonendoscopic browlift. Ophthal Plast Reconstr Surg 2000 Jan;16(1):28-33
[54] Graziosi AC, Beer SMC. pp Browlifting with thread: the technique without undermining using minimum incisions. Aesthetic Plast Surg 1998 Mar-Apr;22(2):120-5
[55] Ahn MS, Catten M, Maas CS. Temporal brow lift using botulinum toxin A. Plast Reconstr Surg 2000 Mar;105(3):1129-35; discussion 1136-9
[56] Serdev, N. Accessories to Face Lifting. II International Symposium of Updating on Skin Aesthetic, Sao Paolo, Brazil, 6-8 May, 1994
[57] Serdev N. Live Surgery Workshop, SMAS Lifting of the face by minimal incision – Brow, Temporal, Medial, Lower - the Serdev Technique. The International Academy of Aesthetic Surgery and Aesthetic Medicine, The Krulig Clinic, Caracas, Venezuela, Nov. 1999
[58] Serdev, N. Scarless Brow Lift Using A Special Suture. Presentations – 3rd World Congress of Cosmetic Surgery with Live Surgical Demonstrations. Int. J. Cosm. Surg. 2002, Volume 2, Number 4
[59] Serdev, N. P. Forehead Subperiosteal Masklift in Combination with McIndoe Facelift Technique and Profile Correction. The 7th IPRAS Congress European Section, Berlin, Germany, June 2-5, 1993.
[60] Serdev N. P. Temporal SMAS lift without skin excision In: Lip Augmentation During Mask and SMAS Lift Procedure, AAARS Annual Meeting, New Orleans, USA, October 5-9, 1994
[61] Serdev, N.P. Temporal SMAS Lifting of the Face. Life Surgery Workshop. Unidad Medica Clinica Del Country, Bogota D.C., Colombia, November 8-10, 1999
[62] Serdev, N. P. SMAS Lifting of the Face by Minimal Incisions – the Serdev Technique. Life Surgery Workshop sponsored by International Academy of Cosmetic surgery and

the Balkan Academy of Cosmetic Surgery, held at the Krilig Clinic in Caracas, Venezuela, November 12-18, 1999.

[63] Serdev, N. P. Principles of Face Beautification, Ier Congresso Internacional de Cirurgia Cosmetica, Buenos Ares Argentina, 31 Octubre – 1 de Noviembre 1999

[64] Serdev, N.P. Temporal SMAS lift, Lecture and Life Demonstration, 1st World Congress of Cosmetic Surgery with Life Demonstrations, Edsa Shangri-La Manila and Quezon City Medical Center, February 25-27, 2000.

[65] ( http://www.mpint.co.jp/apacs/Congress2000/con007.htm ).

[66] Serdev, N.P. Temporal SMAS Lifting of the Face, Combined with Liposuction and Chin Augmentation Using Suture. Life Surgery Workshop, Tel Aviv, Israel, April 20-24, 2000.

[67] Serdev, N. P. Principles of face beautification, The 3-rd World Congress of ISAS, Tokyo, April 8-10, 2000 , 9W58

[68] Serdev, N.P. Lifting del SMAS con Una Pequenna Incision Temporal, VIIIas Journadas Mediterraneas de Confrontaciones Terapeuticasen Medicina y Cirurgia Cosmetica, Sitges, Barcelona, March 16-19, 2000

[69] Serdev, N.P. Facial Rejuvenation by Minimal Skin Incisions, International Congress "Refinements in Aesthetic Surgery" Oradea, Romania, June 22-24

[70] Mitz, V, Peyronie M. The superficial musculoaponeurotic system (SMAS) in the parotid and cheek area. Plast. Reconstr. Surg. 1976; 58: 80.

[71] Miura Y, Moura PD, Ramasastry S, Hochberg J. Can we simplify the nomenclature of the fascial lyers of the temporo parietal region? OnLine J Plast Reconstr Surg, Nov 1997;1: 1.

[72] Stuzin, J. M., Baker, T. J., Gordon, H. L., and Baker, T. M. Extended SMAS dissection as an approach to midface rejuvenation. Clin. Plast. Surg. 1995; 22: 295.

[73] Connell, B. F., and Marten, T. J. The male foreheadplasty: Recognizing and treating aging in the upper face. Clin. Plast. Surg. 1991; 18: 653.

[74] Aston, S. J. Platysma-SMAS cervicofacial rhytidoplasty. Clin. Plast. Surg. 1983;10: 507.

[75] Barton, F. E., Jr. The SMAS and the nasolabial fold. Plast. Reconstr. Surg. 1992; 89: 1054.

[76] Bosse, J. P., and Papillon, J. Surgical Anatomy of the SMAS at the Malar Region. In Transactions of the 9th International Congress of Plastic and Reconstructive Surgery. New York: McGraw-Hill, 1987: 348.

[77] Cardoso de Castro, C. The role of the superficial musculoaponeurotic system in face lift. Ann. Plast. Surg. 1986; 16: 276.

[78] Stuzin JM, Wagstrom L, Kawamoto HK, Wolfe SA. Anatomy of the frontal branch of the facial nerve: The Significance of the Temporal Fat Pad. Plast Reconstr Surg 1989; 83: 265-71.

[79] Ramirez OM, Maillard GF, Musolas A. The extended Subperiosteal Face lift: A definitive Soft-tissue Remodeling for Facial Rejuvenation. Plast Reconstr Surg 1991; 88:227-36.

[80] Tolhurst DE, Carstens MH, Greco RJ, Hurwitz DJ. The Surgical Anatomy of The Scalp. Plast Reconstr Surg 1991; 87: 603-12.

[81] Larrabee Jr., W.F., Makielski, K.H. Surgical Anatomy of the face. New York: Raven Press,1993: 41-48.

[82] Hochberg J, Kaufman H, Ardenghy M. Saving The Frontal Branch during a Low Fronto-orbital Approach. Aesth Plast Surg 1995; 19: 161-163.
[83] Core GB, Vasconez LO, Graham III, HD Endoscopic Browlift. Clin. Plast. Surg.1995; 22: 619-31.
[84] Bostwick III, J., Eaves, F.F., Nahai, F. Endoscopic Plastic Surgery. Quality Medical Publishing, Inc. St. Louis, MO, 1995: 86-129. S.E. The Deep Temporal Lift: A multiplanar, lateral Brow, Temporal, and Upper face Lift. Plast. Reconstr Surg 1996; 5: 928-37.
[85] Bostwick III, J., Eaves, F.F., Nahai, F. Endoscopic Plastic Surgery. Quality Medical Publishing, Inc. St. Louis, MO, 1995: 86-129.
[86] De la Fuente A, Santamaria AB Endoscopic subcutaneous and SMAS facelift without preauricular scars.Aesthetic Plast Surg1999 Mar-Apr; 23: 119-24.
[87] Kamer FM, Frankel SMAS rhytidectomy versus deep plane rhytidectomy: an objective comparison.ASPlast Reconstr Surg 1998 Sep; 102 (3): 878-81
[88] Hagerty RC, Scioscia PJThe medial SMAS lift with aggressive temporal skin takeout.Plast Reconstr Surg 1998 May; 101 (6):1650-6.
[89] Gray H, Goss CM. Anatomy of The Human Body. Philadelphia: Lea and Febiger, 1966: 375-99.
[90] Hamra ST. The tri-plane face lift dissection. Ann Plast Surg 1984 Mar; 12 (3): 268-74.
[91] Casanova R, Cavalcante D, Grotting JC, Vasconez LO, Psillakis JM. Anatomic basis for Vascularized Outer-Table Calvarial Bone flaps. Plast. Reconstr Surg 1986; 78: 300-8.
[92] Abul-Hassan, HS, Ascher, GD, Acland, RD. Surgical Anatomy and Blood Supply of the Fascial Layers of the Temporal Region. Plast Reconstr Surg 1986; 77: 17-24.
[93] Hamra ST. The deep-plane rhytidectomy. Plast Reconstr Surg 1990 Jul; 86 (1):53-61.
[94] Mitz V, Use of deep planes in surgery of rejuvenation of the face Chirurgie 1991; 117 (4): 278-86.
[95] De La Plaza R, Valiente E, Arroyo JM, Supraperiosteal lifting of the upper two-thirds of the face.Br J Plast Surg 1991 Jul; 325 :32- 44.
[96] Caix P, Goin JL, Modschiedler T. "Total SMAS lift" or deep facial lift by temporal approach. Initial eport. Ann Chir Plast Esthet 1992 Jan; 37 (1): 67-74.
[97] Bonnefon ADeep "en bloc" facial lift" Ann Chir Plast Esthet 1992 Jan; 37 (1), 85-94
[98] Hamra ST, Composite rhytidectomy.Plast Reconstr Surg, 1992 Jul; 90 (1): 1-13.
[99] Teimourian B, Delia S, Wahrman A, The multiplane face lift.Plast Reconstr Surg 1994 Jan 93; 1: 78-85.
[100] Campiglio GL, Candiani P. Anatomical study on the temporal fascial layers and their relationships with the facial nerve.Aesthetic Plast Surg 1997 Mar-Apr; 21 (2): 69-74.
[101] Byrd HS The extended browlift. Clin Plast Surg, 1997 Apr; 24 (2): 233-46.
[102] Honig JF Concepts in face lifts. State of the art Mund Kiefer Gesichtschir 1997 May; 1(Suppl): 1S21-6.
[103] Bonnefon A. Deep vertical lift and its development regarding the central facial area and lower two-thirds of the neck. Our technique, Ann Chir Plast Esthet, 1999 Dec: 609-16.

[104] Quatela VC, Sabini P. Techniques in deep plane face lifting. Facial Plast Surg 2000 May; 2: 193-209.

[105] Mittelman H, Newman J. Smasectomy and imbrication in face lift surgery.Facial Plast Surg 2000 May; 2: 173-82.

[106] Maloney BP, Schiebelhoffer J. Minimal-incision endoscopic face-lift. Arch Facial Plast Surg 2000 Oct-Dec; 4: 274-8.

[107] Achauer BM, Adair SR, VanderKam VM, Combined rhytidectomy and full-face laser resurfacing. Plast Reconstr Surg, Dec 2000; 106: 1608-11.

[108] Serdev, N. Glabella muscles ligature using Serdev Suture technique, http://www.youtube.com/watch?v=F7r-W7-kK20

[109] Edgerton, M., Wolfort, F. Technique of Value in the Surgical Treatment of Facial Palsy, Plastic & Reconstructive Surgery: January 1969 - Volume 43 - Issue 1 - ppg 42-52

[110] Montadon, D. A Modification of the Dermal-Flap Canthal Lift for Correction of the Paralyzed Lower Eyelid, Plastic & Reconstructive Surgery: April 1978 - Volume 61 - Issue 4 - ppg 555-557

[111] Yip C-Chew, McCann J. D., Goldberg R. A. The Role of Midface Lift and Lateral Canthal Repositioning in the Managementof Euryblepharon, Arch Ophthalmol. 2004;122(7):1075-1077.

6

# Suture Lifting and Liposculpture Integration in the Creation of Facial Esthetic Harmony

Ronald Feiner and Chedly Bouzouaya

## 1. Introduction

Youthful esthetic facial enhancement can be created with natural and scarless outcomes if innovative and minimally invasive surgical principles are properly employed. Feminine facial beauty can be characterized through mathematical, geometric and architectural constructs. However it is the triad of esthetically revealed eyes, curvaceous undulating cheek-lip landscape and a well defined jawline that hallmarks radiant feminine appeal.

In the contemporary setting numerous minimally invasive and non-invasive treatments are available for facial rejuvenation and beautification. Judicious use of soft tissue fillers, botulinum toxin, skin lasers, photothermics, platelet rich dermal stimulant therapies, chemical peels and bioactive topical applications have variously enabled cosmetic practitioners to exploit an intensifying non-invasive treatment armamentarium. In concert with these treatments, blepharoplasty using radiofrequency technology can be considered as a minimally invasive procedure. In lower lid blepharoplasty, the transconjunctival approach does not result in external scars at all. In the upper lid incision scars are very small and in time barely detectable when hidden in the natural upper eyelid crease.

It can be argued that traditional invasive rhytidectomy is a comparatively overly aggressive and in many circumstances obsolete procedure that should be reserved for relatively elderly case presentations or reconstructive situations. We have found the utilization of percutaneous suture lifting of flaccid or ptotic facial tissues can provide for a natural scarless alternative to invasive rhytidectomy surgery with the added advantage of respecting natural tissue vectors and contours. This is particularly important as the overly common "windswept" appearance associated with outcomes of traditional rhytidectomy can be avoided using percutaneous sutures without excision.

Furthermore, in appropriate cases the disciplines of liposculpture and percutaneous suture lifting can be synergistically integrated to attain a natural and esthetically pleasing facial harmony for the patient.

## 2. History

Historically there has been a steady evolution of percutaneous lift methods. Some techniques unfortunately did not achieve sufficient outcome durability and were accompanied by side effects and complications that included thread migration and extrusion. Rachel et al conducted a retrospective study reviewing 29 cosmetic patients evaluating the morbidity associated with a polypropylene barbed thread lifting technique and its long-term effects. This study demonstrated adverse events in 69% and early recurrence in 45% of the patients. The adverse events that occurred most commonly were pain, dimpling, visible threads, and foreign body reactions. [1]

Abraham et al in their study claimed that thread lift procedures provided only a limited, short term improvement that may have been largely attributed to post procedural edema and inflammation. Furthermore they asserted that the examined thread lifts relied on a similar basic technique involving subcutaneous placement of cogged threads along a planned trajectory, the threads being pulled to achieve the desired skin lift, secured and trimmed at the entry point. [2]

However such studies do not apply to certain well sustained and successful percutaneous thread lift techniques. Technique integrity necessitates methods that must be ingenious in anatomical design, providing for acceptable long term tissue suspension outcomes without significant side effects and risks.

The authors have found the percutaneous suture technique concepts invented by Serdev, N fulfill such requirements. Serdev has devised percutaneous suture lift techniques that are differentiated by the amalgamation of firmly anchored fixation of suspended lax soft tissues and non-barbed polycaproamide sutures with an extended period of absorption delay. [3]

Furthermore Serdev techniques often incorporate relatively deeper anatomical suture passes that enhance outcomes while avoiding impacts and potential injury to critical neurovascular structures. The authors are not aware of any other percutaneous suture lift design constructs that incorporate such innovative features that serve to reinforce the security, viability and extended duration of the desired tissue suspension. *(Detailed descriptions of the Serdev techniques authored by the inventor can be found elsewhere in this book.)*

## 3. Correction of anatomical pathology in midface aging

The authors regard enhancement of the eyes and midface as being critical to successful and youthful facial beautification. However the aging midface has always been a challenging region for cosmetic surgeons. Traditional techniques are complex and variably incorporate invasive rhytidectomy, malar implants and midface elevation with intraoral, temporal incisions or transcutaneous lower blepharoplasty incisions. Wulc & Hartstein wrote that "many of the procedures that have been innovated over the past 20 years are complex and are associated with steep learning curves and new complications. Some of these complications are difficult to manage. Some surgeons are sceptical of the longevity of the procedures designed to correct changes in this area. Many have adopted a particular procedure, only to have abandoned midface surgery altogether for any of these reasons."[4]

However all surgical considerations must take into account the pathological basis for midface aging which is characterised by changes in the central third of the face.[5] Structural changes develop with rhytid formation, progressive soft tissue ptosis and tissue atrophy.

The ideal youthful face is a proportional construct featuring a curvaceous convex into concave "S" shaped facial landscape known by the architectural definition of the "Ogee" curve.[6]

The youthful midface is characterized by prominent cheeks with a smooth transition between the lower eyelid-cheek interface which is an important aesthetic continuum and also a significant indicator of facial beauty. It is important to appreciated the lid-cheek interface is situated above or at level of the orbital rim in youth but with aging descends below the orbital rim. With midface aging the malar fat pad can atrophy and descend inferomedially over the SMAS with the development of a sulcus below the inferior eyelid. Correction involves vertical or superolateral elevation of an adequately volumized malar fat pad in order to restore a youthful midface esthetic.[7], [8]

The retaining ligaments of the malar fat pad and midface consist of the orbital retaining ligaments and lateral orbital thickening.[9] It should also be considered in relation to lower eyelid fat pad herniation that additional to the anterior migration that occurs through a weakened orbital septum, orbitomalar ligament fatigue permits an inferior migration of orbital fat. The diminished integrity of these facial retaining ligaments is fundamental in the pathogenesis of the soft tissue ptosis.

Suspension of the malar fat pad, suborbicularis occuli fat (SOOF) along with reconstitution of the orbibomalar ligament re-mounds the midface and supports (from below) the lower orbital soft tissue structures. With aging, sulcus formation occurs in the osseous insertions of these elongated ligaments, creating sunken appearance in this region.

Laferriere et al reported a percutaneous suspension technique of the malar fat pad anchored to deep temporalis fascia, repositioned it in a more youthful position. It was observed that this minimally invasive technique produced a long lasting elevation that would be a welcomed addition to midface rejuvenation. [10]

However the Scarless Serdev suture[R] percutaneous midface technique ("Cheekbone Lift") appears to be a unique construct on the basis that an inherent percutaneous ligamentous repair is established within the actual procedure. Unlike the case in traditional open surgery where invasive dissection and ligament release is often required before securing tissue elevation, Serdev's percutaneous midface technique does not necessitate ligamentous interruption prior to mobile tissue elevation. The lax mobile tissues to be lifted may include the malar fat pad, SOOF and what Serdev describes anatomically as "mobile muscle-cheek SMAS flap or fascial tube of buccal fat pad (also called Bichat's fat pad)". *(Detailed descriptions of this and other Serdev techniques authored by the inventor can be found elsewhere in this book.)*

It is important to appreciate that these facial soft tissue structures are elevated and suspended by suture fixation variously to the zygomatic periosteum "and in selected cases to orbital rim periosteum or temporoparietal tendon insertion and underlying periosteum, or upper temporal line periosteum and temporal fascia". [11] Thereby ligament laxity is not interrupted but instead effectively repaired with a concurrent elevation and fixation of these lax soft tissues. The procedure is conceptually ingenious while elegant in its simplicity.

Complimentary to the cheekbone lift is the concept of the Serdev Scarless Serdev suture[R] midface lift that sutures loose zygomatic SMAS extension to temporoparietal tendon insertion and underlying temporal periosteum. This technique achieves remarkably firm and secure fixation. [12] Naturally mounded or previously enhanced cheekbone tissues are elevated into a natural and youthfully vectored position. In essence the mid and lower face is securely suspended in a diagonal superolaterally directed elevation. This provides for a naturally inclined correction of the tissue fall induced by aging.

## 4. Synergistic integration of suture lifting and liposculpture

While the suspension of the aging midface is a key region for the restoration of youthful aesthetics, the authors have observed that enhancement of the midface is often more achievable after liposculpture has been performed in appropriate cases of submandibular soft tissue redundancy. This is an important consideration in the quest to optimize esthetic outcomes and was observed recently by Bisaccia et al who described the use of specialized 3-0 polypropylene sutures with absorbable cones to suspend platysma with combined, on occasions, with neck liposuction techniques to elevate sagging tissues of the face and neck, concluding that the technique had proven to be a useful addition to facial rejuvenation. [13]

Liposculpture is a very effective method of rejuvenation in the lower face, particularly in the submandibular region and jowls. It is a viable and minimally invasive alternative to traditional surgical face lifting particularly when combined with well anchored percutaneous suture lifting techniques as in the methods described by Serdev.

From an historical perspective, cosmetic surgeons performing formal face lifting have long recognized the need to consider concurrent neck liposculpture in appropriate cases of submandibular adipose accumulation. Adamson et al. observed that obtaining ideal results with cervico-facial rhytidectomy had frustrated facial plastic surgeons due to the difficulty of removing local excesses of adipose tissue in the submental, submandibular and other facial regions. They noted that open and closed liposuction techniques were being developed in conjunction with face lifting to improve the definition of the facial, mandibular and cervical contours. [14]

Over the several years we have observed that submandibular liposculpture not only improved the target anterior neck and lower face aesthetic but also seemed to improve the midface aesthetic. This is particularly so in younger patients. We have noted that certain other procedural strategies can be synergistic in the attainment of aesthetic facial harmony. Analysis of a patient's potential for an harmonious fascial aesthetic can focus the surgeon's treatment strategy. In suitable cases facial treatment favoring elimination of any prominent anterior neck laxity, ptosis and/or fat accumulation is preferable before attempting other aesthetic procedures for midface and perhaps even upper face enhancement.

This observation is consistent with Fournier's philosophy of esthetic semiology which implies that an interaction or interrelationship may exist between neighbouring tissues. [15] Fournier made particular reference to the contribution of the gravity, weight, hypertrophy or ptosis of the buttocks on the generation of lateral thigh or "saddlebag" deformity. Furthermore in cases where isolated volume reduction of the buttocks alone eliminated the anatomically inferior saddlebag deformity, the term "pseudo-saddlebag" deformity was coined. Fournier indicates that, along with other factors, errors in liposculpture technique can include miscalculation of the exact cause of a targeted fat accumulation. In order to determine the nature or aetiology of age related accumulation or ptosis of fat in many regions of the body, Fournier proposed that an analysis of various passive tissue maneuvers or active muscle contractions should made to assess tissue semiology. As the human body is naturally appreciated in the vertical perspective, the most obvious semiologicical factor to consider is gravity. Fischer, G. described performing liposculpture on a theatre table that is engineered to tilt vertically, enabling the effect of gravity on the tissues to be best appreciated during the actual procedure. Some other practitioners take the opportunity during the procedure to intermittently stand the patient in order to assess this effect. Fischer terms his technique "orthostatic liposculpture". [16]

Accordingly the impact of gravity must always be factored in any treatment plan. Such considerations relate to the expected influence of the gravity and weight of a superior tissue region on inferior location. However we have observed how the reduction of the inferiorly located submandibular adiposity can improve a superiorly located midfacial ptosis or projection insufficiency. We have termed this rather unexpected observation to be an example of "gravity inverted aesthetic semiology". Another example of this "gravity inverted" tissue interrelationship is the creation of the superiorly located "axillary roll" (or perhaps better phrased as "pseudo-axillary roll") in certain cases of the inferiorly located breast hypertrophy.

Zins et al concluded that young patients with minimal sub-platysmal fat can be treated by liposuction alone, reserving surgical skin excision for patients with severe skin excess or laxity. [17] However in most of these circumstances percutaneous suture lifts without recourse to skin excision provide for excellent tissue elevation, minimal trauma and without the imposition of scars for the patient.

## 5. Methodology

Traditional techniques are utilized for submandibular liposculpture with the aspirated fat (platelet rich plasma (PRP) enhanced) for transfer grafting to the midface if there is an indication of significant tissue atrophy in that region.

Fundamentally we have observed that closed suture lifting outcomes can be enhanced due to less strain imposed on the sutures. In other words we are "asking less" of the sutures by lightening the tissue load burden on them, diminishing the risk of suture fatigue and tissue suspension failure. Accordingly in appropriate cases, correction of a coexisting submandibular laxity by liposculpture lays the foundation for improved outcomes in minimally invasive closed suture face lifting and ultimately in other facial enhancement procedures.

Outcomes are readily observed clinically. We postulate that this midface enhancement is perhaps greater than one may expect from subtraction of sub-mandibular weight or the gravity "pull" effect alone. Indeed the subtracted tissue weight loss is generally minimal (20-60 grams fat). As Fournier suggests the totality of the aesthetic improvement is semiologic, possibly influenced by the interplay of factors such as physical mass, muscle tone, vascular, biochemical and hormonal changes in the altered regional tissue balance.

The following outlines our treatment method of a submandibular laxity/adipose accumulation in the aesthetic enhancement of both lowerface and midface disharmony.

All procedures are undertaken in the clinic operating theatre under local anesthetic tumescence (Klein type) alone. [18] Some patients elected to have a pre-med of oral Lorazepam 1mg 1hour before the procedure. We use one and two hole 1.5mm, 2mm & 3mm diameter liposculpture canulae and use a criss-cross (fanning) liposculpture technique. The liposculpture is performed anterior to the platysma. The marginal mandibular nerve and indeed all major vessels, nerves and endocrine gland structure lie deep to the platysma. We have found that the progressive development of a fibrous mesh support that occurs over several months is as important as the actual volume of fat removed. We have encountered no significant infections, bleeding or neural damage with this technique.

Following the liposculpture (either contemporaneously or a later date), suture lifting in the cheek and/or midface is undertaken in manner of the Serdev methods described earlier.

There seems to be a logical advantage when possible in delaying suture lifting until after the maturation of the liposculpture occurs over several months as swelling is diminished and tissue contraction maximized. The ptosed and redundant submandibular neck tissues can be seen to have been elevated and the mentocervical angle generally improved to 90-120 degrees. This is inherently associated with elongation of the neck which in itself is a very pleasing esthetic phenomenon. The soft tissue neck redundancy and ptosis having been corrected allows for powerful and secure percutaneous suture lifting, theoretically possible in all methods. However our own experience favors the combined cheekbone lift and midface lift in the manner of the aforementioned Scarless Serdev Suture[R] methods. *[Figures 1. & 2.]*

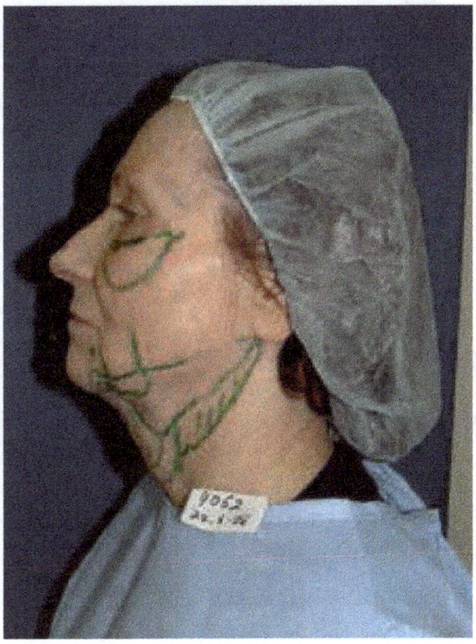

(a)

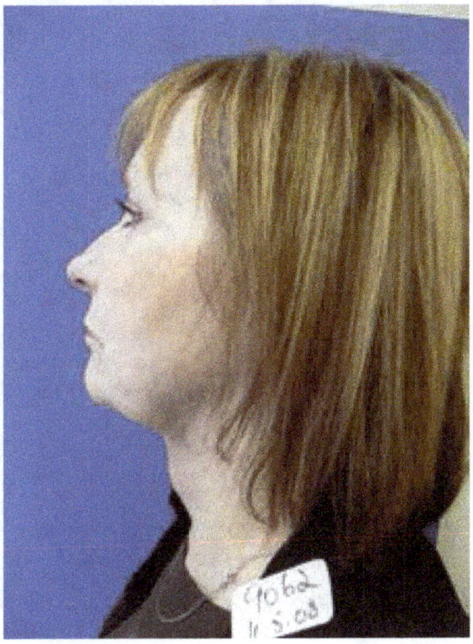

(b)

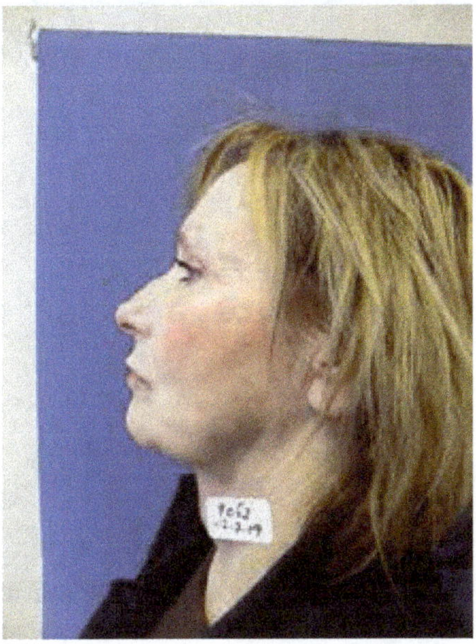

(c)

**Figure 1.** 60 year old patient with midface atrophy and ptosis with associated with submandibular adipose accumulation and laxity. Note natural scarless outcome with esthetic angles and contours.
**(a)** Prior to treatment
**(b)** Post submandibular liposculpture
**(c)** Post subsequent Serdev type percutaneous cheek and midface suture lifts

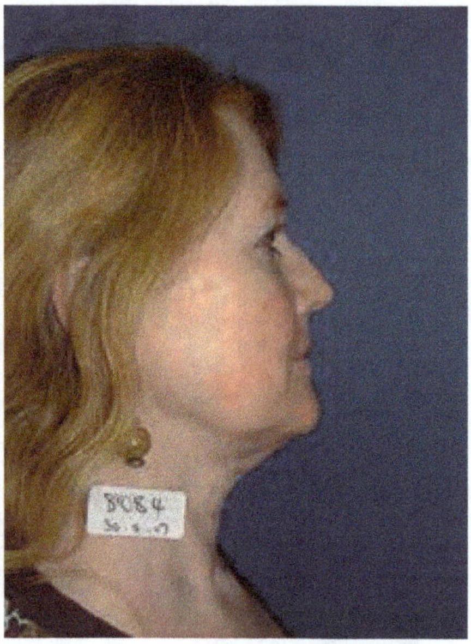

(a)

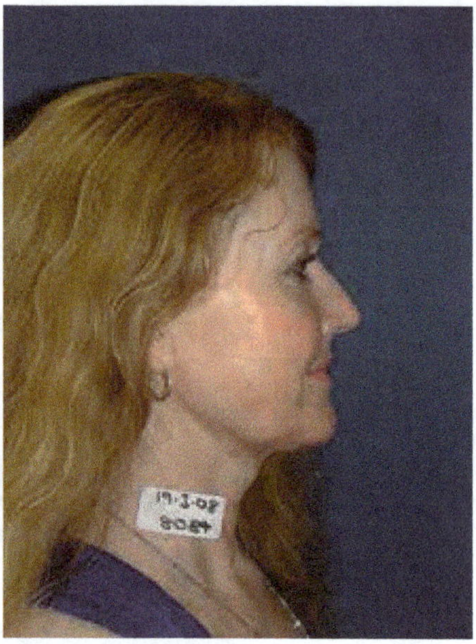

(b)

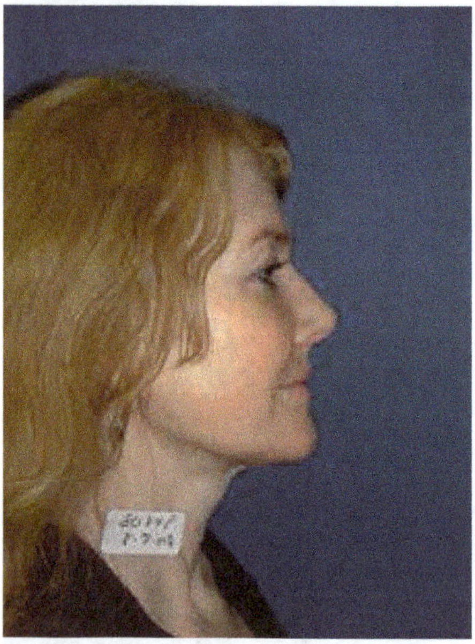

(c)

**Figure 2.** 50 year old patient with midface atrophy and ptosis with associated with submandibular laxity. Note natural scarless outcome with esthetic angles and contours.

**(a)** Prior to treatment

**(b)** Post submandibular liposculpture with fat transfer graft to midface (plus Serdev type percutaneous suture brow lift)

**(c)** Post subsequent percutaneous cheek and midface suture lifts (plus Serdev type percutaneous nasal tip lift and lip augmentation by hyaluronic fillers)

Risks and major side effects are few when these techniques are properly mastered.

The combined risks and side effect profile of both treatment methods include infection, vascular trauma, neurological trauma, endocrine gland trauma and suboptimal outcomes.

In practice we have only experienced very occasional and trivial side effects that have resolved either spontaneously or with minor interventions. Specifically with percutaneous suture lifting, capture of dermal tissue in the sutures can result in skin tethering. However with experience and careful technique this risk can be minimized and if necessary corrected by tissue manipulation or even careful subcision.

Importantly for patient acceptance, both minimally invasive facial suture lifts and liposculpture techniques are easily achievable under local anesthetic alone. If required local anesthesia can be augmented by mild sedation.

## 6. Conclusion

The universal popularity for non-invasive aesthetic facial enhancement using commercial soft tissue fillers, botulinum toxin and skin photothermics/ lasers is well justified with excellent outcomes possible in the hands of creative surgeons. However none of these therapies can significantly elevate or suspend ptotic soft tissues.

Accordingly many surgeons continue to advocate formal invasive face lifting in such circumstances, resulting in permanent scars, significant risks and all too often unnatural looking outcomes. We find such invasive methods unnecessary as well performed and technically advanced percutaneous suture lifting can produce very pleasing and natural outcomes without scars.

While some percutaneous suture lift treatment failures have been reported in the literature, the authors have attained very pleasing outcomes using some of the innovative percutaneous suture lifting techniques in the manner outlined in this chapter. In cases of moderate to heavy submandibular fat accumulation, significantly improved suture lifting outcomes are likely if prior or contemporaneous submandibular liposculpture is undertaken.

Finally it worthy to observe that utilizing minimally invasive techniques places a high demand on the innovative instincts and skills of the treating surgeon. Patient expectations are for a significant esthetic facial enhancement to be achieved without the imposition of scars. Limited surgical field access makes this objective particularly challenging. Non-invasive procedures such as percutaneous suture lifting generate the quest for creative design that inevitably requires review and adaption. Ultimately elegant procedures yielding excellent surgical results predominate and are in turn a tribute to those surgeons who both invent and successfully modify them.

## Author details

Ronald Feiner
*Minimally Invasive Cosmetic Surgeon "Cosmetica Medical Aesthetic Clinic" Shire Central Building, Sydney, Australia*

Chedly Bouzouaya
*Occuloplastic Surgeon Belvedere Centre, Tunis*

## 7. References

[1] Rachel JD, Lack EB, Larson B "Incidence of complications and early recurrence in 29 patients after facial rejuvenation with barbed suture lifting" Dermatologic Surg. 2010 Mar; 36(3):348-54

[2] Rima F. Abraham, Robert J. DeFatta, Edwin F. Williams III "Thread-lift for Facial Rejuvenation: Assessment of Long-term Results" *Arch Facial Plastic Surgery*. 2009; 11(3):178-183.doi:10.1001/archfacial.2009.10

[3] Serdev, Nikolay "Serdev suture techniques in Cosmetic Surgery ". International Journal of Cosmetic Surgery 6 (1): 408–503. (2006).

[4] Morris E. Hartstein (Editor), Allan E. Wulc (Editor), David EE Holck (Editor) Preface "Midfacial Rejuvenation" Pub: Springer Edition: 2012

[5] Yousif NJ. "Changes of the midface with age". *Clin Plastic Surg*.Apr 1995 22(2):213-26.

[6] http://www.merriam-webster.com/dictionary/ogee

[7] Graf R, Groth AK, Pace D, Neto LG.Facial rejuvenation with SMASectomy and FAME using vertical vectors. *Aesthetic Plast Surg*. Jul 2008; 32(4):585-92.

[8] De Cordier BC, de la Torre JI, Al-Hakeem MS, Rosenberg LZ, Costa-FerreiraA,Gardner PM, et al. Rejuvenation of the midface by elevating the malar fat pad: review of technique, cases, and complications. *Plast Reconstr Surg*. Nov 2002; 110(6):1526-36; discussion 1537-40

[9] Gamboa GM, de la Torre JI, Vasconez LO Surgical anatomy of the midface as applied to facial rejuvenation. *Ann Plast Surg*. Mar 2004;52(3):240-5.

[10] Laferriere KA, Castellano RD. Experience with percutaneous suspension of the malar fat pad for midface rejuvenation.Facial Plast Surg Clin North Am. 2005 Aug;13(3):393-9.

[11] Serdev, Nikolay "Serdev Suture Methods on the Face" Int. Journal Cosmetic Surgery Volume 8 No.3 Pages 1504-1553

[12] Serdev, Nikolay "Midface lift-The Protocol" Int. Journal Cosmetic Surgery Vol 11 No. 3 Pages 9-10

[13] Emil Bisaccia et al Dermatologic Surgery Volume 35, Issue 4, pages 645–650, April 2009

[14] Adamson PA; Cormier R; Tropper GJ; McGraw BL Cervicofacial liposuction: results and controversies. ) J Otolaryngol. 1990; 19(4):267-73

[15] Pierre F. Fournier MD, Liposculpture the syringe technique, Arnette, Paris, 1991, Pages 185-187

[16] Giorgio Fischer; Via della Camiluccia, Rome, Italy; "Liposuction Principle and Practice" –"Orthostatic Liposculpture" 10.1007/3-540-28043-X 31_Melvin A. Shiffman and Alberto Di Giuseppe Pub. Springer Berlin Heidelberg

[17] Zins JE; Fardo D "The "anterior-only" approach to neck rejuvenation: an alternative to face lift surgery." Plast Reconstr Surg. 2005; 115(6):1761-8

[18] Klein J.A, Anaesthesia for liposuction in dermatological surgery. J Dermatol Surg Oncol 1988 Oct: 14 (10): 1124-32

# 7

# Mastopexy: How to Reach Consistent Results – New Methods

M. Sulamanidze, G. Sulamanidze and K. Sulamanidze

## 1. Introduction

Ptosis of glandula mammaria is a well-known aesthetic deflection, which gives a woman unpleasant sensations, causing the need for cosmetic surgery in this field to consistently increase over the last several years. The central problem raised by surgeons is the achievement of a longstanding strength of form and a high glandula mammaria position after performing the operation.

There are hundreds of different surgical methods and devices for handling this problem, which are based on more or less significant solution of skin continuity, surgical release of glandula mammaria, cutting out of its parenchymatous tissue in the form of grafts, underrunning for the purposes of getting flexible stroma, cephalic redistribution of glandular tissue and anchoring to structures, such as banding of glandula mammaria musculus or periosteal coverage of feathers. In addition, it is necessary to tolerate the nipple-areola complex to a new higher location, as well as cutting out of glandula mammaria implant proportional to the modified "excipient" for getting stable dermic uplift.

Unfortunately, these approaches are quite often found to be unsuitable and do not clear away the problem of gravity post-operation ptosis over a long-term period. Suspensory skin sags, overcast seams decrease and on the back of the remained nipple-areola complex in the high position, the whole stroma of the glandula mammaria sinks down gradually, making the previously achieved rather good results ineffective (figure 1a, b, c) [1, 2, 3, 4, 5, 6].

In this case there occurs a relative desolation of the glandula mammaria top hemisphere, an overflow of the lower hemisphere, a flattering of glandula mammarias and its spreading on the chest wall. Visible seams aggravate the aesthetic failure of the performed operation.

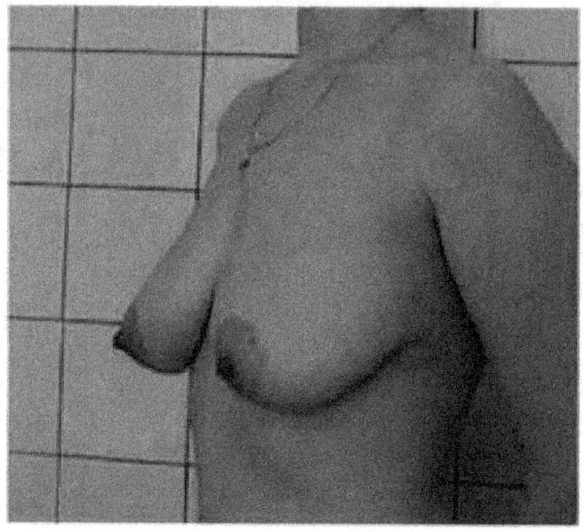

a

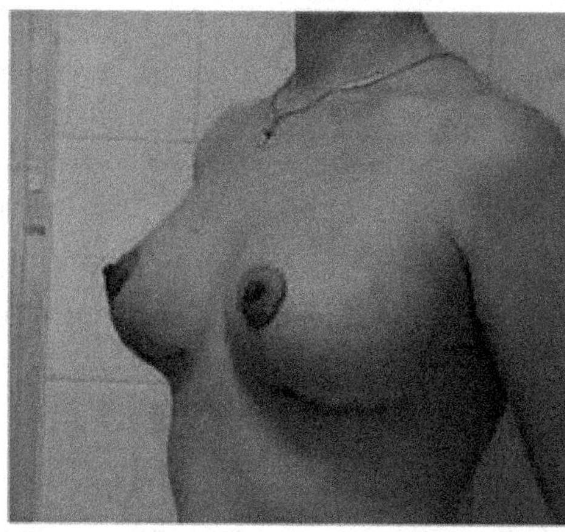

b

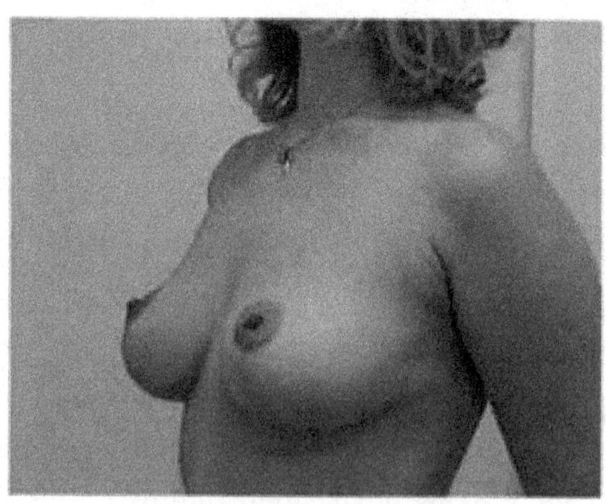

c

**Figure 1.** The result of classic mastopexy. The sight of the patient before (a); after 2 weeks (b) and a year after the operation (c)

Such results can satisfy neither the surgeon nor the patient and make us doubt the worthiness of the classic mastopexy surgery in most cases of mastoptosis.

Long experience, watching the patients in the post-operation period, analysis of the performed surgeries made it possible to reveal the following reasons of the poor results:

- weakness of architectonics to which the pulled glandula mammaria is attached (banding of glandula mammaria masculus, a periosteal coverage of the feathers);
- incompetence of the overcast surgeon's seams;
- weak effectiveness of the devices which are aimed at supporting the pulled glandula mammaria from the bottom and the sides.

A logical decision was prompted – it is necessary to fix the pulled glandula mammaria to more indurated stable architectonics and provide a strong, steady cradle of the formed glandula mammaria in the lower and lateral portions. Such ideas were put into practice - the original technology was worked out: for the stable anchorage of the glandula mammeria, the technique of hanging the glandula mammeria on the collar bone with the use of special suture material was used, as for the improvement of a glandula mammaria form, strengthening and supporting of the pulled glandula mammaria in the remote post-operation period, cellular endoprosthesis or sutured under-running of the grandula mammaria were used. [7, 8].

The method, which we called "hypodermic bodice", has been successfully used since May 2002 for treating mild glandula mammaria ptosis. The suggested techniques of aesthetic mammoplasty gives an opportunity to get a satisfactory form of a glandula mammaria without post-operation cicatrices or with scarcely noticeable cicatrices in natural places and also to reach the longstanding strength of its form and high catastasis.

## 2. Materials and methods

### A. Materials

During the performance of mastopexy in accordance with the offered method, the following surgical instruments and surgical materials are used.

**Aptos Needle DRN 60** is a blunt-ended reflexive needle with an adherent polypropylene needle USP 0, 100 centimeters long. This tool is employed for instilling of the needle around the collar bone and stable anchorage of the glandula mammaria.

**Aptos Needle 2/0** is a double-edged needle with a smooth retention suture of prolene 2/0, 100 centimeters long, fixed to the needle in the middle part of it. This unit has a knack for a double-sided patency, it allows to instill the needles under the skin and to perform subdermal under-running of soft tissues according to the broken or the lengthen boundary without skin dimpling with the result of the even pulled boundary (figure 3).

**Mersilen specimen-grid holder Ethicon** (Johnson & Johnson, USA) is a holder in the thickness of 0.25 millimeters, the diameter of the stroma is 120x85 micron (figure 4).

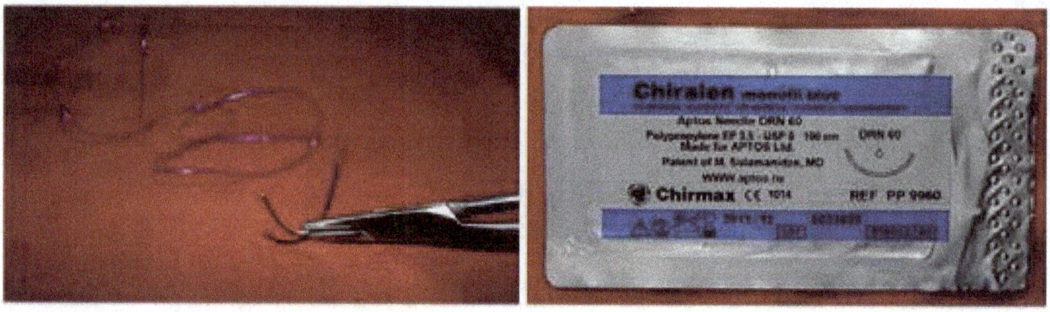


a b

**Figure 2.** The needle with the suture Aptos Needle DRN 60 for instilling of the needle around the collar bone.

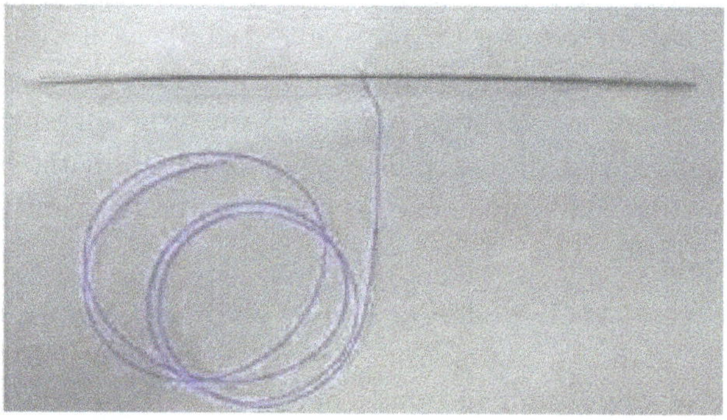

**Figure 3.** Aptos Needle 2/0 is a needle with the suture for instilling of the glandula mammaria.

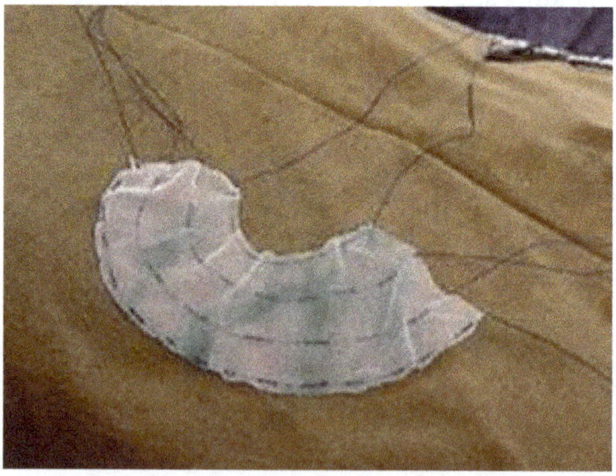

**Figure 4.** Mersilen speciment-grid holder Ethicon for instilling in the subdermal spatium of glandula mammaria.

**Specimen-grid holder Breform** (Breform™ Limited, RSA) which is made from a multifilament polyether in the form of a glandula mammaria (figure 5). It allows to make the result of the operation stable.

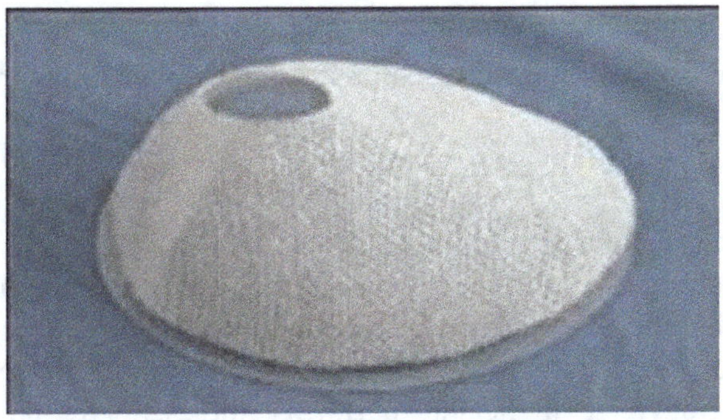

**Figure 5.** Polyether specimen-grid holder Breform made for anchoraging the results of mastopexy.

## B. Methods

Our methods of minimally invasive breast mastopexy consist of anchoring the breasts (with the use of a cellular implant or under-running the breasts with sutures) and the follow-up mastopexy and hanging the breast on the clavicle.

*Operational technique of suturing around the clavicle*

The operation was performed under general anesthesia. The patient was laid down in a semi-sitting position. Two discissions, of 2-3 millimeters long each, were made along the midclavicular line: one was above the clavicle to its periosteal coverage, the second was lower, at the level of the second intercostal space to the banding of the greater pectorial muscle. The soft tissues were separated by a thin fastener like "mosquito" and hydropreporation of the soft tissues around the clavicle was performed as well (normal saline with epinephrine in amount of 20 ml).

A clavicular acus (Aptos Needle DRN 60) was taken with a heavy acutenaculum. It was inserted in the lower discission by its blunt end, instilled upward subdermal towards the clavicle and agested through the upper discission together with the suture. The suture was pulled with the acus, but the "tail", 10 centimeters long, was left in the lower maim. The acus was turned in the upper maim and the end of the acus was instilled around the collar bone, not separating from the bone. The acus with the suture was egested in the lower maim, where the nodosity with the left "tail" was tied.

Therefore, the path of the clavicular acus went from the lower maim subdermally in the adipose layer to the clavicle, then the path went behind it (postclavicular spatium) and next - under the banding of the internal surface of the greater pectorial muscle to the view of the lower maim, where the acus was egested to the maim through the fibers.

Two interrupted stiches of prolene 6/0 closed the maim over the clavicle at the end of the operation.

The most important stage of the whole operation is instilling of the acus behind the clavicle. In order to do it without any complications, it is necessary to perform the following actions:

- make hydropreporation of the tissues behind and under the clavicle. This will allow moving the attached prescalenic musculus from the bone and enlarge the postclavicular spatium;
- turn the patients' head to the opposite side from where the operation is performed. For the pecroral arch, turn it below maximal. It will allow putting the clavicle forward and providing comfortable position for performing the operation;
- use only the recommended acus for instilling the suture, the bending and the length of which are aimed at the safe performance of the operation;
- move the end of the acus exactly along the bone without stopping the process; the surgeon can achieve it if he/she performs the semicircular movement of the acutenaculum carefully.

***Technique of the surgery on insertion of a reticular implant in the hypodermic spatium of the breasts (the method of the "hypodermic bodice")***

The surgery was performed under general anesthesia with the infiltration of the hypoderm by means of isotonic solution with adrenalin added.

*The respective marking was made beforehand.*

The patient was put in the semi-sitting position. Reticular implant was installed through the inframammar and the periareolary access. The length of the discission depended on the method of the surgical release of the cellulocutaneous flap. If this part of the operation was performed with the copper bent blunt-pointed scissors without endoscopic maintenance, the discission was made with the length of no less than 5 centimeters, while with the use of endoscopic equipment or a wire scalpel the length of the discission was no more than 2-3 cm.

Detachment of the flap was done within the lower lateral and medial quadrants of the milk gland. A net was implanted and spread in the underflap area after hemostasis, which was later sewed with the interrupted stitch in the projection of the inframammar fold and the lower edge of the areola. 3-4 pairs of threads which had been sewed to the lateral and medial edges of the net were taken to the wound in the intercostal spatium under skin, where the thread had already been taken around the clavicle. Here they were taken out, pulled, and tied to the ends of the clavicularis thread, lifting the breasts as the result.

At the end of the operation two interrupted sutures were put on the wound in the area of the second intercostal space, while the main wound (under the areola and in the inframammar fold) was sewed in three stages by continuous method.

The important features of this operation are the following:

- the selection of the patients by indication;
- surgical release of the cellulocutaneous flap of such area which allows the net to seize a sufficient volume of the breasts subsequently, especially from the lateral side;
- the installation and straightening of the inserted net in the way that no "recesses" and roughness emerge, and only after that its fixation by the side seams;
- even alternating tightening of the threads with the control of the form of the lifted breasts and their stable tightening to the clavicular thread;

*Technique of ligature sawing of the breasts (method of thread lifting of the breasts)*

The operation was performed under the general anesthesia with the patient in the semi sitting position.

The respective marking was made beforehand.

The middle clavicular line was drawn from top to bottom through the nipple to the inframammar fold, marking pints on that line: on the level of the second intercostal space (point A), the upper and lower edges of the areola. The distance from the lower edge of the areola to point A was divided into halves, this is where point B was marked, the segments A-B and B- the upper edge of the areola were also divided into halves, where points C and D were marked.

By analogy points A1, B1, C1, D1 were marked below the areola. Oval lines were drawn through these points which outlined the breasts in different levels.

The operation was started with bayonet incisions, 1-1.5 centimeters in depths in points A, B, C, D, which were widened by blunt method with the use of the "mosquito".

Under-running of the breasts was performed with Aptos Needle 2/0. To perform that the point of the needle was inserted in the wound in point A and the thread was taken through under the skin according to the marking. The needle was partially taken out and turned if it was needed, moving it further according to the line of the marking until reaching the point of insertion, and it was taken out in point A. Then the thread was pulled out with its 5-7 centimeters ends left out and taken to the holder.

Under-running of the breasts according to the rest of the lines which had been drawn through points B-B1, C-C1, D-D1 of marking was done by analogy. Therefore, the breasts were fringed with threads in four levels. After that the threads were lifted and the ends were bound together alternately in the form of knots starting from point A to point E.

Afterwards, with the use of the same blunt-pointed needle, the thread for under-running the clavicle (Aptos Needle DRN 60) was tied to the thread from point A to the thread from point C, the thread from C to point B, the thread B to the thread A, and the thread from this point to the thread which was fixed to the clavicle. In this way the breasts were lifted to the aesthetically acceptable form and position.

The important features of this operation are the following:

- the selection of the patients by indication;
- the insertion of the needle hypodermically at the necessary depths without visualization of the thread through the skin;
- under-running of the breasts in the way that in the areas of the entrance and the exit of the turn of the needle there are no retractions of the breasts left;
- even lifting of the threads and their tying together at the same level with the control of the required form.

82 operations of aesthetic mammoplasty of breasts applying the method of sewing the breasts with threads, their lifting, and their suspension to the clavicle, 11 operations with the use of reticular implants have been performed in Total Charm clinics since 2002, in total 93 operations.

## 3. Results

The indications for undergoing such operations were considered to be:

- a small or a moderate ptosis of milk glands (I-II degree);
- a small size of the milk glands (relative size 1-2.5);
- a small or a moderate excess of skin;
- a small extent of involuntary changes of breasts tissues;

Operative intervention with these methods took place in cases of primary ptosis of breasts or of the recurrence of ptosis in the post-operation period. We have resorted to these methods for preventing the post-operation ptosis of breasts and in the presence of post-operation scars.

In practice, we have applied the first and the second or the first and the third operation.

In any plastic surgery when it is necessary to reduce the area of the skin one of the two well-known methods are used. The first one – resection of the necessary amount of skin in the process of operational intervention, the second one – expecting its retraction, as long as the skin is known to shrink as the result of its release from the function of the long-lasting support of the substructural adipose, parenchymal, and other tissues, the value and the weight of which usually increases with the lapse of time. The second method in particular lies in the basis of some of endoscopic aesthetic operations and methods of thread face lifting. The same characteristic of the skin is taken into account and applied in the operation of "hypodermic bodice".

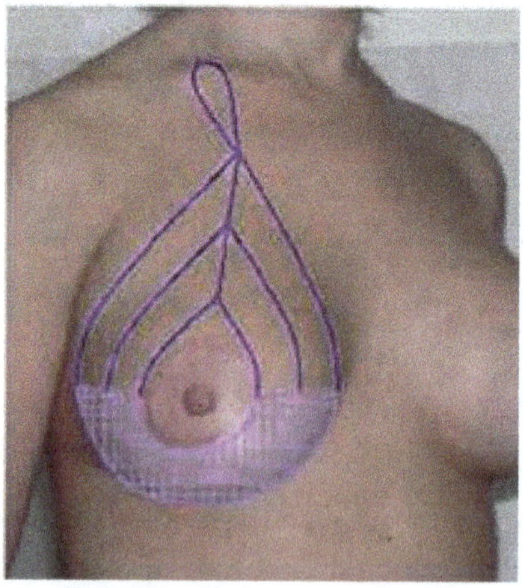

**Figure 6.** Scheme of marking the breasts for insertion of a reticular implant (the method of "hypodermic bodice").

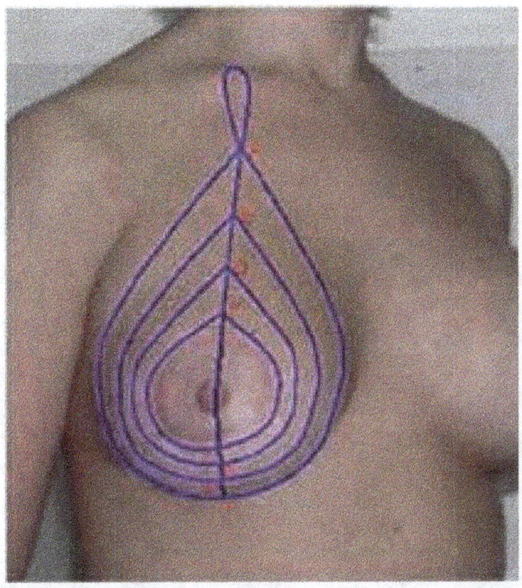

**Figure 7.** Scheme of marking of the breasts for under-running with the needles and the further lifting of the breasts (the method of the needle breast lifting).

The operational interventions were performed easily without extra trauma, the post-operation period in most cases did not show any after effects, while the aesthetic results were good and stable. In all cases the above mentioned method provided consistent, long-lasting mastopexy.

The presented clinical results confirm the effectiveness of the operations performed (figures 8-13).

## 4. Complications

During the whole period of performing the operations we witnessed the following complications and unpleasant evidences:

- the case of failure of the hypodermic knot in point B from the left side on the 3rd day after the operation. As a result, ptosis recurrenc of the left breast and obvious skewness of the milk glands occurred (figure 14a);
  Under the infiltrational anesthesia the wound in this place was opened, the ends of the threads were found and a new stable knot was put in place. The post-operation period did not show any complications and the final result was satisfying (figure 14b);
- the case of acquiring an atrophic indrawn scar, which was resolved with the method of lipofilling (figure 15a);
- some cases of skin indrawing in the places of the needle turns or of the skin-deep needle conduction. The defects were eliminated with the help of massage and the method of lipofilling;

We try to examine regularly the patients who were operated with these methods, as long as the methods are new and require special attention. We are usually interested in the following issues in the post-operation period: the condition of the milk gland near the reticule; the invasion of the reticule by the fibrous tissues; the condition of the clavicle; its stability, and the condition of the milk glands during menses, pregnancy, labour, lactation, and during the following period (figure 16).

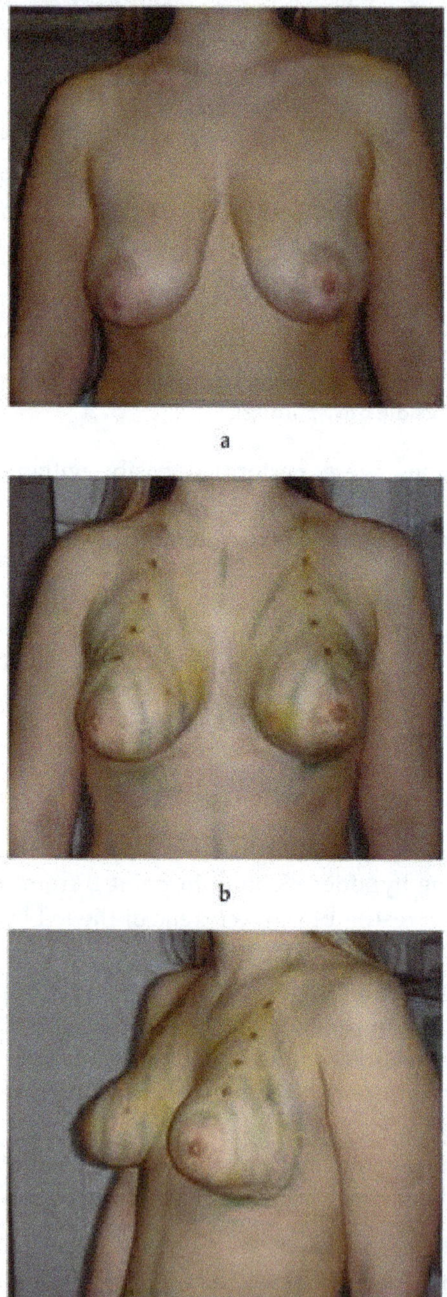

a b c

**Figure 8.** Patient A., 32 years old, before (a,b) and in 2 days after (c,d) the thread breasts lifting.

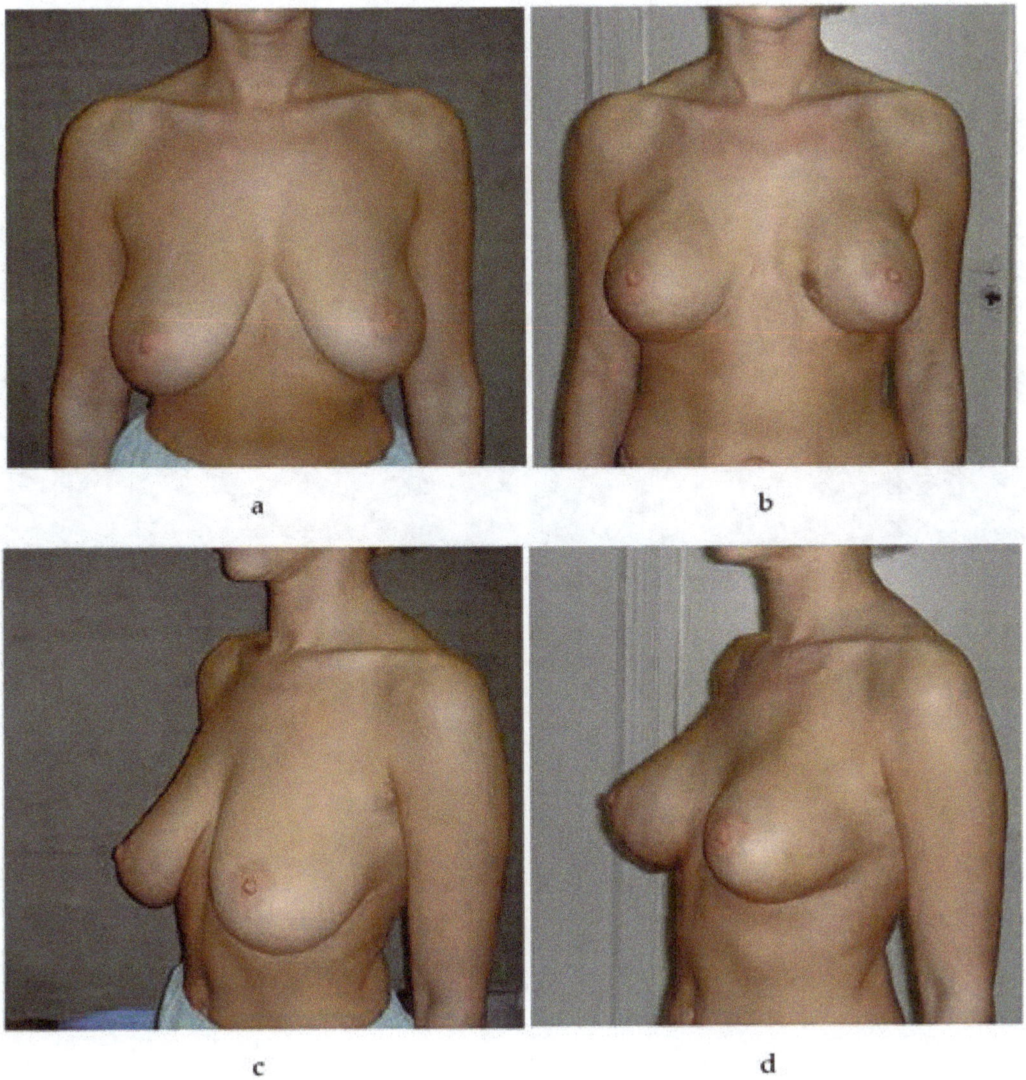


**Figure 9.** Patient B., 44 years old, before (a,b) and in 10 days after (c,d) the thread breasts lifting;

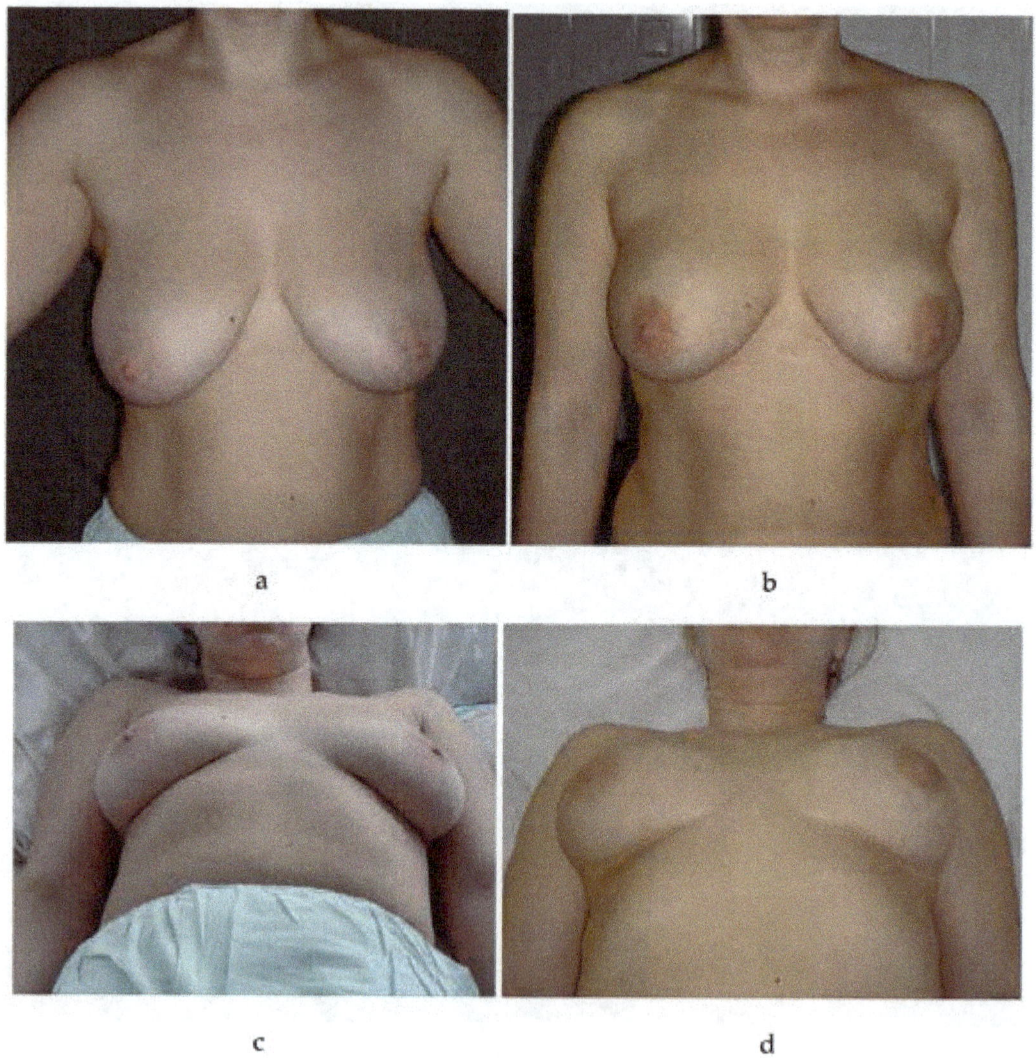


**Figure 10.** Patient C., 34 years old, before (a,b) and in 2 years after (c,d) the thread breasts lifting;

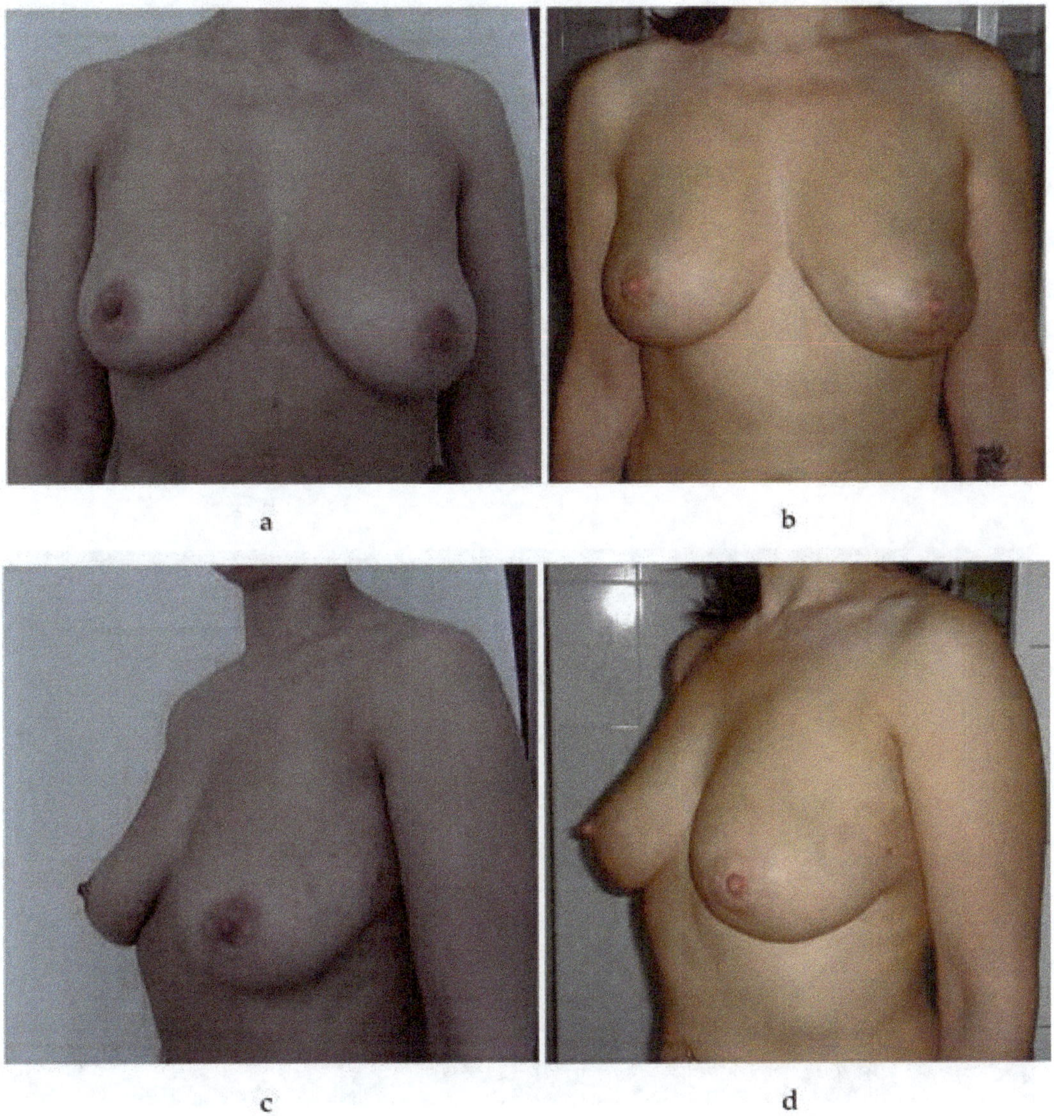


**Figure 11.** Patient D., 34 years old, before (a,b) and in 5 years after (c,d) the operation with the use of a reticular implant.

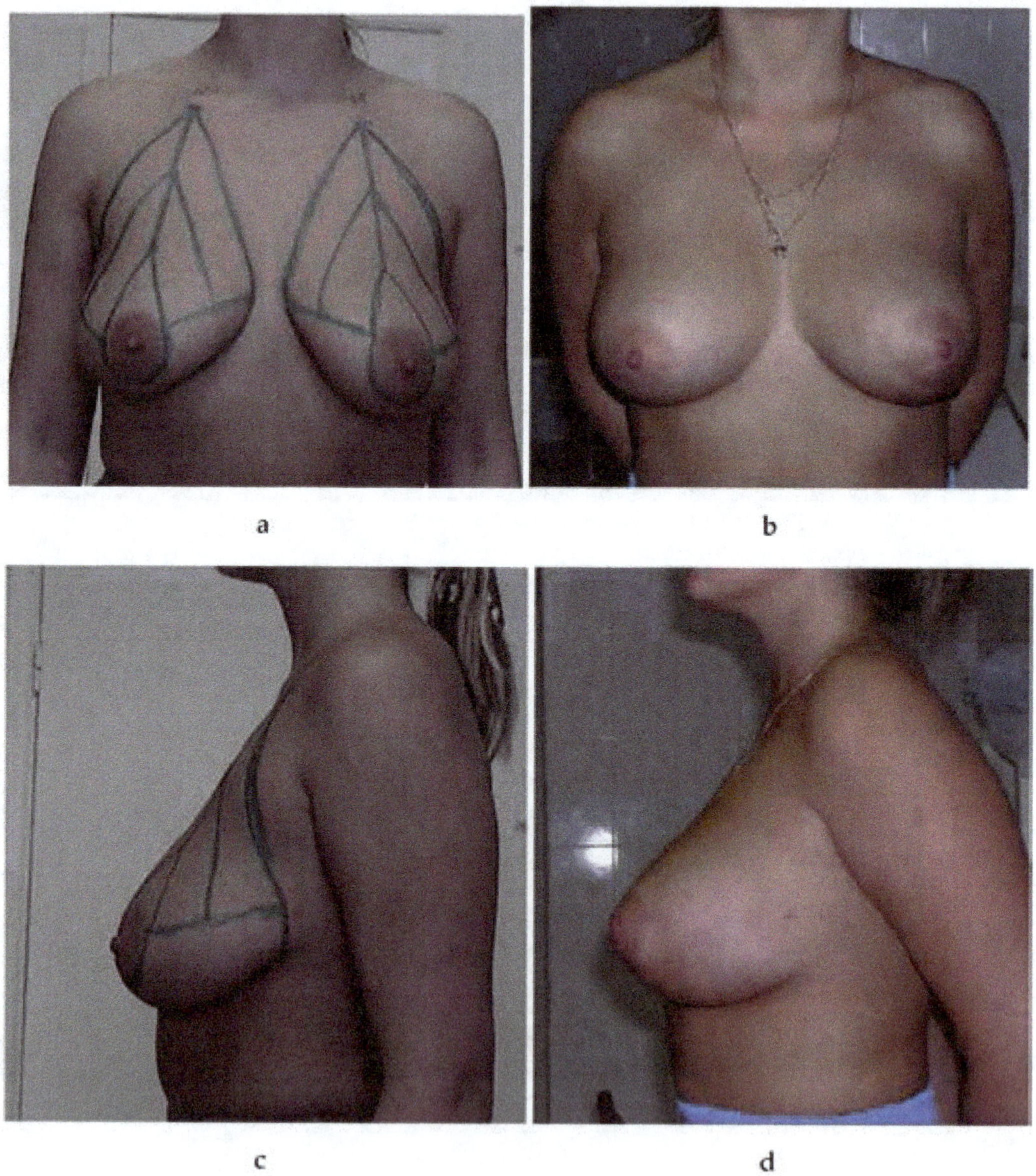


**Figure 12.** Patient E, 35 years old, before (a,b) and in 2.5 years (c,d) after the breasts lifting with a reticular implant.

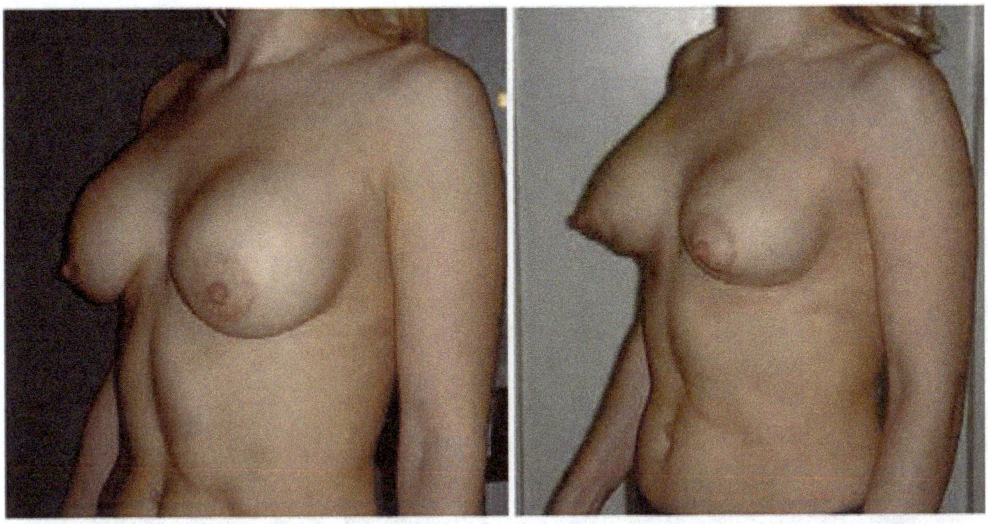

a b

**Figure 13.** Patient F, 30 years old. Some years ago the patient underwent augmentational mammoplastic in a different clinic. At the admission to our clinic she complained about the dissatisfying condition of her breasts. During the examination capsular contracture was observed. The implant remained in its place, while the tissue of the gland shifted down (glandulus ptosis). The patient underwent a thread breast lifting. Before (a) and in two months after the intervention (b).

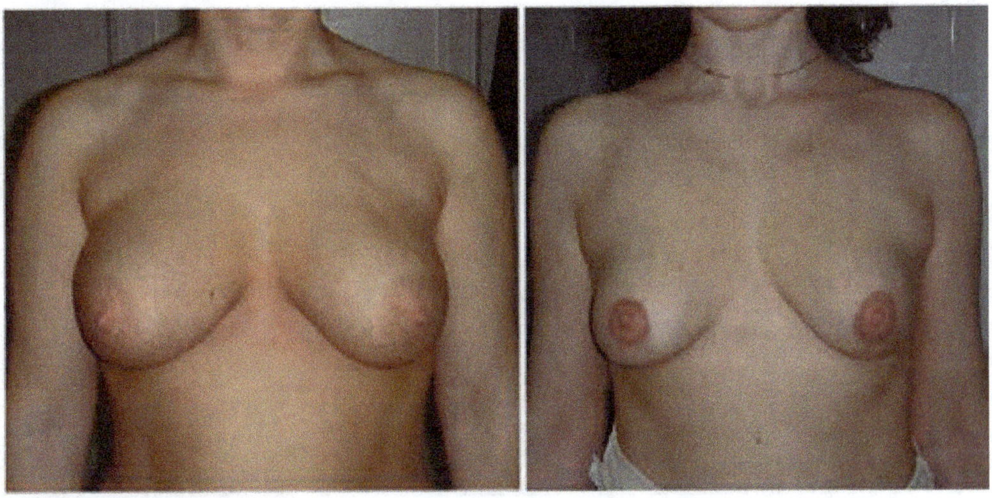

a b

**Figure 14.** Patient G, 38 years old. Complication – failure of the thread knot in three days after the thread lifting recurrence of the left breast ptosis. Before (a) and in a year after the re-operation (b).

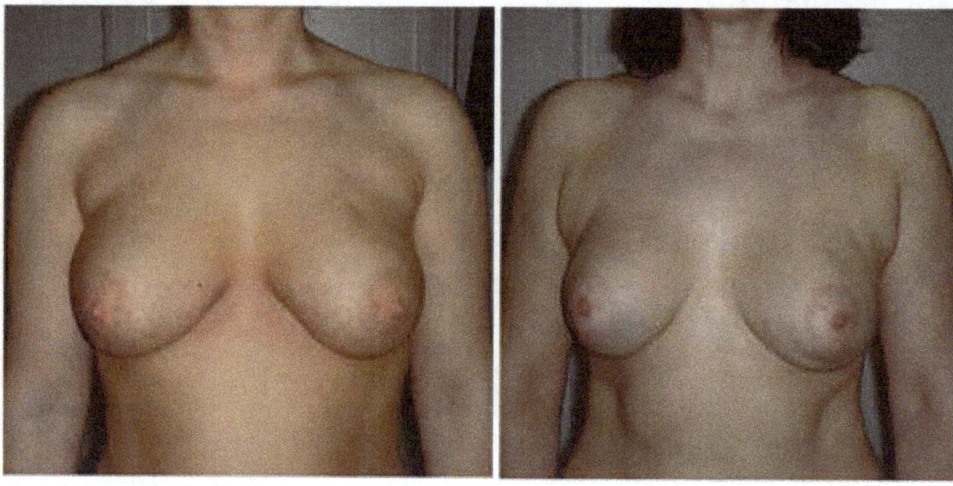

a b

**Figure 15.** Complication - atrophic scarring (a); visualization of the threads – indrawing of skin in the areas of the turns of the needle and skin-deep needle conduction (b).

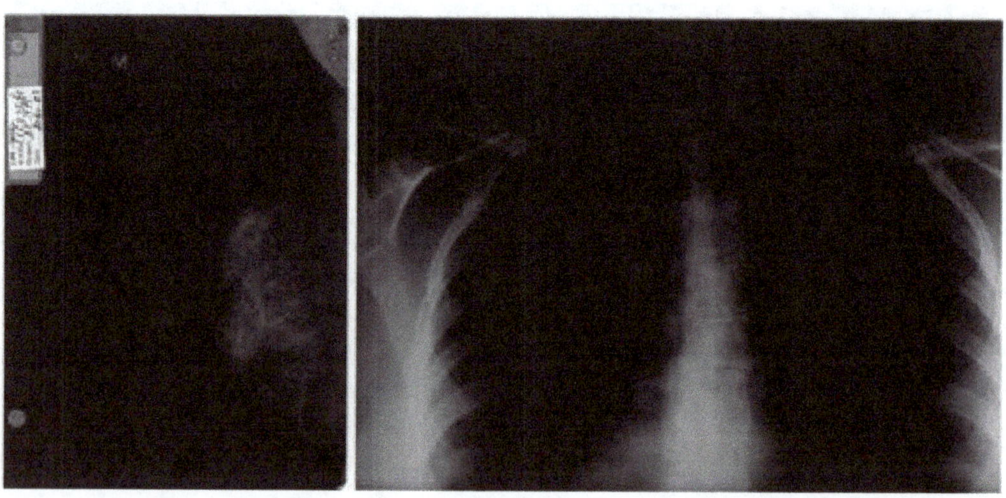

a b

**Figure 16.** Patient E. X-ray examination of the breasts (a,b) and the chest in two years after the breast lifting with installation of a reticular implant.

Besides, in our practice there have been two cases of pregnancy, delivery, and further lactation. No problems were observed (figure 17).

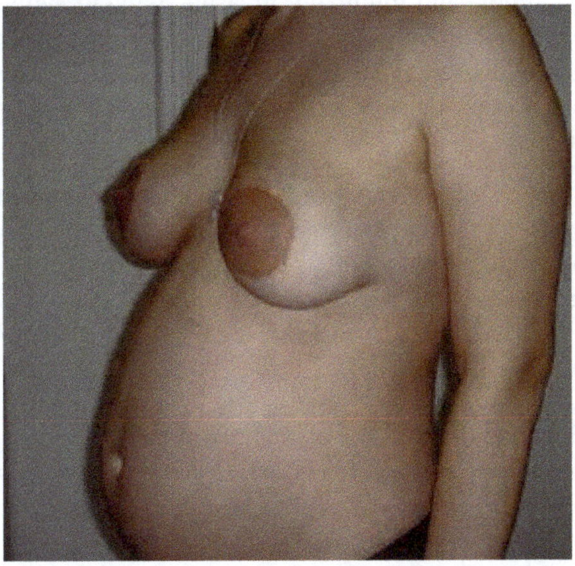

**Figure 17.** Patient K, 28 years old, in 2.5 years after the thread breast lifting, pregnancy period.

## 5. Conclusions

A group of surgeons of Total Charm clinic have presented the following methods and techniques, which serve to improve the results of mastopexy:

- suspension of the lifted breasts to the clavicle providing its stable attachment to the firm osteal structure, which does not allow the breast to move down gradually in the long run;
- insertion of a reticular implant in the hypodermic area of the lower and lateral segments of breasts, envelopment of these areas of the milk gland and its suspension to the clavicle, which leads to strengthening of the breasts and acquiring of the necessary aesthetically accepted form;
- thread sewing of the breasts through the cuts in the skin and its further suspension to the clavicle – girth of the milk gland from all the sides with solid surgical sutural material with application of hypodermic seams without incisions in order to create a resilient stroma of the gland with conical shape and to prevent its cephalic movement.

The first two methods are widely known in plastic surgery, but have been considerably modified by our group, the latter method is original and has been developed by the group.

Six-year period of performing mastopexy using "hypodermic bodice" method by underrunning of the breasts with Aptos threads, numerous examples and accumulated experience have shown that the method has justified the hopes. During the post-operation period, no patients have shown abnormal changes of milk glands, substructure, and the clavicle. No cases of dissatisfaction complaints have been reported.

Also attention should paid to the method of hypodermic dissection of the soft tissues (to create a cellulocutaneous flap) which is performed with the use of wire scalpel (Aptos Wire). The operation is easy, simple and minimally invasive, without significant hemorrhage. In comparison with the endoscopic method, it does not require costly equipment and special training of the surgeon, while the post-operational rehabilitation of the patient is reduced. The acquired cellulocutaneous flap has even thickness, good blood supply, and survives well in the donor wound.

The presented methods of milk gland ptosis correction in combination with the use of reticular endoprosthesis for mastoptosis correction are regarded as promising areas in aesthetic surgery of minimal invasion, and they require further examination and accumulation of experience.

## Author details

M. Sulamanidze, G. Sulamanidze and K. Sulamanidze
*Clinic of Anaplastic and Aesthetic Surgery Total Charm, Moscow, Russia - Tbilisi, Georgia*

## 6. References

[1] Adamyan A. A., Romashov Y.V., Kopiltsov A.A. Mammoplast in postlactational involution. Annals of plastic, reparative, and aesthetic surgery, 1997; (4);47-54.
[2] Borovikov A.M. Ter-Nokogosiyan G.A. Aesthetic mamoplast. What we talk about. Annals of plastic, reparative, and aesthetic surgery, 2002; (3);41- 46.
[3] Borovikov A.M. Milk gland ptosis. Selected issues of plastic surgery, 2005; 1(12).
[4] Burdin V.V. Beliyaev M.V. To the question of the choice of operational intervention in the postlactational involution of the milk glands. Annals of plastic, reparative, and aesthetic surgery, 2001; (2); 16-20.
[5] Milanov N.O., Startseva O.I., Chausheva S.I. Analysis of experience in single-stage mastopexy and endoprosthesis replacement of milk glands. Annals of plastic, reparative, and aesthetic surgery, 2005; (1); 44-51.
[6] Frishberg I. A. Surgical correction of cosmetic deflection of women's breasts. – Moscow, 1997.
[7] Sulamanidze M.A., Savchenko S.V., Vozdvizhenskiy I.S., Sulamanidze G.M., Osipov A.G.. Horisontal mammoplast. Annals of plastic, reparative, and aesthetic surgery, 2002; (3); 40-46.
[8] Sulamanidze M.A., Vozdvizhenskiy I.S., Sulamanidze G.M., Sulamanidze K.M. Application of reticular endoprosthesis in mamoplast. Our experience. Thesis collection II International Conference "Modern technologies and opportunities of reconstructive and reparative aesthetic surgery". October 19-20, 2010 – Moscow, 2010.

Section 2

# Barbed Thread Lifts

# 8

# Experience in Preventive Measures and Treatment of Complications at Face and Neck Thread Rejuvenation

M.A. Sulamanidze, I.S. Vozdvizhenskiy, G.M. Sulamanidze,
K.M. Sulamanidze and E.G. Azizyan

## 1. Introduction

Face and neck soft tissues lift with the use of special threads is a relatively new and not a thoroughly studied approach to aesthetic surgical and cosmetological correction. Aptos method (anti ptosis) occupies a special place here, because its subjacent conception differs crucially from other thread methods as well as classical surgical ones. Seeming simplicity of intrusion in Aptos method, availability and cheapness of necessary materials and instruments brought a lot of doctors to the point of start in using it, but, unfortunately, without special training. The fact that the doctors do not have special training in Aptos method practice is the main cause of complications and unpleasant aftereffects, the information about which has recently started to appear in literature.

After having studied all the available sources, we have predominantly found the reports about successful results with a minor number of complications and side effects. In the majority of articles both the indications and the intrusion technique are described incorrectly, as well as causes of complications (without considering the anatomical facial special features and kinetics of different groups of muscles), and consequently, this leads to incorrect results.

That is why we have decided to analyze the complications, side-effects and unpleasant aftereffects at face and neck soft tissues thread lift application using Aptos method in various ways. We have analyzed the long-term Aptos method correction experience gained by the surgeons of our clinics (by now there have been performed up to 7000 operations), complications after the application of Aptos among the patients that came from other clinics, and the data presented by doctors from different countries.

*The aim of the conducted work* is to diagnose the causes of complications and work out recommendations for the treatment and preventive measures.

## 2. Materials and methods

Out of 900 medical case records taken arbitrarily from the clinical archives of the period from 2002 to 2010 (100 histories per year) only those have been chosen that have data about different complications, problems, and patients' discontent (75 records). According to these documents and the voluminous photo archives of our clinics, a statistical inquiry has been conducted, the results of which are presented in this report along with the commentaries and conclusions. The main products and the corresponding strategies used in our clinics are the following: Aptos thread, Aptos Needle, Aptos Spring, Aptos Thread 2G, Aptos Needle 2G. The manufacturer (Aptos-pro company) usually produces threads from non-absorbable (Prolene) as well as from absorbable (Caprolactone) material. Description of the product, procedure and surgery techniques is given in our numerous publications and presentations [2-5, 10], that is why in this article we present short basic information about Aptos methods. This is necessary for understanding the causes of complications, different in nature and severity, and negative manifestations.

Aptos Thread – the first generation of Aptos products – is a thread, 12 cm long, with convergent angle-wise pins; the thread is fixed subcutaneously with the help of a special hollow needle (figure 1a).

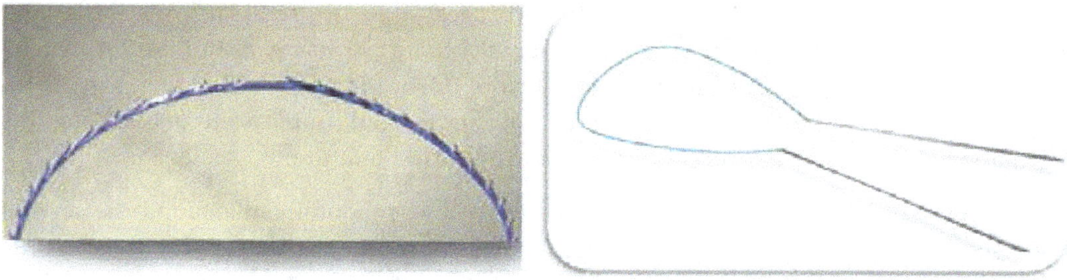

a b

**Figure 1.** a Aptos Thread, b Aptos Thread 2G

Aptos Thread 2G is the same kind of thread, but 25 cm long, the ends of which are connected with needles; the needles are sharpened in a special way, their points are joined and put together with temporary glue (figure 1b). This permits to stick the both needles with the jointed points subcutaneously, separate them at the required depth, and move each needle with the thread along the trajectory, marked beforehand.

Aptos Needle is a unit with a thread, without pins, which is connected with a double-edged needle in its middle part; such a construction permits to put a needle with a thread subcutaneously along the straight, arched or round (tobacco pouch shaped) contour without skin dimpling. The manufacturer produces three types of these needles (figure 2a).

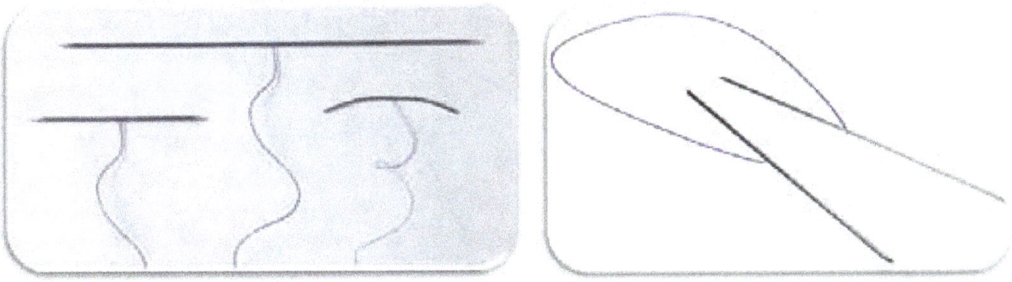

a b

**Figure 2.** a Aptos Needle, Aptos Needle 2G

Aptos Needle 2G combines advantages of Aptos Thread 2G and Aptos Needle. The thread in this case is exactly the same as Aptos thread 2G, but up to 50 cm long and with convergent pins, connected with two double-edged needles in its middle part (like Aptos Needle), the points of which are put together with temporary glue. That is how the subcutaneous implementation of the thread with pins is performed, and notably, along any contour.

Aptos Spring is a helical elastic thread with "memory" which is used for the lift of the tissues with the most active facial movements.

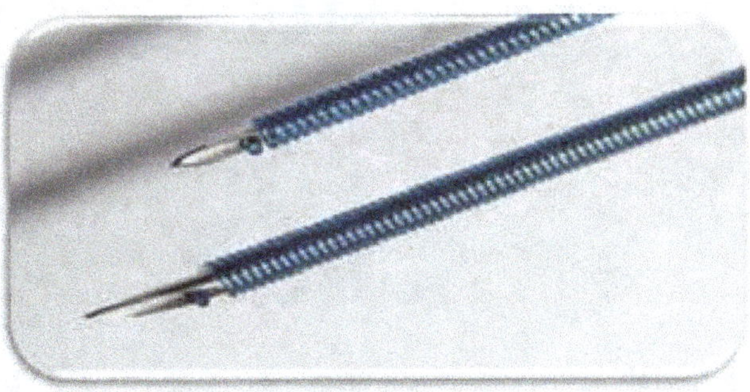

**Figure 3.** Aptos Springs

## 3. Research results and discussion

Carrying out the research, we have clearly decided on the definitions of complication and inevitable accompanying interference effect. Besides, it was important to understand which complications and disadvantages are characteristics for all aesthetic surgery interferences and which ones are characteristics only for thread lift methods (scheme 1).

For example, we do not regard light paraesthesia, pain, asymmetry and shallow indrawings in the needle puncture places to be complications. Overcorrection is a necessity, a mandatory operation attribute, we have tried to achieve it on purpose in order to stabilize the interference result and make it as long-term as possible (picture 4 a, b, c, d).

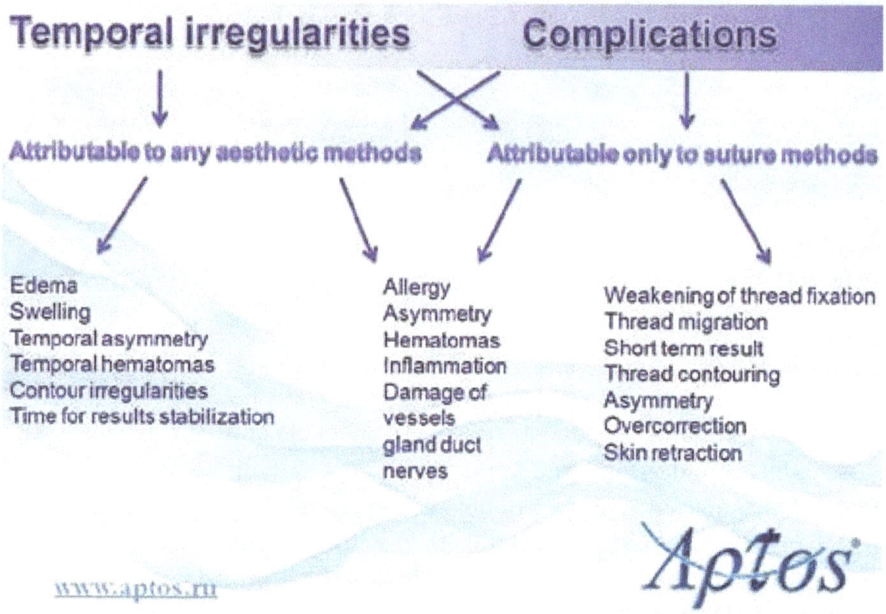


**Scheme 1.** Classification of Complications and Attendant Thread Lift Negative Factors

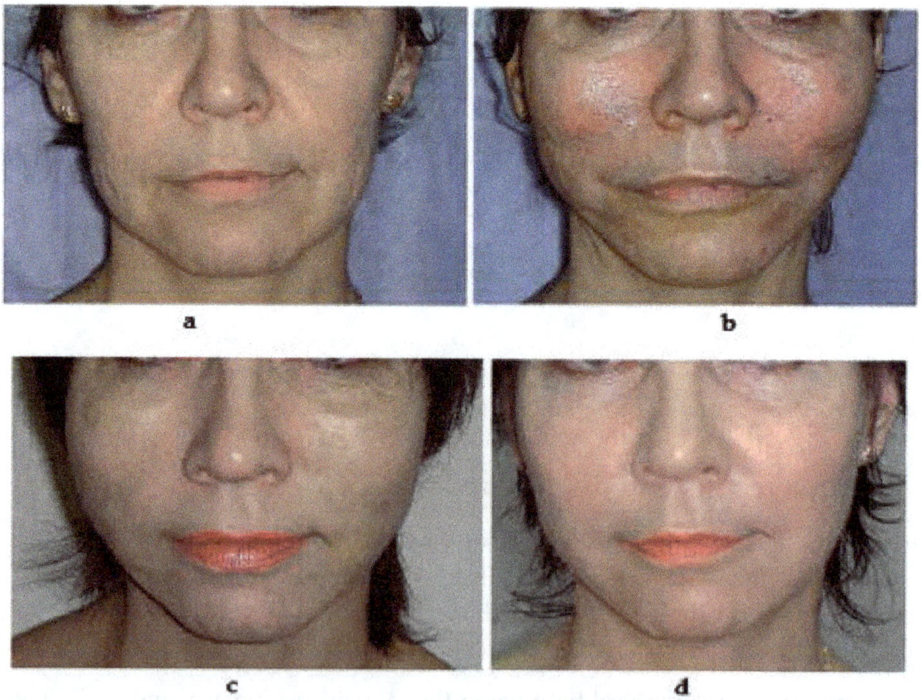

**Figure 4.** Patient N., 38 years old. Middle facial area lift – Aptos Needle 2G, mental area – Aptos Thread 2G, labiomental wrinkles – Aptos Springs: a – before; b – right after the correction; c – in 2 weeks; d – in 2 years after the interference

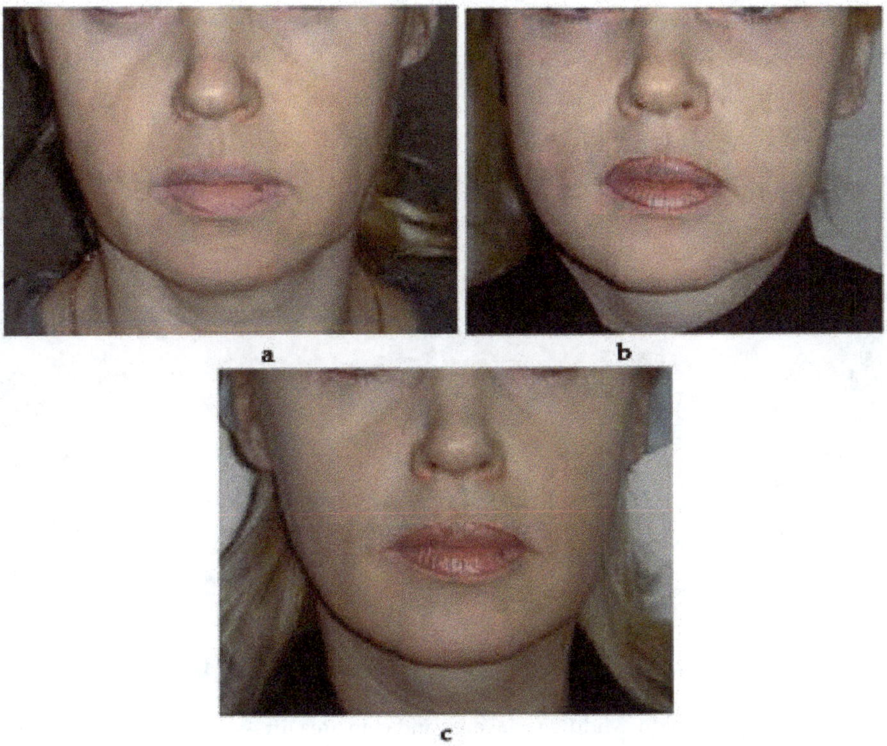

**Figure 5.** Patient A., 44 years old. Middle facial area and mental area lif – Aptos Thread 2G, labiomental wrinkles – Aptos Springs, submandibular and neck areas – Aptos Needle 2/0: a – before, b – in12 days, c – in 3 months after the interference

The interferences can be accompanied by moderate constraint of mimic, masticatory, swallowing and other facial movements, we do not regard these manifestations to be complications either. All the enumerated disadvantages usually go away on its own in dynamics, or you can use common resolving drug therapy or physiotherapy. We present a picture of a patient who had these unpleasant manifestations for 2 weeks, but subsequently the results stabilized and she was satisfied with the performed correction.

We regarded persistent edemata (more than 2-3 weeks), wrong contour, asymmetry, thread visualization, allergy, infection, bleeding along the thread trajectory, thread migration and thread protrusion onto the skin surface, early relapse of soft tissues ptosis, solution of vessels continuity, nerve trunks continuity, and other anatomical structures continuity to be complications.

We threat persistent edemata with additional general clinical methods. Probably, such cases were connected with patients' individual characteristics as it was not always possible to correlate long-term edemata with the severity of undergone surgeries.

In case of wrong contour, indrawn skin areas, if they were not corrected after massage we employed resolving drug therapy and physiotherapy, and eliminated the problem with the method of undercutting with the use of a wire scalpel, or corrected it with fillers. The asymmetry was corrected with additional thread lift or, on the contrary, with weakening excessively tight threads (figuree 6 a, b). It is most likely that the cause of asymmetry is the surgeon's work fault.

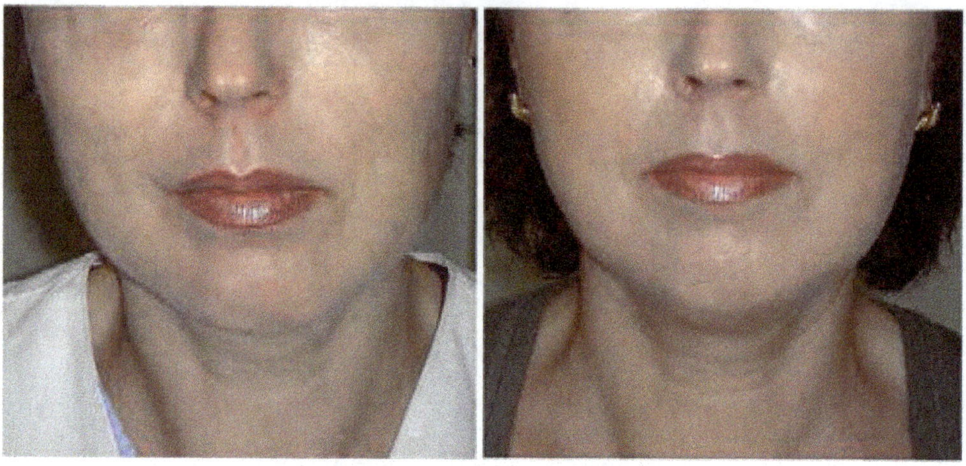

a b

**Figure 6.** Patient L., 47 years oldd. Middle facial area and chin area lift – Aptos Needle 4/0, mental area – Aptos thread 2G, labiomental wrinkles – Aptos Springs.

Two cases of late allergy to the intruded absorbable thread have been marked: the first one is in 10 days, the second one is in 2 months. In the first case the process was terminated with medications, in the second case the threads were removed. (figure 7).

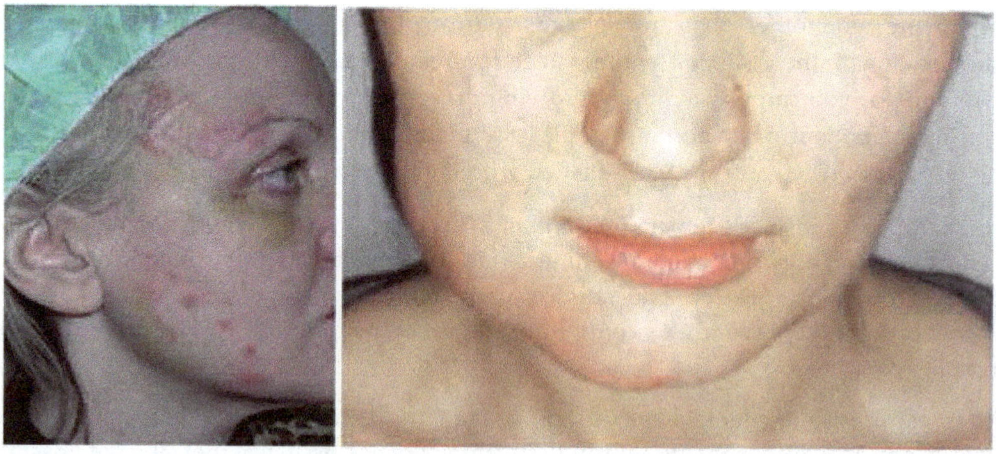

a b

**Figure 7.** a Allergic reaction to absorbable threads implementation in 10 days after the interference b. Allergic reaction to absorbable threads implementation in 2 months after the interference

Migration threads and threads with the end protruded onto the skin surface were also subject to removal (figure 8).

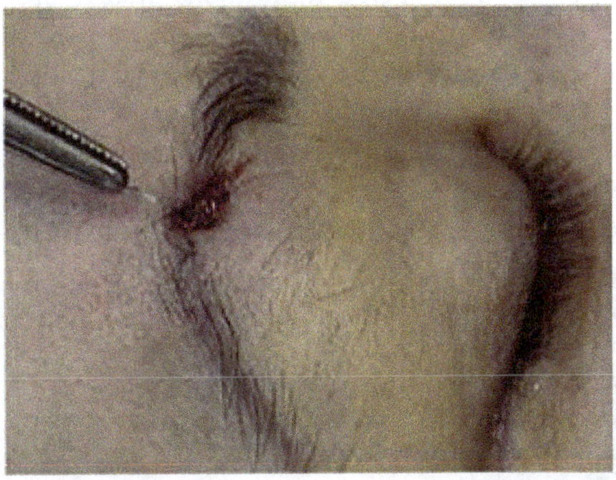

**Figure 8.** Thread migration case

Since 2008 the usage of prolene Aptos Thread has been stopped and replaced with more modern, second generation threads. And since that time we have not come across any similar unpleasant effects. Such a complication as thread vizualisation has always been connected with its shallow intrusion (except for the eyebrow lifting where this is a necessity). In most cases this problem was successfully eliminated by vigorous massage movements. In rare cases these threads were removed (figure 9).

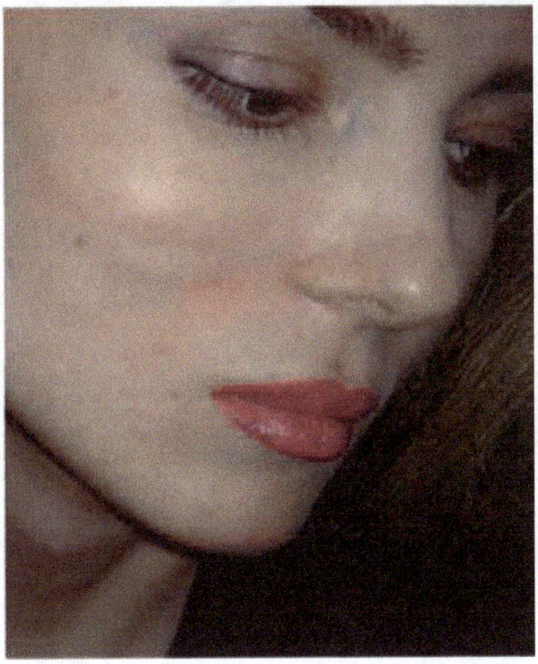

**Figure 9.** Thread visualization case

The appearance of complications of inflammatory nature is presumably connected with the infection intrusion into subcutaneous layers during the surgery or post-operative period (figure 10). Preventive measures for such complications involve observation of aseptic and antiseptic rules, following to the doctor's prescription in the post-operative period (taking antibiotics, proper skin care and other recommendations). The treatment is medicamental and general surgical; in case of indication the threads are removed. In our clinic we use noninvasive subcutaneous thread detection methods (US, bright main light visualization, diaphanoscopy) and its mini intrusive removal with the use of a special glover's needle (figure 11). This procedure does not present any technical difficulties for an experienced specialist.

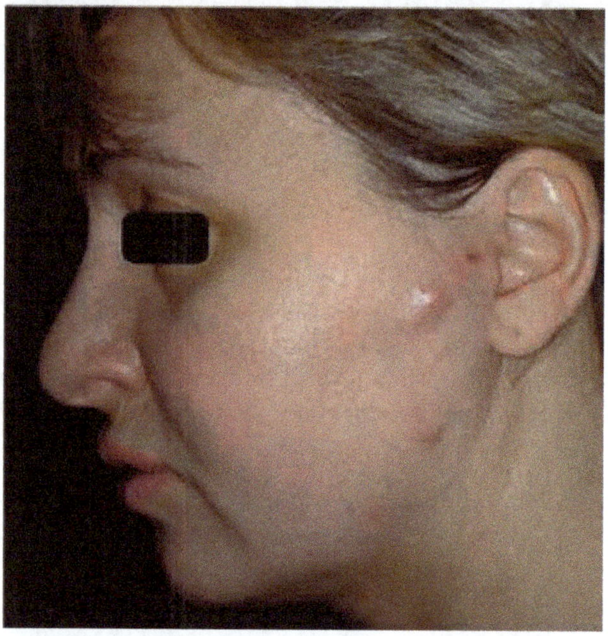

**Figure 10.** Pus abscess case around thread implementation

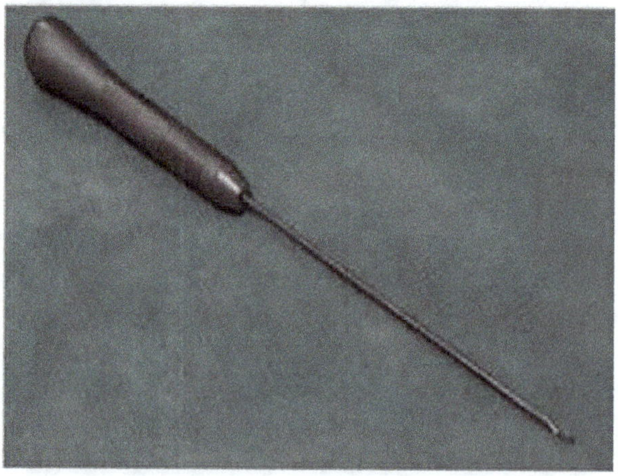

**Figure 11.** Glover's needle

In our clinical practice we have not come across the hematomas that needed emptying, macrovessel and nerve trunk continuity solution. However, there is a case of Stenon duct continuity solution described in literature that needed operative surgical intervention in order to be treated [13]. The cases of early soft tissues ptosis relapse are especially worth noticing.

The experience shows that sustainability and stability of thread lift results depend on the observation of a number of rules.

1. **Strict selection of patients according to the indications**

The best face tissues lift results in our clinics are achieved with patients under 50 years old with a slightly thick skin, without pronounced atrophy of subcutaneous fat, with moderate soft tissues ptosis manifestation (feebly marked nasolabial folds and soft-tissue bolsters above them; slightly wrong contour of infraorbital areas in the form of lacrimal grooves; presence of "jowls"), after the preliminary cosmetological deep skin cleansing procedure. For a variety of reasons these patients refused to do classical face lift operations and preferred light and medium face tissues lifts, imperceptible for the others. These were also the patients who were discontent with the previous results of rhytidoplasty, as the face tissues lift was feebly marked in the medial parts and the high volume of bucco-zygomatic areas was not reached.

2. **Preoperative Determination of the Interference Goal**_(tissue lift, tissue redistribution, creation of a new high volume or combination of these effects)

Aptos methods permit to reach the enumerated goals. For example, eyebrow tail lift and thread canthopexy are performed by Aptos Needle 2G method, while new high volume of the middle part of the face is performed by Aptos Needle 4/0 or Aptos Needle 2G. These methods permit to "border" the lifted tissues area and fix them rigidly to rigid structures.

3. **Fixation of Threads With Pins is Effective Only in the Kinetically Inert Zones**

Eyebrow, bucco-zygomatic, mental, and submandibular areas are among these zones, as they do not have active muscles and soft tissue layers can be easily shifted. That is why rigid lift methods are recommended only in the range of these zones. For the soft tissues lift of the kinetically active zones ("grief wrinkle" correction, mouth corners ptosis) we used an elastic lift – Aptos Springs method.

Simultaneous movement of soft tissue layers of two or more zones is a complicated action, as these zones are separated from each other by dense bands of fibrous tissue that do not allow a long-term lift of all the zones to be performed simultaneously [1, 8].

A number of colleagues in their practice ignore these circumstances and employ long threads from temporal or even parietal regions through the whole cheek down to the submandibular area (figure 10a). Of course, during masticatory and mimic movements parts of protuberances or the whole thread are easily destroyed and, consequently, the lift stability declines. Poor results of linear lifts performed by long threads from temporal areas down to the nasolabial triangle and "Marionette Line" can be explained in the same way (figure 10b).

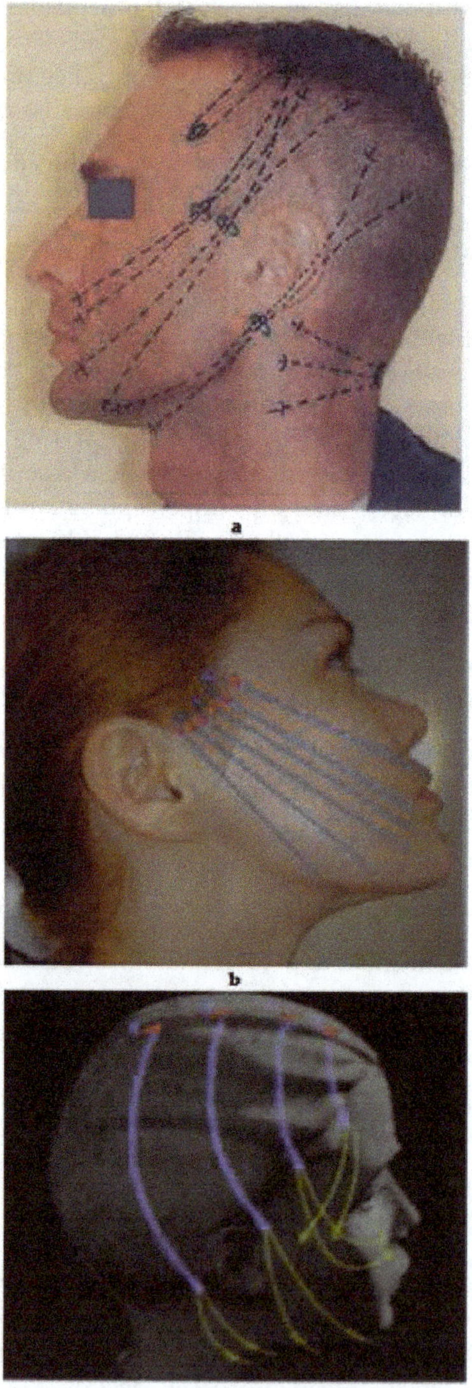

a

b

c

**Figure 12.** a. Marking before long threads implementatio, b. Linear thread direction for the middle facial zone lift, c. Whole face thread lift marking by the method of putting threads over the scalp

One of the doctors during the performance of the Aptos Thread surgery put long threads from one part of the face over the whole patient's scalp on the other in order to have the threads intruded on the right part of the face could support the threads on the left part of the face and vice versa (figure 10 c). It is not difficult to imagine the whole operation technology, the process of the practical thread implementation along such a long and difficult contour and the severity of the injury of the tissues along the thread implementation way. Of course, this is not a minimally-invasive intrusion any more [7, 14].

### 4. Thread Fixation Depth

It is determined by the stated objectives, the facial area, the skin depth and the chosen lift thread method. For example, in the case of eyebrow and "jowl" lift threads are fixed rather superficially, while in the bucco--zygomatic and infraorbital areas they are intruded rather deeply into the subcutaneous layer in order to create high volume of the middle facial zone.

Thereby it is possible to confirm that the preventive measures of complications and early relapse cases possible in applying Aptos method are based on the doctor's knowledge of the causes of age and contour facial deformations, the right understanding the idea of Aptos tissue lift, selection of patents according to the indications, the right method choice, irreproachable mastery of equipment, and the delicate intrusion performance. Complication and long-lasting side effects treatment include the achieved results correction (undercutting, implementation of absorbable fillers), elimination of eased and migrating threads, repeated thread or classical lift, physiotherapy, and massage [11, 12].

## 4. Conclusions

The absolute advantages of the Aptos thread method at the lift surgery performance are:

- Simplicity, easiness, efficiency;
- Minimal invasiveness and slight injuring procedures;
- Reliability, sufficient sustainability, and high quality lift;
- Possibility of combination with other interferences;
- Short rehabilitation period.

Complications and unpleasant side effects are not inherent in the very nature of the Aptos method; they are so rare, slight and easily corrected that aesthetic surgery specialists do not have to refuse the usage of lift thread methods.

Some authors present only negative results in their articles about thread lift [6, 9]. However, it must be emphasized that the results of our long-term work absolutely do not agree with the statistics of these publications (Diagrams 2 and 3). The unreasonably suspicious attitude towards the method does not assist the development and improvement of the thread lift methods, and minimally-invasive aesthetic surgery in whole like alternatives to classical lift methods and contour facial surgery.

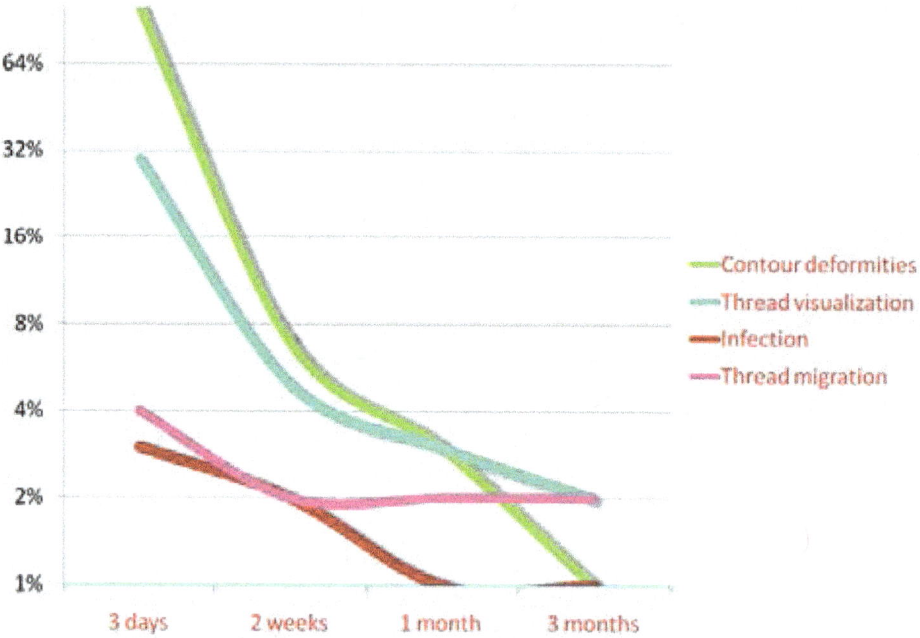


**Scheme 2.** Frequency and Appearance Dates of Complications in Thread Lift Case

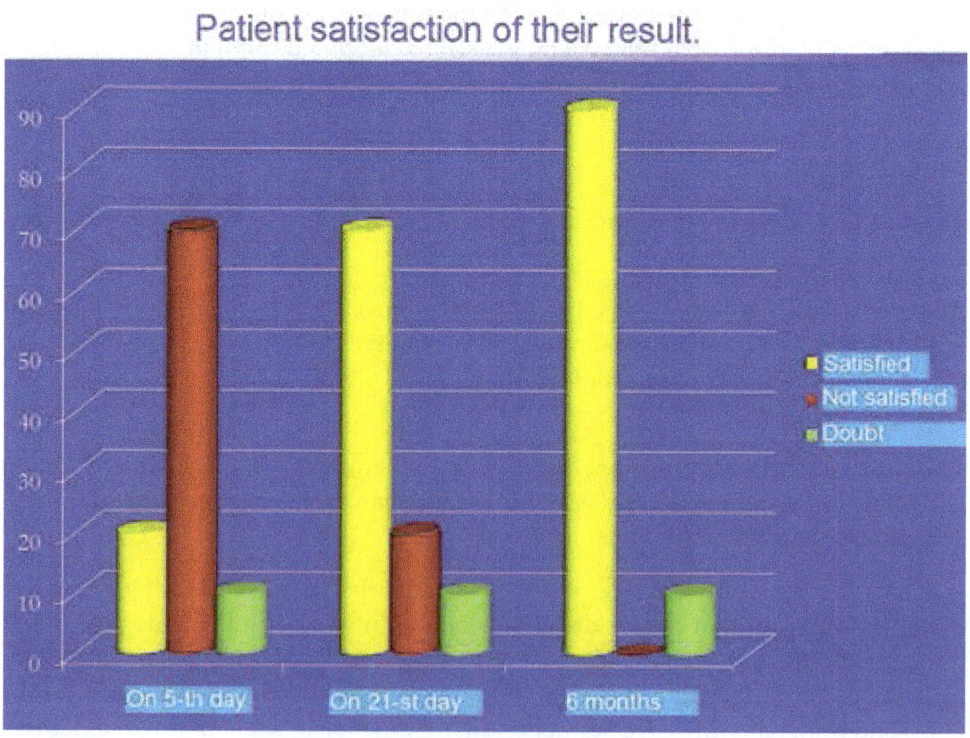


**Scheme 3.** Patients' Satisfaction with the Results of Thread Lift

## Author details

M.A. Sulamanidze, I.S. Vozdvizhenskiy, G.M. Sulamanidze,
K.M. Sulamanidze and E.G. Azizyan
*Clinic of plastic and Aesthetic Surgery and Dermatocosmetology TotalCharm, Moscow (Russia), Tbilisi, Georgia*

## 5. References

[1] Kazinnikova O.G., Adamian A.A., Age specific changes in facial and cervical tissues // Annals of plastic, reparative, and aesthetic surgery, 2000, 1, 52-61.

[2] Sulamanidze M.A., Sulamanidze G.M. Flabby, ageing face. New approaches // II Congress on aesthetic and restorative surgery, Moscow, 1998:15

[3] Sulamanidze M.A., Sulamanidze G.M. Soft tissues lift: old philosophy, new approach - a method of internal stitching (Aptos Needle) // Annals of plastic, reparative, and aesthetic surgery, 2005, 1, 15-29.

[4] Sulamanidze M.A., Sulamanidze G.M. Aptos methods: past, present, future // Aesthetic Medicine Newsletter, 2007, 3, 23-32.

[5] Sulamanidze M.A., Sulamanidze G.M., Vozdvizhenskiy I.S., Sulamanidze K.M., Kadzhaya A.A. New Method of Elastic Thread Face Lift // Aesthetic Medicine, 2010, 3, 275-280.

[6] Aesthetic byers guide. – 2006
www.miinews.com

[7] Guillo D. Fils Aptos implantation en X. Surginevs 2005, 8, 10-13.

[8] Mendelson B.C., Muzaffar A.R., Adams W.P. Surgical Anatomy of the Midcheek and Malar Mounds // Plastic. And Reconstruct. Surgery. – 2002, September. – Vol. 110, №3. – P. 885-896.

[9] Rachel, J.D., Lack, E.B., Larson, B. Incidence of complications and early recurrence in 29 patients after facial rejuvenation with barbed suture lifting // Dermatol. Surgery. – 2010. - №36. – P. 348-354.

[10] Sulamanidze M.A., Fournier P.F., Paikidze T.G., Sulamanidze G.M. Removal of Facial Soft Tissue Ptosis With Special Threads// Dermatol. Surgery. – 2002, May. - №28. – P.367-371.

[11] Sulamanidze M.A., Sulamanidze G.M. Aptos Suture Lifting Methods. 10 Years of Experience // Clinics in Plast.Surgery. – 2009, April. – Vol.36, №2. – P.281-306.

[12] Sulamanidze M.A., Sulamanidze G.M., Sulamanidze C.M., Vozdvizhensky I.S. Lifting of Soft Tissues With Barbed Threads. Side Effects, Complications. // 11-th ESPRAS Congress Plastic, Restorative and Aesthetic Surgery, 20-26 September 2009, Rhodes, Greece. – Book of Abstracts. – P.25

[13] Winkler E., Goldan O., Regev E. Stenssen duct rupture (sialicele) and other complications of the Aptos thread technique // Plast. Reconstr. Surgery. – 2006. - №118. – P. 1468-71.

[14] Woffles Wu. Advances in Stitch Lift // 2-nd Regional Conference in Dermatological Laser and Facial Cosmetic Surgery. – 2006, 20-22 January, Hong Kong. – Programme Book. – P.30

9

# New Method of Face Elastic Thread Lift

M. Sulamanidze, G. Sulamanidze, I. Vozdvizhenskiy,
K. Sulamanidze and A. Kadzhaya

## 1. Introduction

Within the last few decades the priorities for the treatment of facial ageing and sagging, especially in the paraoral area, have changed dramatically. Patients demand this interference to be performed with minimum risk to their health, minor injury, short postoperative rehabilitation period, and, above all, long-term aesthetic effect.

However, during the process of lifting operation on the mentioned facial zone mobilization and hypodermic soft tissues transfer (subcutaneous tissue, SMAS, muscles) into a new higher position and applying interrupted sutures through the soft tissues are regarded as key points of the long-term effect, that is impossible to achieve without a considerable operational trauma. Besides, the strongly pronounced mobility of this facial area brings the results of the interference to the relapse of the aesthetic deformation.

## 2. Classical methods of face lift and their disadvantages

It is known that traditional face lift methods are not effective enough to eliminate aesthetic age manifistations in the paraoral area, as these zones are at the maximum distance from the section and face lift line. That is why during face lift operations some surgeons make a wide separation of face skin up to the nasolabial folds and mouth corners, and then raise the skin fold upwards and laterally to the maximum possible extent, removing considerable skin surplus. Performance of such surgeries quite often leads to unnaturally stretched faces, alopecia in the temple area and hypertrophy of postoperative cicatrices, appearing deceitfully under auricula lobes and stretching them down (picture 1). Even deep plane lift methods (so called SMAS- and intraperiosteal lifts) do not always eliminate the aging face signs in its medial parts.

In picture 2 we can see a skin area with marking, in picture 2(b) – the same area after mobilization in the course of rhytidoplasty. It is clearly seen that the skin area that had been

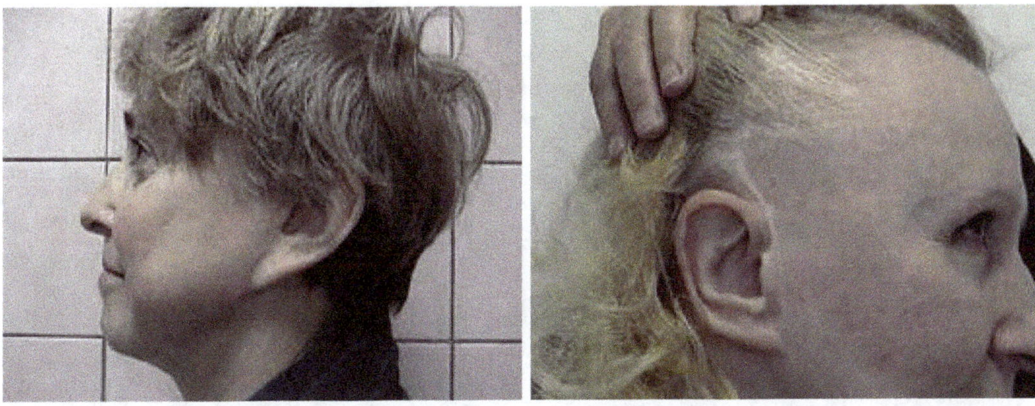

a b

Figure 1.

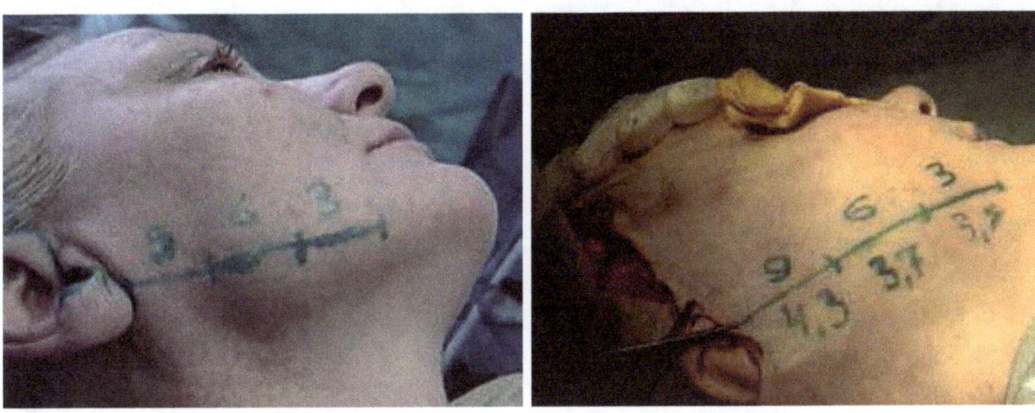


a b

Figure 2.

the furthest from the place of the force application stretched out insignificantly – only to 0.4 cm, while the nearest skin graft stretched considerably – it became 1.5 cm longer.

Furthermore, paraoral facial areas are in the zone of active influence of masticatory and mimic muscles, and in the nearest postoperative period the areas around the mouth corners, smoothed out as the result of the surgery, become sagged again. This factor also interferes with the stabilization of the face lift result [1].

In the last few years, despite the anatomic and functional features of the paraoral area, different methods of hard thread lifting have been used quite often for mouth corner soft tissue lift. Such an approach cannot give consistent long-term effect, as in this case the presence of highly developed and active masticatory and mimic muscles, which quickly destroy the achieved result (in 2-3 months a relapse is expected), is underrated.

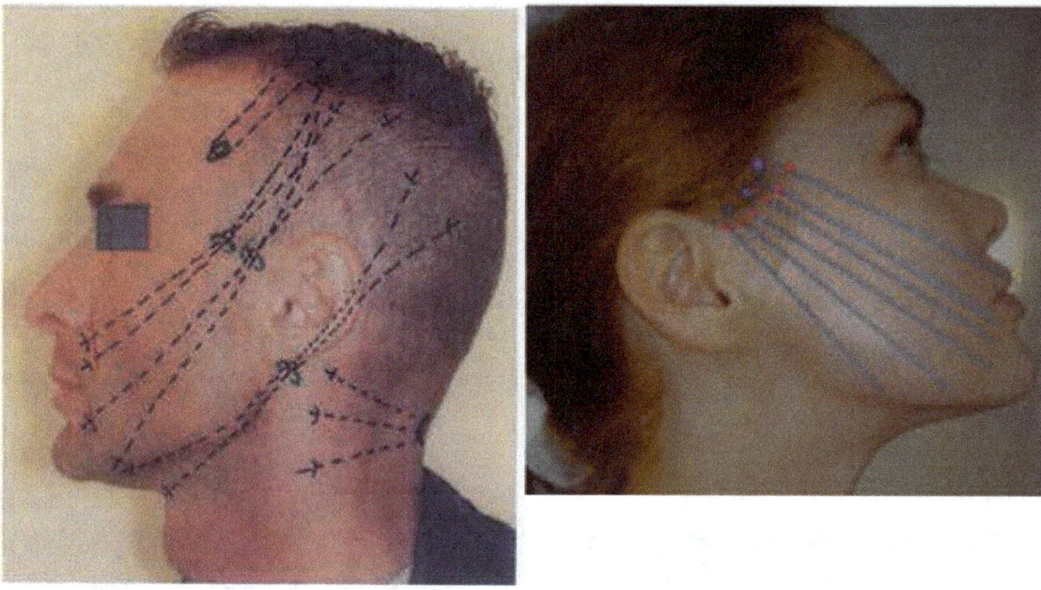

a b

**Figure 3.**

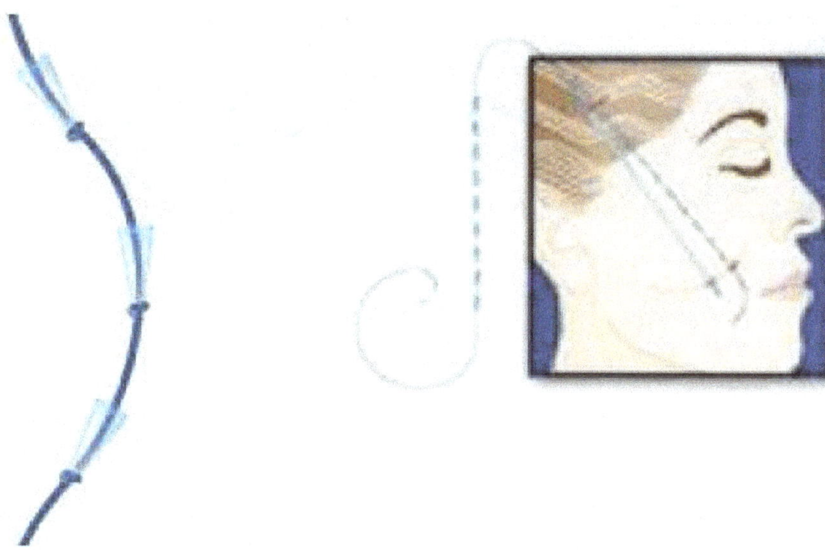

a b

**Figure 4.**

Even such powerful lift constructions as Silhouette Sutures, as they can seem at first glance, cannot resist kinetics of these muscles and cannot save lift results in such areas for a long period of time (picture 4), as the direction of threads' position resists muscle contraction and relaxation.

## 3. Elastic thread lift of the paraoral area. Aptos Springs Method

In 2004 elastic thread lift of the paraoral area – Aptos Springs Method – was developed in our clinic. Both the method and the threads developed for using in this technique have Russian and international patents [6, 7].

Aptos Springs thread is a special twisted in form of a spring polypropylene (non-absorbable) thread 2/0, which has a "memory". In the course of production this thread undergoes a special processing which provides it with spring type characteristics. A spring in a compressed position is wound around an injection needle of 1.1x100 or 0.9x90 mm (picture 5). There are two Aptos Springs threads of each size in one package, and one package usually is enough for one procedure.

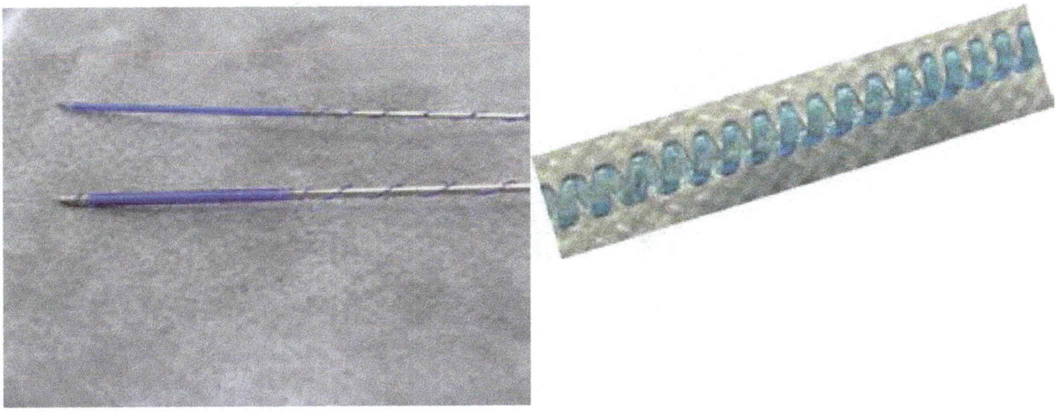

a b

**Figure 5.**

The manufacture produces Aptos Springs threads made from polypropylene (non-absorbable) as well as from absorbable Kaprolac threads (Light Lift), which gets fully absorbed in the tissues within a year, and the fibrosis, which appears in this place, keeps on "working".

In the clinical practice Aptos Springs threads are used for:

- labiomental fold elimination (Marionette Line) (variant I);
- mouth corners lift (variant II).

During the consultation the patient is informed about the method possibilities, details of the surgery performance, its duration, rehabilitation period special characteristics, and the duration of the lift effect. The patient decides on his/her own with the use of which product (absorbable or non-absorbable threads) the surgery is to be performed.

## 4. Variants of the surgery performance

### 4.1. Labiomental fold elimination (surgery technique, variant I)

The "marionette line" is marked and two parallel lines, 1 cm distant from each other, are drawn perpendicularly to the wrinkle (picture 6). The Aptos Springs thread of the bigger thickness is usually fixed above, and the one of the smaller size is fixed below.

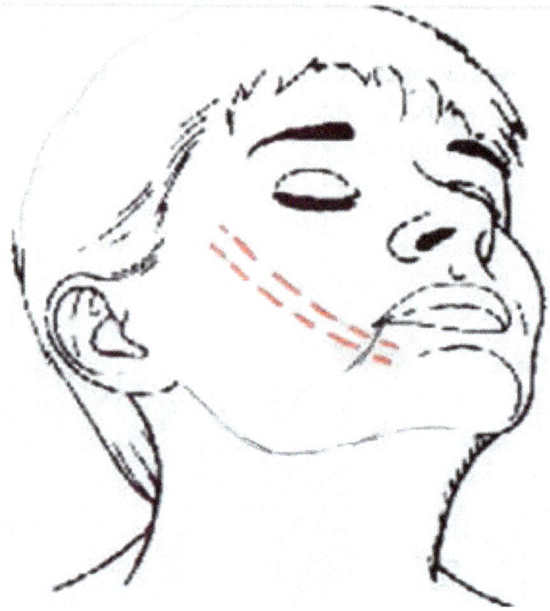

**Figure 6.**

Before it is fixed the spring is stretched along the length of the needle and is inserted subcutaneously in this position. The needle is inserted at the upper point and pushed towards the wrinkle; in the first half of the way it is deepened to the SMAS limits, in the second half it is shifted closer to the skin and crosses the fold at this depth. The needle is taken out from the skin 1.5 cm past the Marionette line, while the spring is left subcutaneously. After a slight lifting of the spring thread from the both sides, its surplus is cut off and the ends are buried under the derma. In this case there is no need to use any special thread ends' fixing as it is evenly and rigidly fixed in the tissues with the help of its coils.

Right after the fixation, on the operating table, you can see a lift effect and elimination of the labiomental folds and the soft tissue folds over them. By compressing Aptos Springs threads lift sagging soft tissues, and stretch and shrink in synchrony with facial muscles in the process of mimic, masticatory or other facial movements (picture 7).

Subsequently fibrous tissue appears around the thread, which in its turn provides strengthening of the lifting and spring type effect with a long-term consistent result (picture 8,9,10).

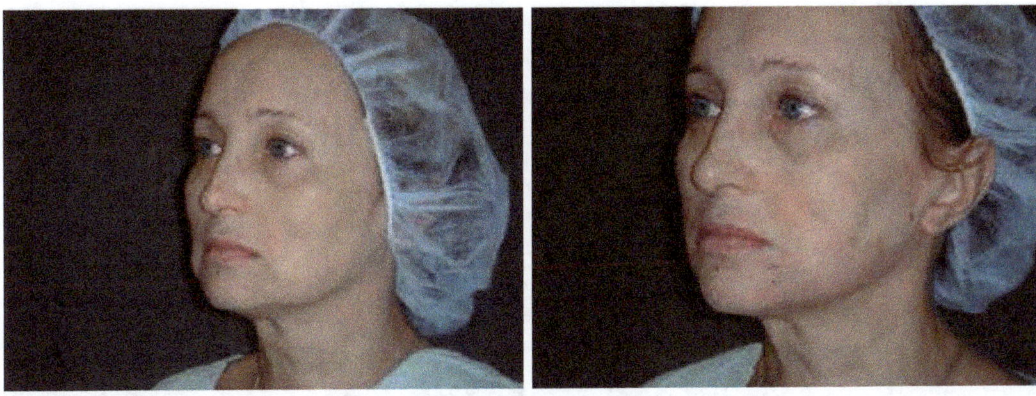

a b

**Figure 7.**

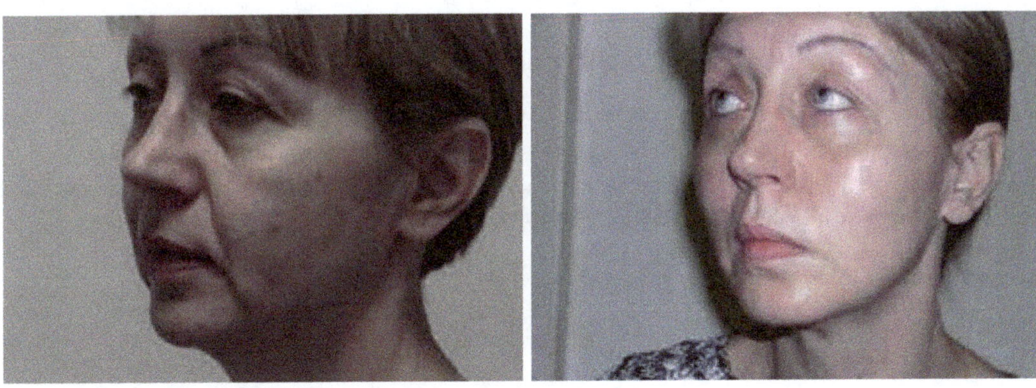

a b

**Figure 8.**

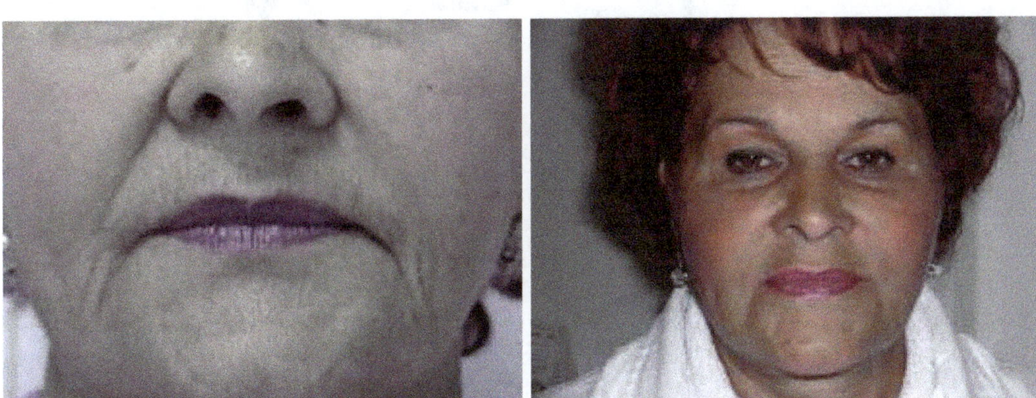

a b

**Figure 9.**

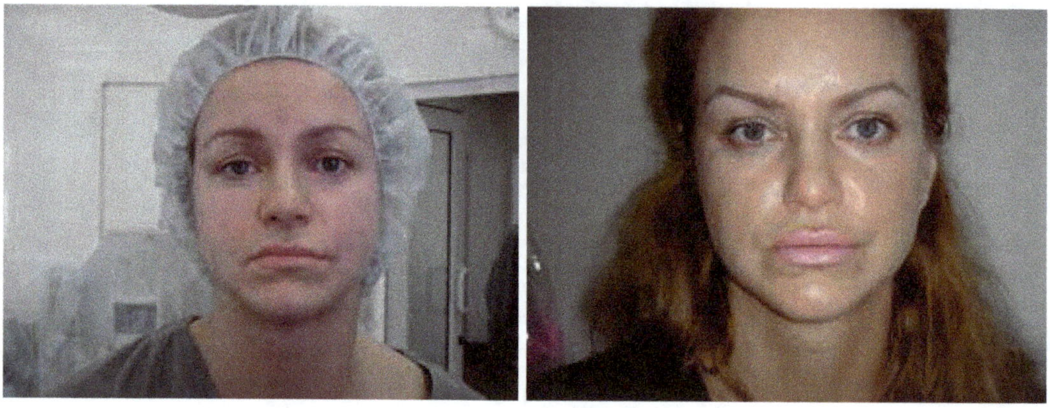

a b

**Figure 10.**

## 4.2. Mouth corners lift (surgery technique, variant II)

The marking used for the mouth corners lift surgery is made in the following way: one line is drawn perpendicularly to the "marionette line", just like in Variant I, while the second line is drawn parallelly up to the mouth corner, and then up and angle-wise, sideward the red border of the upper lip at a distance of 1.5-2.0 cm (picture 11).

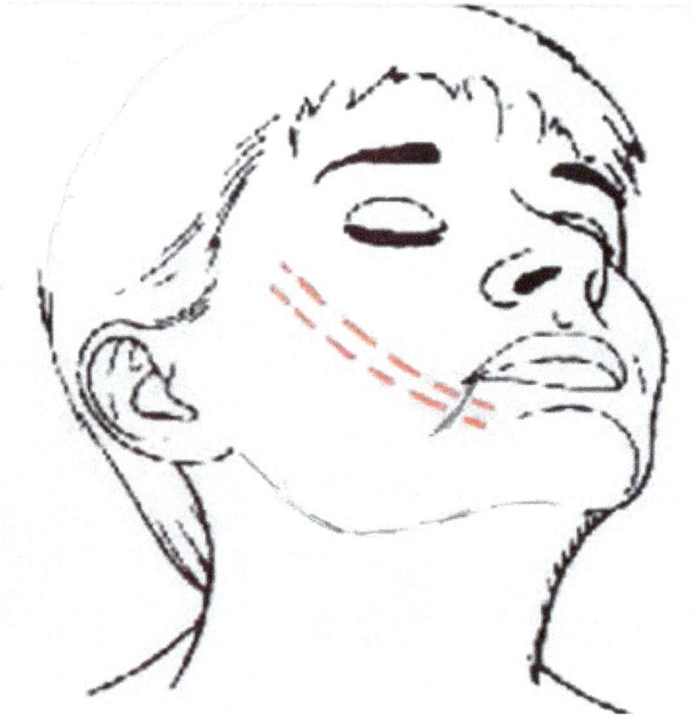

**Figure 11.**

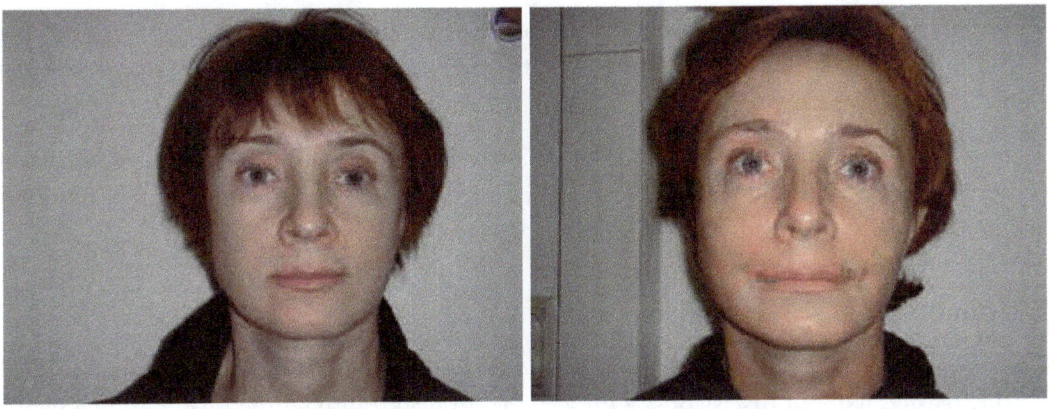

a b

Figure 12.

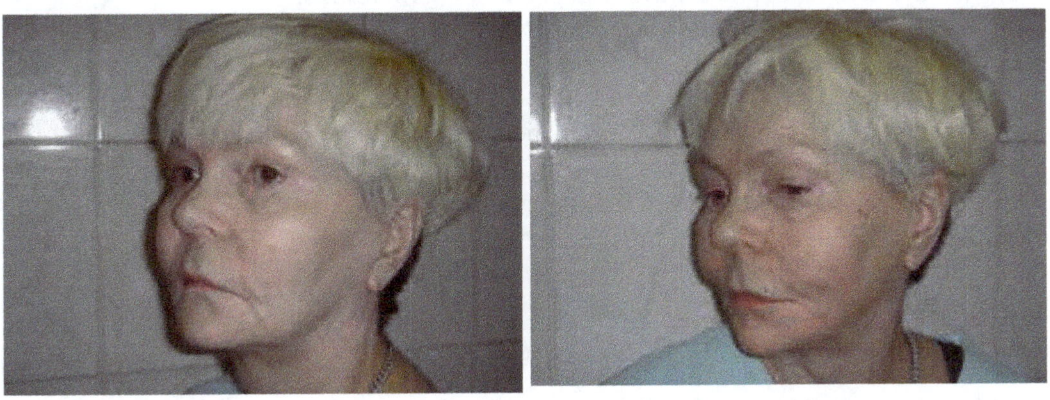

a b

Figure 13.

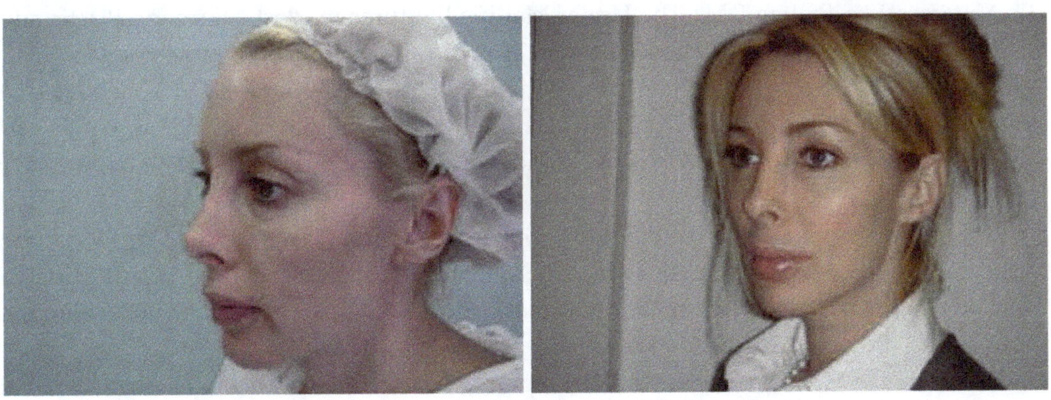

a b

Figure 14.

The Aptos Springs thread of the bigger thickness is fixed sideward the "marionette line", the thread of the smaller thickness is brought to the mouth corner and then inserted under the skin of the red lip border.

Right after the threads fixation (as early as on the operating table) we can see the mouth corner lift effect ("constant smile" effect), slight eversion of the lateral areas of the upper lip and labiomental folds elimination of slight expressiveness (picture 12, 13, 14).

## 5. Conclusions

Operations by Aptos Springs method are performed under local infiltration anaesthesia quickly, easily, without discissions, with a slight surgical trauma, little postoperative pains, and a short rehabilitation period. Since 2003 more than 2000 similar operations have been carried out in our clinic both in the form of monotherapy and simultaneously with other rejuvenation interference and always with good long-term results.

## Author details

M. Sulamanidze, G. Sulamanidze, I. Vozdvizhenskiy,
K. Sulamanidze and A. Kadzhaya
*Clinic of Plastic, Aesthetic Surgery and Dermatocosmetology, Total Charm,*
*Moscow, Russia*

## 6. References

[1] Mendelson B.C., Muzaffar A.R., Adams W.P. Surgical Anatomy of the Midcheek and Malar Mounds // Plastic. And Reconstruct. Surgery. – 2002, September. – Vol. 110, №3. – P. 885-896.

[2] Guillo D. Fils Aptos implantation en X. Surginevs 2005, 8, 10-13.

[3] Matarasso A., Pfaifer T.M., The Use of Modified Sutures in Plastic Surgery. Plastic and Reconstructive Surgery, 2008; 122 (issue 2):652-658.

[4] Sasaki G.H., Komorovska-Timek E., Bennet D.C., Cabriel A. An Objective Comparison of Holding, Slippage and Pull-Out Tensions for Eight Suspension Sutures in the Malar Pads of Frech-Frosen Human Cadavers. Aesthetic Surgery Journal, 2008; 28 (4): 387-396.

[5] Sulamanidze M.A., Sulamanidze G.M., Sulamanidze C.M., Vozdvizhensky I.S. Lifting of Soft Tissues With Barbed Threads. Side Effects, Complications. // 11-th ESPRAS Congress Plastic, Restorative and Aesthetic Surgery, 20-26 September 2009, Rhodes, Greece. – Book of Abstracts. – P.25

[6] Sulamanidze M.A., Sulamanidze G.M. Aptos Springs – a new concept of lifting. Journal of the Japan Society of Aesthetic Surgery, 2005; 42(5):183.

[7] Sulamanidze M.A., Sulamanidze G.M. Surgical Thread and Cosmetic Surgery Method. WO, 2005/087283.

# 10

# Morphological Foundations of Facelift Using APTOS Filaments

A.A. Adamyan, M.A. Sulamanidze, N.D. Skuba and Z.R. Khusnutdinova

## 1. Introduction

Correction of earlier involutional changes of the face, in the first place facial skin ptosis, encounters some difficulties. On the one hand, these changes are not serious enough to serve as an indication for radical aesthetic surgery. On the other hand, traditional minor surgical interventions fail to ensure well-apparent beneficial effect.

Moreover, many women are reluctant to undergo extensive surgery since it entails prolonged rehabilitation which may sometimes take one and a half months to be completed.

No wonder, many plastic surgeons tend to resort to a combination of minor invasive interventions that are apt to significantly shorten the rehabilitation period and are possible to perform in an outpatient setting.

## 2. Materials and methods

Recent years witnessed wide implementation into clinical practice of aesthetic surgery of an effective, atraumatic method of treatment of facial involutional alterations – lifting of the soft tissues with the help of specially designed "APTOS" threads [1, 4, 5, 6, 7, 8].

The method is based on the use of specially designed polypropylene APTOS filaments and is recommended for managing moderate involutional changes in the facial soft tissues and local face lifting. One side of an APTOS thread bears barbs that extend forward in the direction of its movement through the tissue, on the other side the barbs extend backward, i.e. in the opposite direction. Barb length - 1 mm, barb angle thickness could vary from 30 to 50 degree depending on the barb resistance force. Such a design ensures that the filament gently glides through soft tissues in a desired direction but resists drawing in the opposite one, i.e. remains fixed as appropriate. As a result, subcutaneously implanted filaments keep in place the lifted facial tissues uniformly drawn into puckers, do not allow them to slip down, and thus maintain a new facial contour.

However, until now it remains unknown how the APTOS threads behave within the tissues in time and what are the local and morphological processes maintaining the tension and creating the rejuvenating effect.

In an attempt to clarify the mechanism of tissue reactions to subcutaneous implantation of APTOS filaments, an experimental study of the resulting morphological changes was undertaken at the A.V. Vishnevsky Institute of Surgery. A group of 20 white rats was used as a model from which 72 tissue samples were obtained for histological studies [3]. Morphological findings were compared with the results of examination of tissue samples following implantation of smooth polypropylene filaments to another group of animals that served as control.

The material for histological analysis included implants, their capsules, and the surrounding tissues.

Relative vascular bed density (RVBD) at different time intervals after implantation was estimated and compared with RVBD of intact rats to evaluate changes of blood supply to the tissues surrounding implanted polypropylene filaments [2].

Relative vascular bed density was calculated by the following standard formula

$$RVBD = \frac{\text{Number of points in the blood vessel field}}{\text{Total number of points in the examined field}} \times 100\%$$

## 3. Results and discussion

On day 3 after subcutaneous implantation, the filament was found to be isolated from the surrounding tissue mass by an immature connective tissue capsule (fig. 1a) the lateral sides of which gave rise to connective tissue bands. The capsule wall was much thicker close to the barbs than near the smooth thread portions. Also, the capsule wall facing epidermis was significantly thicker than its remaining part, probably due to mechanical pressure exerted by the integumentary tissues on the filament and the capsule developing around it. Such variability of the capsule wall thickness is considered to be beneficial for the final face lifting effect and improve its stability.

The histological study revealed marked hyperemia of the microvascular bed. It was especially pronounced where barbs rose from the shaft of the thread. The barbs looked braided with tissue cells. The inner capsule layer at the base of the barbs was composed of fibroblasts dominated by young cells. Connective tissue bands growing from the capsule wall were readily apparent as well as inflammatory reaction that resulted in fibroblast accumulation around the barbs and thickening of the capsule wall where it faced epidermis. There were practically no signs of inflammation in the form of infiltration around the implanted filaments.

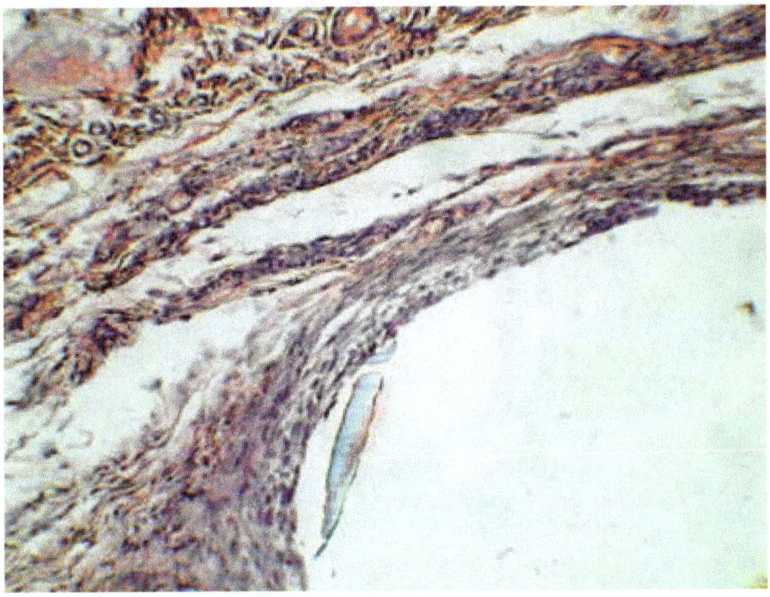

a

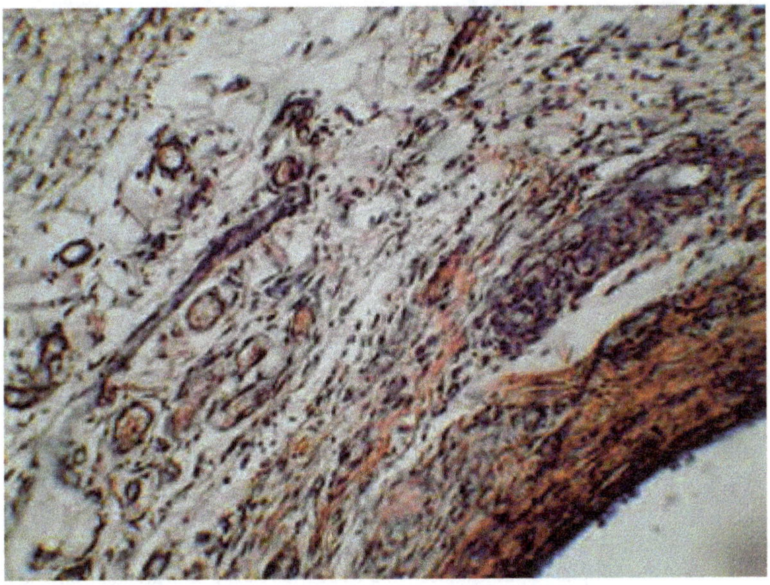

b

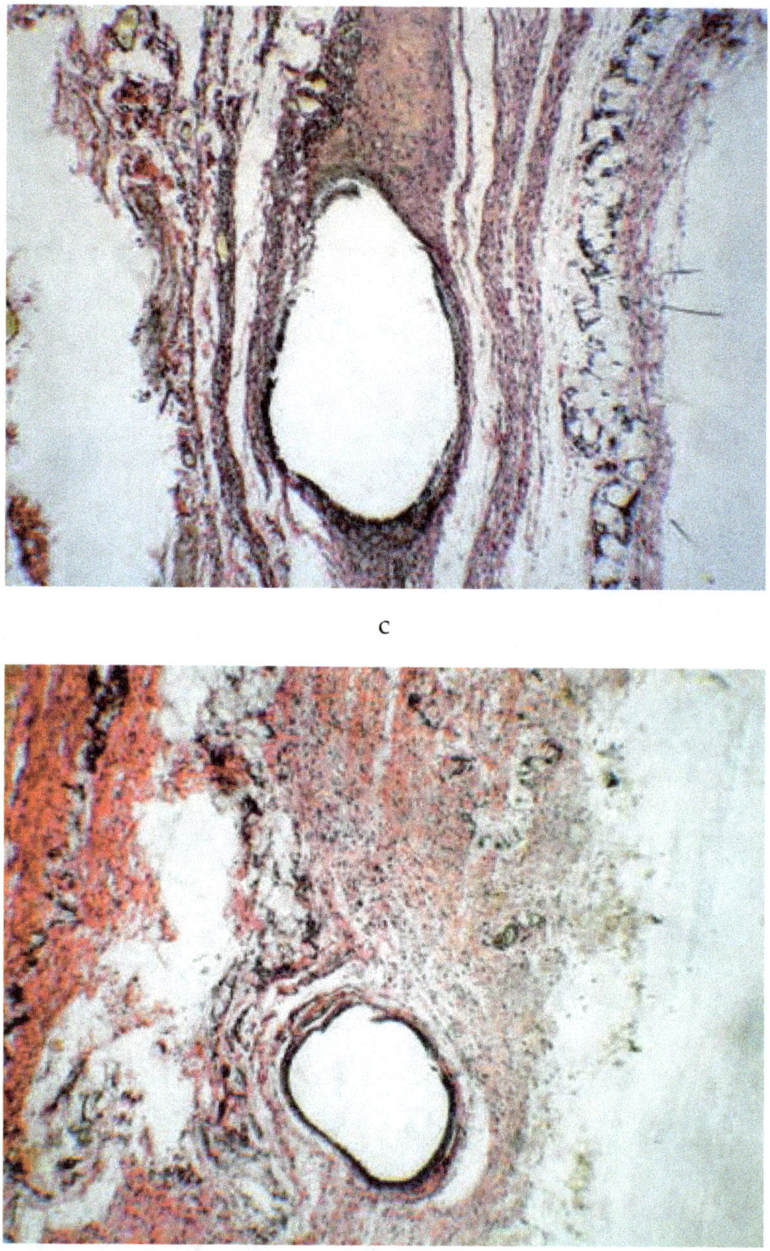

c

d

a - 3 days after implantation. Cellular elements predominate over fibrous ones, the number of microvessels increases (x100); b - 7 days after implantation. The capsule has a bilayer structure, persistent hyperemia develops due to marked vasodilation (x100); *c*-*7* days after implantation. Connective tissue bands can be seen arising from the upper poles of the capsule (x40); *d* - *7* days after implantation (x40)

**Figure 1.** Microphotographs of the capsule surrounding APTOS filament (a-c) and smooth polypropylene thread (d). Van-Gieson pyrofuchsin staining

The structure of the capsule surrounding a smooth polypropylene filament on day 3 after implantation was not substantially different from that formed around a barbed APTOS filament. Only the wall thickness was smaller, being 19.25 mem on the side facing epidermis and 23.5 mem on the side facing the subcutaneous fat layer. A thinner capsule around smooth filaments was due to the absence of barbs and the respective less injurious effect of the implanted material.

The shape of the capsule developing after the implantation of both APTOS and smooth filaments was that of a rhombus. However, the capsule around smooth filaments gave out no connective tissue bands arising from their lateral walls.

On day 7, the capsules around APTOS filaments became thicker due to a rise in the number of collagen fibres. Each capsule exhibited two distinct layers characterized by different cell to collagen fibre ratio (fig. 1b):

1. inner layer enclosing the filament and dominated by young cells and
2. outer layer in which collagen fibres predominated.

The capsules assumed the rhomboid shape while their lateral apices gave rise to connective tissue bands that became thinner as the distance from the capsule increased (fig. 1c). The total length of a band (the capsule wall inclusive) was 886 mem, the width ranged from 108 to 187 mem. The capsules remained well-vascularized despite a progressive rise in the number of collagen fibres within 7 days after filament implantation. The capsule walls were penetrated by a large number of capillary vessels, microvascular hyperemia persisted both in the immediate proximity to the filaments and at a certain distance from them. No signs of pyogenic inflammation could be seen.

The outer capsule layer, although rather thin, always contained a large number of capillary-type vessels.

Isolated lymphoid and plasma cells as well as swollen fibroblasts were readily apparent close to microvessels. The amount of blood congestion in the microvascular bed decreased with the distance from the filament.

The thickness of the capsule formed around a smooth polypropylene filament by day 7 after implantation was 17.75 mem on the side facing epidermis and 17.25 mem on the side facing the subcutaneous fatty layer. Lateral walls were as thick as 54.5 and 25 mem (fig. 1c).

On the whole, the major morphological characteristics of the tissues surrounding smooth filaments on day 7 after implantation underwent significantly smaller modification compared with the tissues responding to APTOS filaments.

On day 40, further thickening of the capsule wall around both the shaft and the barbs of APTOS filaments took place; however, the capsule development was not completed. The capsule wall facing epidermis was significantly thicker than that facing the subcutaneous fat layer (58 and 18.75 mem, respectively). Connective tissue bands arising from the capsule walls, shafts and barbs of APTOS filaments became thicker and longer than before. Simultaneously, the number of microvessels increased. Most of them underwent hyperemia, but no signs of exudation were documented.

A peculiar morphological finding on day 40 was parallel bands composed of connective tissue fibres and extending towards the subcutaneous fat layer. According to micrometric measurements, the bands were from 5,000 to 8,000 mem long and from 900 to 300 mem wide. They occupied a total area of 4,200 mem.

Characteristic changes in loose connective tissue close to the implanted filaments included:

- an increased number of vessels in the microcirculatory system (arterioles, venules, pre- and postcapillaries, and capillaries) compared with tissues located farther from the implants;
- microvessels looked overfilled with blood, i.e. had an open lumen, any time after the implantation of APTOS filaments; in other words, implantation induced persistent hyperemia and therefore stimulated blood supply to the tissues surrounding APTOS filaments;
- fibroblasts of loose connective tissue had enlarged nuclei and plasma volume and finely dispersed chromatin which suggested a functionally active state.

Staining with toluidine blue revealed an increased number of mast cells in the loose connective tissue layer surrounding APTOS filaments. These cells were concentrated in perivascular space of the microcirculatory system (fig. 2).

The tissue response to smooth polypropylene filaments on day 40 after their implantation was not significantly different from that to APTOS filament. However, the capsule

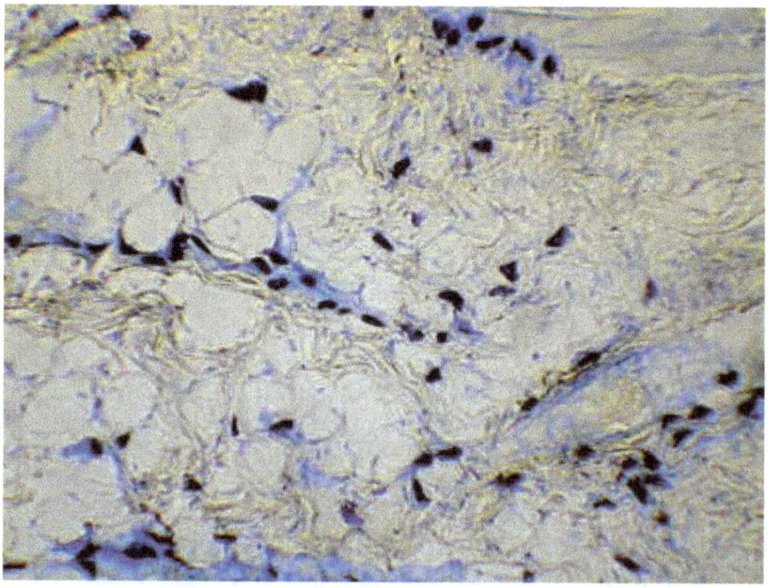

**Figure 2.** Microphotograph showing accumulation of mast cells around APTOS filament. Staining with toluidine blue (x 40)

developing around smooth polypropylene threads had thinner walls and matured quicker than around APTOS filaments, evidently due to less severe irritating effect on the tissues.

The capsule wall thickness varied from 52,5 mem on the side facing epidermis to 42.75 mem on the side facing the subcutaneous fat layer. The lateral walls of the capsule were approximately 400 mem thick. The width of the middle part of the lateral walls was around 136.75 mem. Tissues surrounding smooth filaments contained an increased number of microvessels, but hyperemia and vascularization were less pronounced than around APTOS filament.

On day 90 after the implantation of APTOS filaments, the inner capsule layer was composed of functionally active cells, each containing a large amount of cytoplasm. The outer layer consisted of collagen fibres and a small number of fibrocytes (fig. 3a).

Fibrous capsule structures and similar structures of the surrounding tissue merged into one another giving rise to a continuous network.

In the course of time, the fibrous capsule became more and more tightly integrated with the surrounding tissue which promoted solid fixation of the implanted filaments. Both the shaft and the barbs of the filaments were braided with fibrous tissue structures. The capsule wall near the barbs was thicker but less mature than around the shaft of the filaments; it contained more cellular elements than fibrous ones. Simultaneously, the number of mast cells increased. Giant cells close to the filaments were very rare and localized near the barbs.

Smooth polypropylene filaments had better developed capsules than APTOS filaments on 90 days after implantation. Fibrous elements in their walls predominated over cellular ones. The capsules displayed neither inflammatory reaction nor signs of resorption. Tissue vascularization in the immediate proximity to smooth polypropylene threads was less pronounced than around APTOS filaments.

The capsule had a rhomboid shape. However, unlike the capsule around APTOS filaments, it gave out no laterally extending connective tissue bands. This confirms that smooth polypropylene threads are unsuitable for facelift.

On day 210 after implantation, the connective tissue capsule around APTOS filaments continued to develop having the wall thickness of 39.6 and 35.4 mem on the sides facing epidermis and subcutaneous fat layer, respectively.

The capsule became thinner, fibroblasts underwent conversion into fibrocytes, collagen fibres predominated over cellular elements. Capsular fibrous structures merged with the fibrous structures of the surrounding tissue, i.e. their further integration occurred.

The capsule around filament barbs looked less mature than around the shaft (fig. 3b) due to irritating effect of the former on the adjacent tissue.

No giant cells indicative of resorptive macrophagal reaction could be seen in the capsule.

Prolonged period of capsule development around barbs ensured stronger adhesion between implanted filaments and the surrounding soft tissues (fig. 4a).

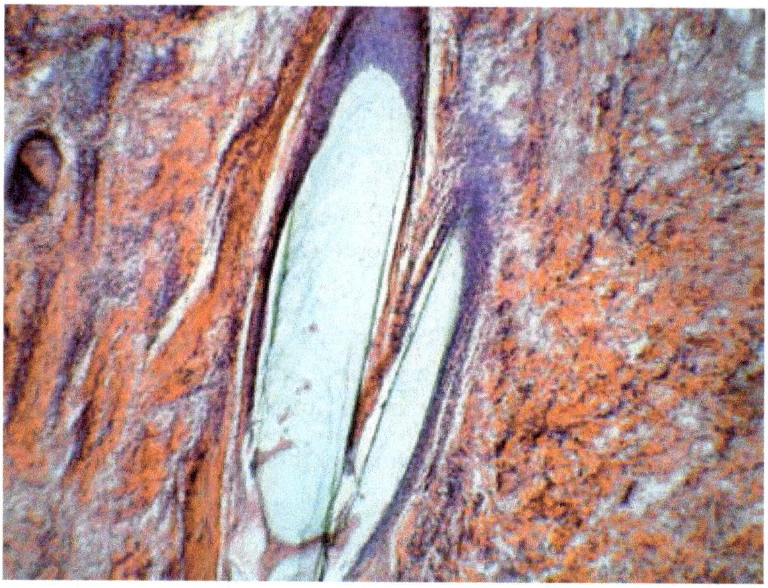

a

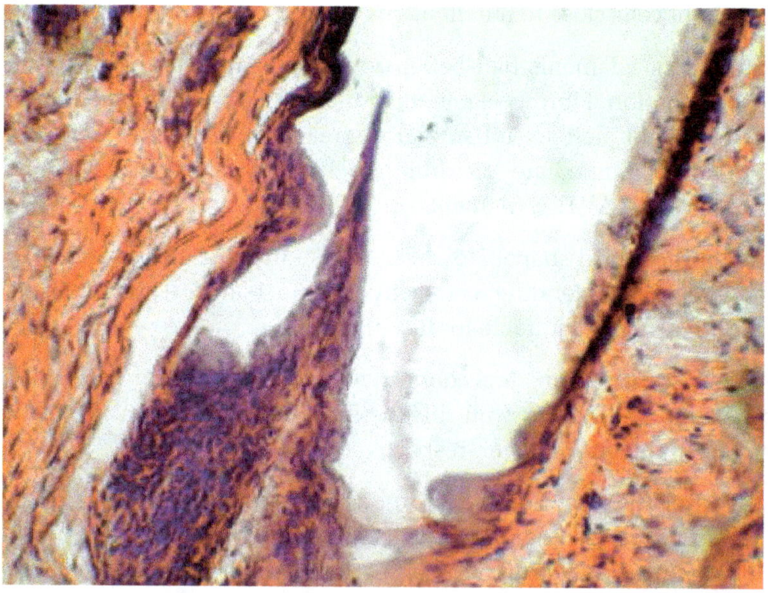

b

a - 90 days after implantation. The capsule wall around the barb is much thicker than around the shaft. Cellular elements predominate (x 40); *b* - 210 days after implantation. The capsule wall around the shaft is thin and contains few cells. The capsule around a barb contains many cellular elements (x 40)

**Figure 3.** Microphotographs of the capsule surrounding APTOS filament and its barb. Van-Gieson pyrofuchsin staining *(a-b)*

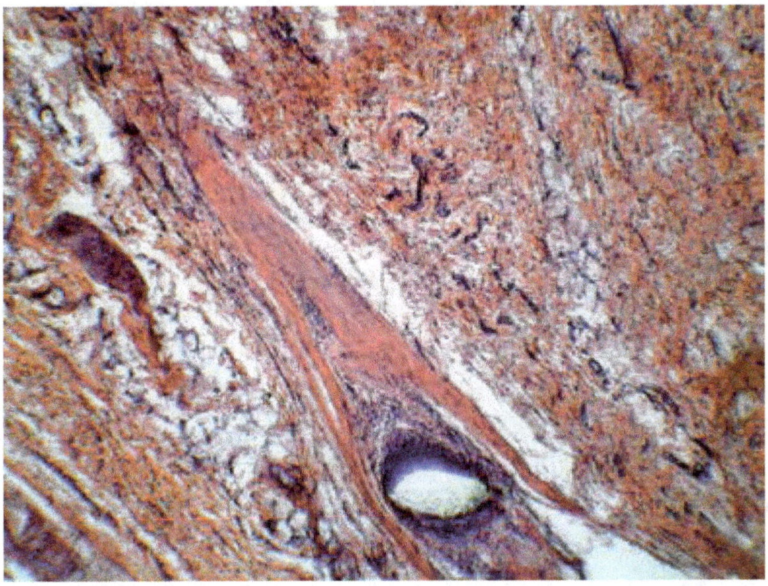

a

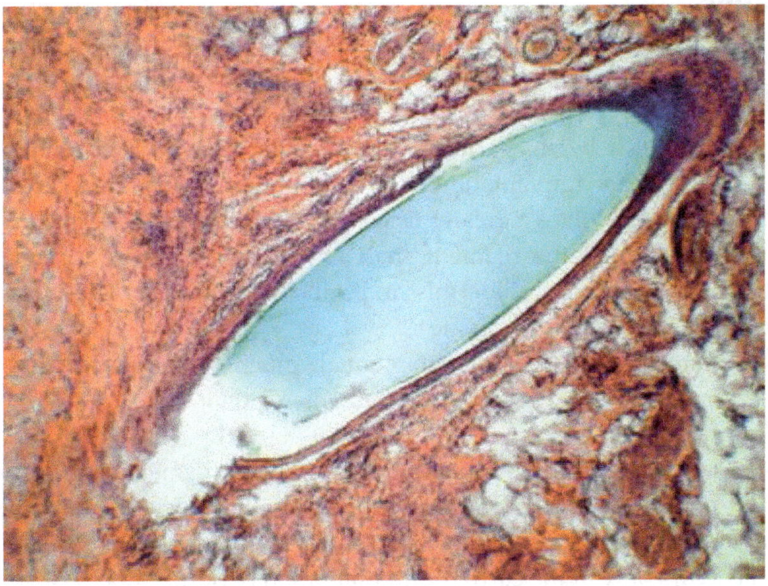

b

a - the capsule gives rise to well-apparent connective tissue bands. Collagen biosynthesis continues (x 40); b - the capsule contains few cellular elements throughout its length. Cellular elements in the right top corner show themselves as a result of oblique section across the filament and the surrounding capsule (x 40)

**Figure 4.** Microphotographs of the capsule surrounding a barb of APTOS filament (a) and a smooth polypropylene thread (b) 210 days after implantation. Van-Gieson pyrofuchsin staining

The capsule wall thickness around the barbs varied from 150 to 54.2 mem, the lateral walls were 220 mem long and 133 mem wide.

The structure of the capsule that developed around smooth polypropylene thread by day 210 after implantation was practically identical with that of the capsule around APTOS filament, but its maturation was about to be complete, and fibrous elements predominated over cellular ones (fig. 4b).

A study of blood supply to the tissues surrounding implanted filaments based on the estimation of relative vascular bed density has demonstrated its 20% increase on day 3 after implantation of APTOS filaments compared with only 6% in case of smooth polypropylene threads (a 8.1 and 7.9% rise, respectively from the baseline level in intact rats).

A maximum increase of the relative vascular bed density occurred on day 40 after implantation (11.0 and 9.1% in tissues surrounding barbed filament and smooth thread, respectively).

In the course of further follow-up, the relative vascular bed density remained constant in the tissues surrounding both APTOS filaments and smooth polypropylene threads.

## 4. Conclusions

To summarize the results of comparative histological study of the soft tissues surrounding implanted filaments, the following conclusions can be drawn:

- Collagen biosynthesis begins earlier and ends later after the implantation of APTOS filaments than after the implantation of smooth polypropylene threads; moreover, it is more extensive and involves a greater tissue volume in the former case.
- Fibrous capsule around the filament shaft and barbs gives rise to connective tissue bands that extend towards epidermis and subcutaneous fatty layer and merge with connective tissue fibres of these tissues.
- Tissues surrounding APTOS filaments contain much more microvessels than tissues enclosing smooth threads where the microcirculatory system extends but insignificantly.
- Microvessels formed after the implantation of APTOS filaments have an open lumen. This feature referred to as «phenomenon of persistent hyperemia» can be seen at any time after the implantation, unlike the case of smooth polypropylene threads when hyperemia occurs only in the early postimplantation period.
- Barbs of APTOS filaments are enclosed in their own connective tissue capsule having significantly thicker walls than the capsule around the shaft of the filament. This greatly contributes to solid fixation of APTOS filaments in the surrounding tissues.
- A capsule around the barbs is less mature than around the shaft of the filament. This suggests a stronger stimulatory effect of the barbs on the surrounding tissues which in

turn accounts for prolonged collagen biosynthesis and thus promotes fixation of both the filaments and the lifted tissues.

- Tissues surrounding APTOS filaments contain mast cells, the number of which remains virtually constant throughout the postimplantation period. These cells contribute to vasodilation in the microcirculatory system and transportation of hyaluronic acid to the tissues around the filaments. The number of mast cells in the tissues surrounding smooth polypropylene threads is signiicantly smaller.
- Implantation of APTOS filaments induces no phagocytic reaction.
- The relative microvascular bed area increases by 26% after the implantation of APTOS filaments leading to a marked improvement of local tissue oxygenaion and blood supply. Implantation of smooth polypropylene threads causes a much smaller increase of relative vascular bed density.

## Author details

A.A. Adamyan, M.A. Sulamanidze, N.D. Skuba and Z.R. Khusnutdinova
*Clinic of Anaplastic and Aesthetic Surgery Total Charm, Moscow, Russia - Tbilisi, Georgia*

## 5. References

[1] Adamyan A.A., Skuba N.D., Sulamanidze M.A., Khusnutdinova Z.R. "Morphological substantiation of facial skin lifting with APTOS threads" International Congress on Plastic, Reconstructive and Aesthetic Surgery, Abstracts of Papers, Moscow., 2002, p. 9 – 10.

[2] Avtandilov G.G., Fundamentals of pathoanatomical practice, Moscow, «RMAPO», 1998, 505 p.

[3] Bykov V.L., Cell biology and general histology, St. Petersburg, - "Sotis", 1998, 364 p.

[4] Sulamanidze M.A., M.D., Fournier P.F., M.D., Paikidze T.G., M.D., Sulamanidze G.M., M.D. Removal of Facial Soft Tissue Ptosis With Special Threads. DERMATOLOGIC SURGERY, Vol. 28 No. 5, May 2002.

[5] Sulamanidze M., Paikidze T., Sulamanidze G., Utilisation du fil "APTOS" dans le lifting facial. La revue de chirurgie esthetique de langue Francaise. T. XXV, N103, May 2001, Pp. 17-22.

[6] Sulamanidze M., Paikidze T., Sulamanidze G., Lifting facial con hilos APTOS. International Journal of Cosmetic Medicine & Surgery. Volumen 3 Numero 3. Diciembre 2001, Pp. 139-142.

[7] Fournier F.P., Reflexions sur les fils tuteurs APTOS de Sulamanidze. La revue de chirurgie esthetique de langue Francaise. T. XXV, N104, septembre 2001, Pp. 23-27.

[8] Fournier F.P., Fils et fillings. La revue de chirurgie esthetique de langue Francaise. T. XXV, N105, decembre 2001, Pp. 3-6.

Section 3

# Barbed Threads Sutured One Side

# 11

# Minimally Invasive Face and Neck Lift Using Silhouette Coned Sutures

Peter Prendergast

## 1. Introduction

Over the last decade, the number of patients opting for minimally invasive procedures has increased [1]. In the US, noninvasive cosmetic procedures have increased by more than 350% since 1997, compared to about 70% for cosmetic surgical procedures. Although open facelift is still indicated for patients who have moderate or severe ptosis of the lower face and neck, younger patients with mild ptosis and patients who do not want to undergo open surgery or general anaesthesia are often suitable candidates for suture of thread lift techniques. Patients favour minimally invasive procedures because they are quick, relatively inexpensive, and do not require prolonged recovery time. Additionally, less invasive procedures typically produce less dramatic results compared to excisional surgery, so the result is subtle and natural looking (Fig.1). Although the story of barbed sutures probably began with Alcamo's design of a roughened suture in 1956, the concept of lifting the face or neck through minimal incisions or punctures using sutures or threads is relatively new. Buncke, a microsurgeon, referred to "facelifts and other cosmetic operations where the sutures would provide lines of tissue support beneath the skin" [2]. Following this, various sutures using different materials, morphologies, and designs were developed by surgeons in USA, Russia, Bulgaria, and elsewhere. Isse, an American surgeon, initially embraced the idea of using barbed sutures to lift soft tissues. He developed the Isse Endo Progressive Facelift Suture, a barbed suture similar to the sutures developed in Moscow by Sulamanidze, and Singapore by Wu. He later abandoned this design in favour of a novel approach—using cones instead of barbs to spear subcutaneous tissues. Isse designed these so-called Silhouette sutures for a number of reasons. He felt that the morphology of the cones or 'trumpets' along the suture would have superior holding power compared to barbs. He also believed that using cones made of an absorbable material (poly lactide) would incite an inflammatory reaction that would in turn stimulate neocollagenesis around the cones and potentially provide a longer lasting effect. Silhouette sutures are now FDA approved and distributed worldwide. The author utilizes these sutures for minimally invasive lifting of the brow, midface, and neck. The procedure is performed in an office setting under local anaesthesia without sedation. This chapter details the Silhouette suture morphology, important anatomy, indications, technique, and potential complications.

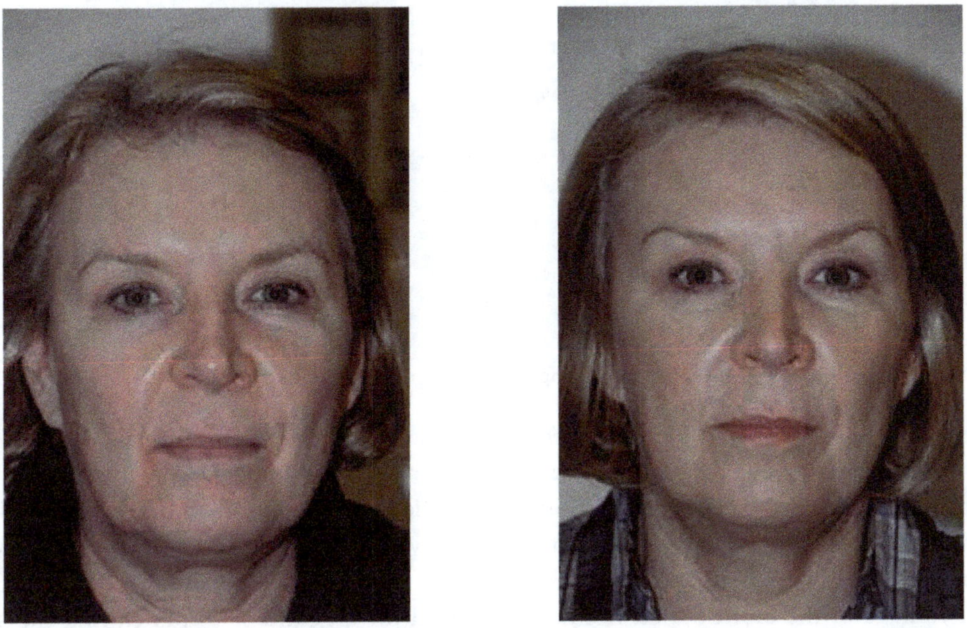

(a) (b)

**Figure 1.** a Before, b After Silhouette suture lift. With kind permission from Springer Science+Business Media: Aesthetic Medicine. Art and Techniques, Suture lifting techniques, 2011, p.413, P.M. Prendergast, fig. 34.15.

## 2. Silhouette suture morphology

The Silhouette suture consists of a dyed polypropylene suture with six regularly spaced transparent cones or trumpets along its length. There is a 20.3cm 20 gauge straight blunt-tipped needle swaged to the distal end of the suture and a 26mm half-circle needle to the proximal end. The cones are made of absorbable poly-L-lactic acid and are held on the suture by six regularly spaced knots (Fig. 2).

As the sutures are inserted the cones slide proximally and cover the knots. When the proximal end of the suture is retracted, the cones slide distally as they purchase on the tissues, and are held on the sutures by the more distally placed knots. Included with Silhouette sutures are 2 x 0.5cm polypropylene mesh patches for anchorage to deep fascia. The biomechanics of the cone morphology provides excellent lifting and holding ability and less propensity to "cheesewire" through friable or soft fatty tissues compared to barbed sutures [3]. The knotted suture means there has been no compromise to the structure of the main body of the suture, unlike barbed sutures where linear shredding can occur when

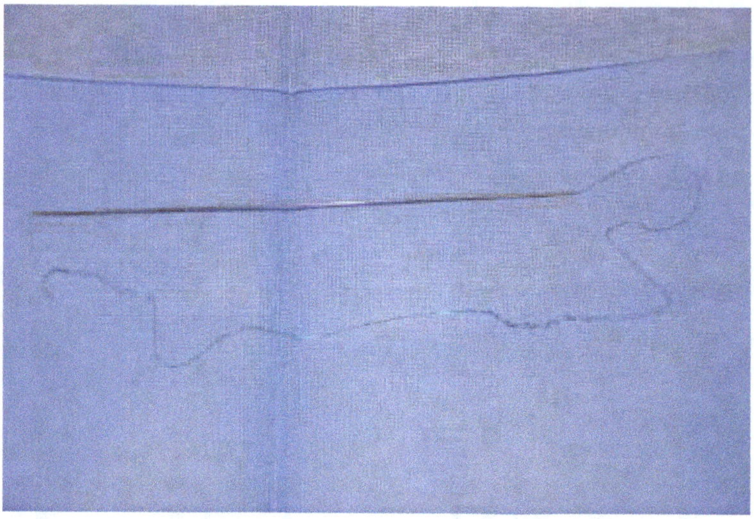

**Figure 2.** The Silhouette suture with blunt-tipped straight needle for placement

tensions are applied to the barbs. Coned sutures are somewhat bulkier than barbed ones, leading occasionally to irregularities or visibility in patients who have a thin soft tissue envelope. This softens out quickly without intervention. Although the original sharp straight needle is available for suture passage, a blunt one was recently introduced, presumably to reduce the chance of nerve or vascular injury during deployment of sutures. The disadvantage of the blunt-tipped needle is the need for an extra step: puncturing the skin with a needle prior to exiting the skin. Also, more force is required to pass the blunt needle through fibrous tissues such as the lateral neck area and temporal area. Haematoma is rare using either a sharp or blunt tipped needle provided the needle is passed through the correct plane, particularly when lidocaine with epinephrine is used for infiltrative anaesthesia.

## 3. Clinically oriented anatomy

A thorough knowledge of facial anatomy is essential for any surgeon who performs suture or thread lift techniques. The thread lift techniques described in this chapter require small incisions, and the passage of blunt-tipped needles blindly through the subcutaneous fatty and fibrofatty tissues of the face and neck. Care must be taken to avoid inadvertent injury to important structures, including vessels, sensory nerves, and motor nerves. Understanding the anatomy of the soft tissue planes is also important for Silhouette suture lift techniques since different planes are traversed with the sutures, and anchorage to deep fascia in the temporal area or neck is required to secure the lift and prevent slippage.

In the temple behind the hairline, the temporalis muscle is covered with a tough, shiny white, adherent deep temporal fascia (DTF). An anchor patch can easily be sutured to this fascia through a small (3cm) temporal incision. Loosely attached to the DTF lies the superficial temporal fascia (STF). This thin layer is continuous with the superficial musculoaponeurotic system (SMAS) in the face beyond the hairline and the galea aponeurotica medially over the forehead. At the hairline, the STF splits into two separate leaves that envelop branches of the temporal branch of the facial nerve. Close to the zygomatic arch, the DTF splits to envelop an intermediate fat pad and facial nerve branches.

The facial nerve emerges from the stylomastoid foramen 6-8mm medial to the tympanomastoid suture of the skull. The posterior auricular nerve and nerves to the posterior belly of digastric and stylohyoid branch from the main trunk before the facial nerve enters the substance of the parotid gland. Within the parotid gland, the facial nerve divides into its main branches: temporal branch, zygomatic branch, buccal branch, marginal mandibular branch, and cervical branch (Fig. 3). The temporal branch exists as 3-4 rami as it exits the superior part of the parotid gland and courses superficially over the zygomatic arch. From the zygomatic arch to the point where the nerve fascicles enter the orbicularis oculi above the brow, these nerve branches are susceptible to injury. Invariably, the temporal branch fibres cross the zygomatic arch between 0.8cm and 3.5cm anterior to the bony external acoustic meatus. They travel enveloped in two leaves of the superficial temporal fascia and enter fibres of frontalis and orbicularis oculi about 2cm superior to the brow. A danger zone exists in the plane of the superficial temporal fascia from the zygomatic arch to the temporal area where the temporal nerve branches are susceptible to injury by suture-passing needles [4].

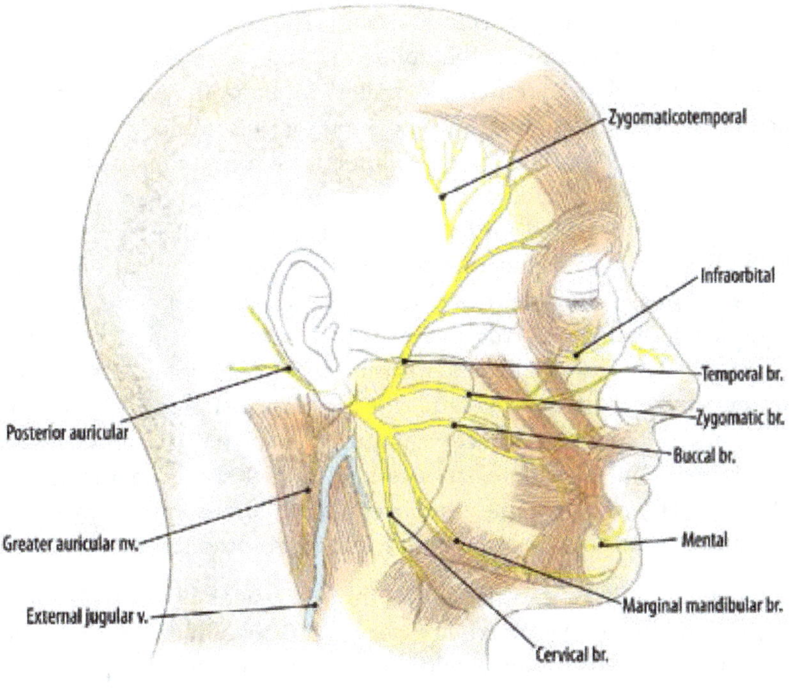


**Figure 3.** The five branches of the facial nerve: temporal, zygomatic, buccal, marginal mandibular, and cervical. With kind permission from Springer Science+Business Media: Advanced Surgical Facial Rejuvenation, Facial anatomy, 2012, p.11, P.M. Prendergast, fig. 1.11.

There may be up to three zygomatic branches of the facial nerve. One usually passes above the eye to innervate fibres of frontalis and orbicularis oculi. The lower branch passes under the origin of zygomaticus major and supplies this muscle, lip elevators, and the lower orbicularis oculi. Smaller branches also supply depressor supercilii and the superomedial orbicularis oculi. The buccal branch of the facial nerve is closely adherent to masseter within the parotidomasseteric fascia. It travels anteriorly over the buccal fat, below and parallel to the parotid duct. This nerve innervates the buccinators and muscles of the upper lip and nose. Injury to the buccal branches of the facial nerve during a Silhouette thread lift is unlikely since the needles pass in a more superficial plane to retract the superficial soft tissues and fat compartments.

The marginal mandibular nerve exits the inferior aspect of the parotid and travels anteriorly above the mandibular border, although it may drop to up to 4cm below the mandibular border. About 2cm posterior to the corner of the mouth, the nerve courses upward over the mandibular border, just deep to the wafer-thin platysma muscle. At this point, it is prone to injury during liposuction or surgical techniques in this area. Silhouette suture exit points are situated superiorly for midface lifting, although passage of the needles in the neck close to the mandible could theoretically injure this nerve.

Silhouette suture face lifting employs small absorbable cones to retract soft tissues of the midface. These soft tissues are essentially superficial fat compartments, separated from one another by condensations of connective tissue. The superficial fat compartments, as described by Rohrich [5] comprise the following: the nasolabial fat compartment, the medial, middle, and lateral temporal-cheek "malar" fat pads, the central, middle, and lateral temporal-cheek pads in the forehead, and the superior, inferior, and lateral orbital fat pads (Fig. 4). During midface elevation using Silhouette sutures, the nasolabial, medial, and middle cheek fat pads are retracted and elevated, compressing them somewhat against the inferior orbital and lateral orbital fat compartments. The result is volume restoration and softening of the nasolabial fold and tear trough deformity. Irregularities can occur where cones tether the ligaments that occur between these fat compartments. This is particularly true of the zygmoatic ligament, a true ligament that arises from the zygomatic periosteum and inserts into the dermis near the lateral canthus. As described later, cones should be excised from the suture to prevent irregularities in this area. False retaining ligaments are more diffuse condensations of connective tissue that connect superficial and deep facial fasciae [6]. The cones on Silhouette sutures also retract these ligaments, increasing the stability of the lift. The mild waviness or irregularity that occurs immediately following suture lifts is transient and softens out within a few days without intervention.

The sensory innervation of the face is via the three divisions of the trigeminal nerve (fifth cranial nerve) ophthalmic nerve, maxillary nerve, and mandibular nerve. The ophthalmic nerve supplies the forehead, upper eyelid, and dorsum of the nose via the supraorbital, supratrochlear, infratrochlear, lacrimal, and external nasal nerves. The maxillary nerve supplies the lower eyelid, cheek, upper lip, ala of the nose, and part of the temple, through the infraorbital, zygomaticofacial, and zygomaticotemporal nerves. The mandibular nerve has motor and sensory fibres. Its branches include the inferior alveolar nerve, lingual nerve, buccal nerve, and auriculotemporal nerve. These supply the skin over the mandible, lower cheek, part of the temple and ear, the lower teeth, gingival mucosa, and the lower lip (Fig. 5). The greater auricular nerve, derived from the anterior primary rami of the second and third cervical nerves, supplies the skin over the angle of the mandible.

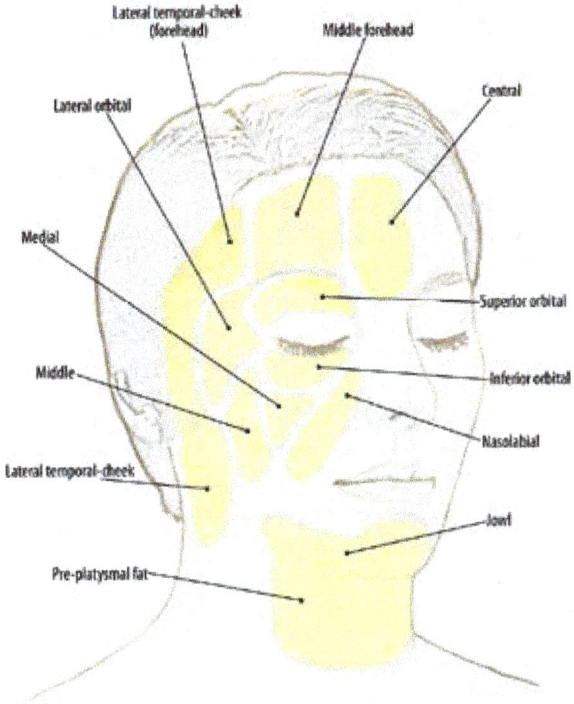


**Figure 4.** The superficial fat compartments of the face

Silhouette suture lifts are performed under local anaesthesia: infiltrative, regional, or a combination of both. Infiltrative anaesthesia provides a "hydrotomy" or fluid plane through which suture needles can easily pass. Infiltrative anaesthesia also provides local vasoconstriction, via epinephrine, and potentially reduces bruising and the risk of haematoma. Newer blunt-tipped needles are designed to reduce the likelihood of vascular (and neural) injury. Regional nerve blocks anaesthetize large areas of the face and cause less localised tissue distortion than infiltrative anaesthesia. Tissue filling and distortion with anaesthetic solution can make it difficult to assess the soft tissues intraoperatively and the degree of retraction required for a satisfactory lift. Regional blocks of the main nerves providing sensation to the temples and midface are described here.

The zygomaticotemporal nerve emerges from its foramen on the deep surface of the zygomatic bone and supplies the anterior temple. It is blocked by injecting 1-2ml anaesthetic behind the junction of the lateral orbital rim and the upper border of the zygomatic arch. The zygomaticofacial nerve arises from its foramen below and lateral to the inferolateral border of the orbital rim and supplies the soft tissues and skin over the malar eminence. To block this nerve, anaesthetic is injected over the periosteum at the site of the zygomaticofacial foramen.

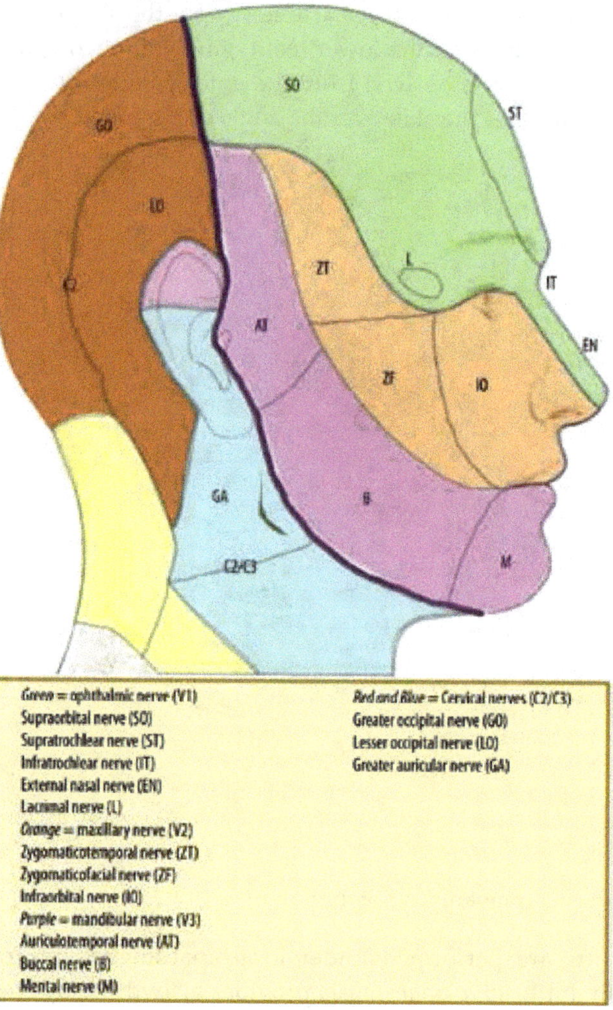


**Figure 5.** Sensory innervation of the face and neck. *With kind permission from Springer Science+Business Media: Advanced Surgical Facial Rejuvenation, Facial anatomy, 2012, p.12, P.M. Prendergast, fig. 1.12.*

The infraorbital nerve is the largest branch of the maxillary nerve. It enters the face through the infraorbital foramen 2.7-3 cm from the midline in men and 2.4-2.7 cm from the midline in women, about 7 and 6 mm inferior to the inferior orbital rim in men and women respectively. It supplies the lower eyelid, ala of the nose, medial cheek, nasolabial fold, and upper lip. To block the infraorbital nerve, about 2 ml anaesthetic solution is injected over the foramen. To reach the foramen, a transdermal or intraoral approach is used.

With proper placement of blunt-tipped Silhouette needles in the correct plane, bleeding is uncommon. Infiltrating small volumes of anaesthetic with epinephrine along the proposed suture paths provides a bloodless field and further reduces ecchymosis. It is important for the surgeon who performs suture lifting techniques to have a knowledge of the vascular supply to the face. The arterial supply is outlined here.

The skin and soft tissue of the face receive their arterial supply from branches of the facial, maxillary, and superficial temporal arteries—all branches of the external carotid artery. The ophthalmic arteries, arising from the internal carotid system, supply a masklike area including the central forehead, eyelids, and upper part of the nose (Fig. 6).

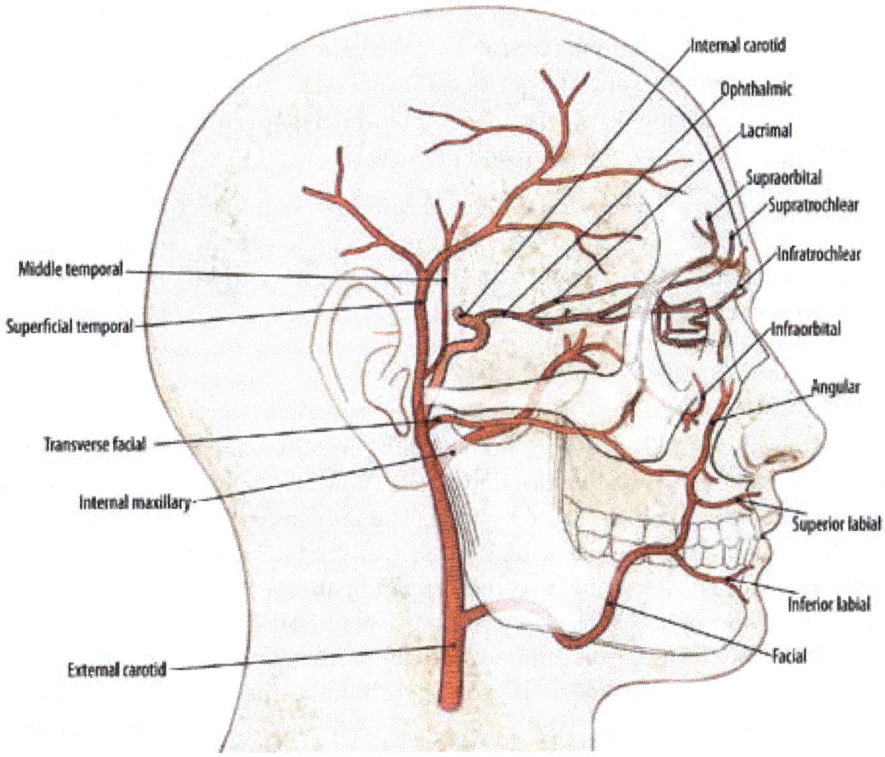


**Figure 6.** The arterial supply of the face. With kind permission from Springer Science+Business Media: Advanced Surgical Facial Rejuvenation, Facial anatomy, 2012, p.13, P.M. Prendergast, fig. 1.13.

The facial artery arises from the external carotid and loops around the inferior and anterior borders of the mandible, just anterior to masseter. It pierces the masseteric fascia and ascends upwards and medially toward the eye. It lies deep to the zygomatici and risorius muscles but superficial to buccinator and levator anguli oris [7]. At the level of the mouth the facial artery sends two labial arteries, inferior and superior, into the lips where they pass below orbicularis oris. The continuation of the facial artery near the medial canthus beside the nose is the angular artery.

The maxillary artery is a terminal branch of the external carotid with three main branches, mental, buccal, and infraorbital arteries. The mental artery is the terminal branch of the inferior alveolar artery that passes through the mental foramen to supply the chin and lower lip. The buccal artery crosses the buccinators to supply the cheek tissue. The infraorbital artery reaches the face through the infraorbital foramen and supplies the lower eyelid, cheek, and lateral nose. It anastomoses with branches of the transverse facial, ophthalmic, buccal, and facial arteries.

The superficial temporal artery is the terminal branch of the external carotid artery. In the substance of the parotid, just before reaching the zygomatic arch, it gives off the transverse facial artery which runs inferior and parallel to the arch and supplies the parotid, parotid duct, masseter, and skin of the lateral canthus. The superficial temporal artery crosses the zygomatic arch superficially within the superficial temporal fascia. Above the arch, it gives off a middle temporal artery that pierces the deep temporal fascia and supplies the temporalis muscle. Thereafter, about 2cm above the zygomatic arch, the superficial temporal artery divides into anterior and posterior branches. The anterior branch supplies the forehead and forms anastomoses with the supraorbital and supratrochlear vessels. The posterior part supplies the parietal scalp and periosteum.

The ophthalmic artery is a branch of the internal carotid system (Fig. 6). Its branches include the lacrimal, supraorbital, supratrochlear, infratrochlear, and external nasal arteries. There is significant communication between the external and internal carotid artery systems around the eye through several anastomoses.

## 4. Indications

Patients who may benefit from the Silhouette lift procedure include those with mild to moderate heaviness or ptosis of the face and neck. Typically, patients are 35 to 45 years old with normal or slightly excessive facial volume. The fat compartments in the midface have fallen slightly, accentuating the nasolabial crease. As the fat falls away from the lid-cheek junction, the tear trough deformity becomes apparent under the eyes. The anterior cheek flattens and the shape of the face changes from a youthful heart-shape to a more aging rectangular-shape. By elevating the midface fat compartments using the Silhouette sutures, all of these aging features can be improved. Repositioning the midface in a vector that is mostly superior improves the shape of the face, softens the nasolabial crease, and ameliorates the lid-cheek junction. It is important to remember that a Silhouette lift is not an excisional procedure, but one that merely repositions ptotic soft tissue. As such, if there is marked laxity of skin, a Silhouette lift is not indicated. Similarly, if the patient's face is very thin, Silhouette sutures are not appropriate. Where there is a very thin soft tissue envelope, lifting the fat with Silhouette sutures will simply bunch up the skin and create irregularities over the cones.

A Silhouette suture lift improves mild ptosis of the neck and helps restore an optimum mentocervical angle, which should be 80-95º. For more pronounced signs, including excessive laxity, heavy platysmal bands, and submental fat, other procedures may be more appropriate, including excisional surgery, platysmaplasty, liposuction, or chemodenervation.

Before any suture or thread lift procedure, the patient's expectations should be assessed. If the patient expects dramatic results, or a powerful lifting effect that could only be achieved through open surgery, the procedure should not be performed unless the patient can readjust their expectations. Suture lifting techniques do not replace open excisional surgery. The author explains to patients that suture lifts usually provide more lifting that external tissue tightening devices, but do not replace invasive surgery. They reposition tissue, but do not remove them. Once a patient has realistic expectations and appreciates that the aim is a natural-looking enhancement rather than a dramatic transformation, the likelihood of a successful outcome is high. Additionally, it should be explained to the patient that no intervention provides permanent results. Suture lifts can be repeated over time if necessary. The Silhouette sutures described here may be retightened during a secondary procedure.

## 5. Step-by-step technique

The author administers 1mg lorazepam and one solpadol (paracetamol 500mg, codeine 30mg) preoperatively for anxiolysis and moderate analgesia. Preoperative photographs should be taken in front, oblique, and side views.

### 5.1. Midface

Markings are made with skin markers with the patient in the sitting position. First, a guide line is marked from the corner of the mouth to the angle of the mandible. Exit points should not be made inferior to this line to prevent disruption of the sutures during facial animation. Next, the proposed exit points are marked. For midface lifting, the standard exit points are as follows: 1 cm lateral to the midpoint of the nasolabial fold, 1.5 cm inferior to the first point, 1.5 cm lateral to the previous point at or just above the guide line, and 1.5 cm lateral to this point (Fig. 7). Depending on the desired lifting vector, the suture paths are estimated using a dashed line from these exit points to a point where the lines converge behind the temporal hairline. A line is marked behind the hairline in the temporal scalp, measuring about 3 cm, where the incision is made.

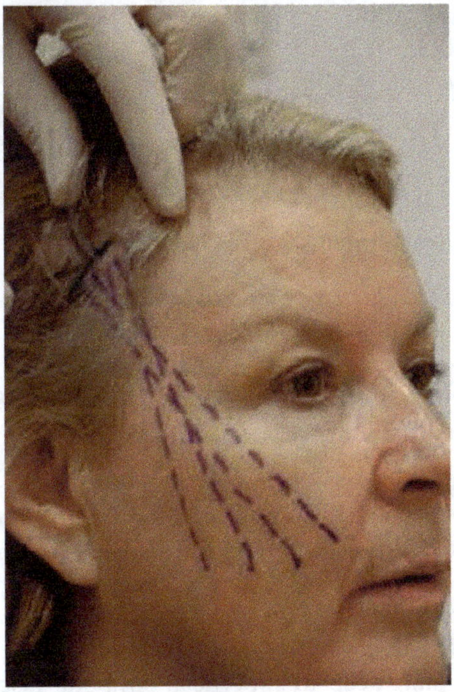

**Figure 7.** Preoperative markings for Silhouette midface lift

The patient is positioned supine for the procedure. Sterile technique is used, with formal skin preparation and surgical draping, exposing the operative field. The instruments and materials required for lifting using Silhouette sutures are shown in figure 8. A solution of 2% xylocaine (lidocaine 2% with epinephrine 1:200,000) and 0.9% sodium chloride is used for infiltrative anaesthesia. Using a combination of 30 gauge and 27 gauge short and long needles, the incision site and proposed suture paths are infiltrated. Adding sodium bicarbonate to the solution reduces discomfort on infiltration. A maximum of 7mg/kg lidocaine (with epinephrine) should not be exceeded to avoid lidocaine toxicity.

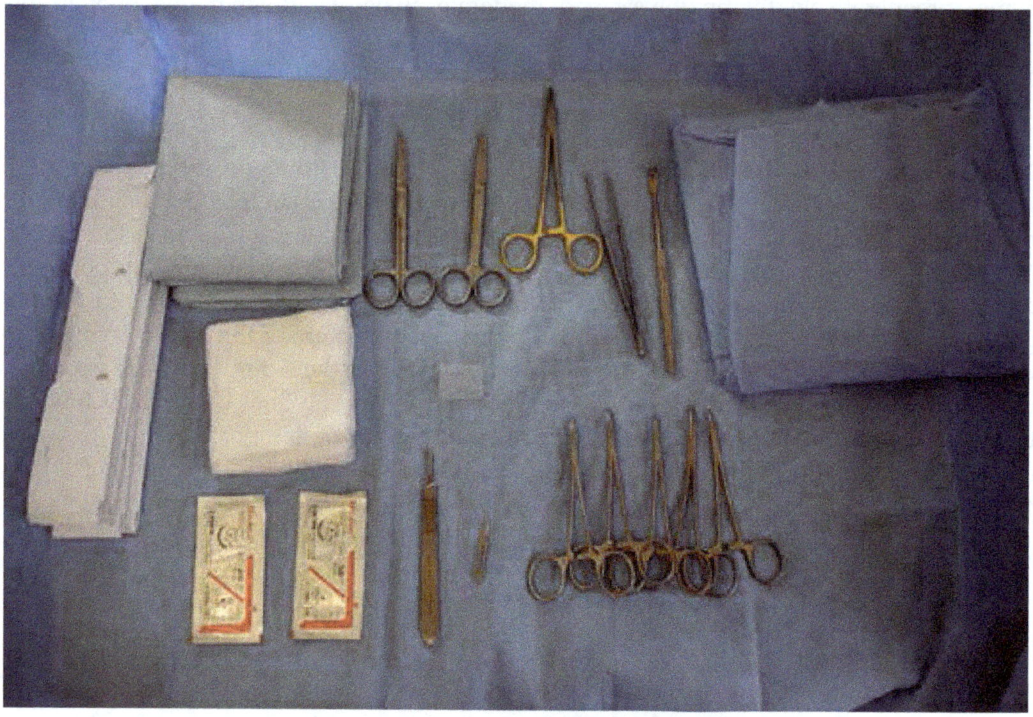

**Figure 8.** Instruments and materials required for Silhouette suture lift procedure

A 3 cm incision is made in the temporal area. Since this area is particularly vascular, diathermy is essential for adequate haemostasis. Once the skin is opened, the subcutaneous fat is gently retracted, exposing the superficial temporal fascia (STF). This thin layer is opened to expose the white, shiny deep temporal fascia (Fig. 9). A space is created by bluntly dissecting over the deep temporal fascia.

A small, 1 cm x 0.5 cm patch of polypropylene mesh (Suramesh) is placed on the deep temporal fascia and secured using a single vicryl suture. In order to delineate the planes before suture placement, sharp dissection above the superficial temporal fascia separates the subcutaneous fatty plane and the superficial temporal fascia (Fig.10). To avoid placing the needles close to the temporal branch of the facial nerve beyond the hairline, the needles are placed in the subcutaneous fat above the superficial temporal fascia. It is best to start in the correct plane, rather than start deep to superficial temporal fascia (STF) and then change course at the hairline to come superficial to the STF blindly.

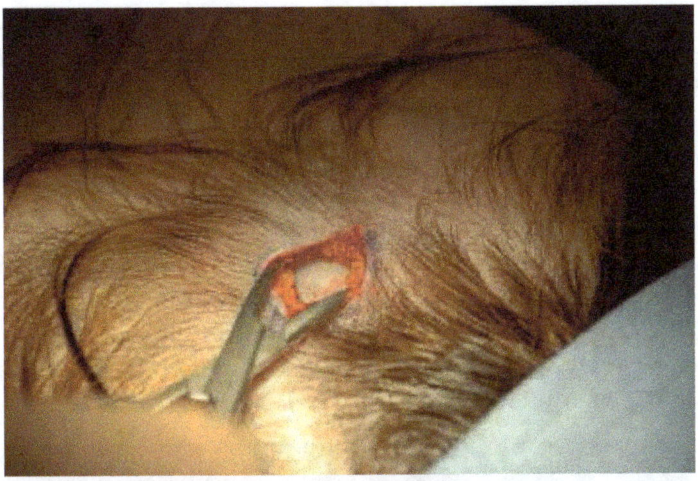

**Figure 9.** Temporal incision with exposed deep temporal fascia.

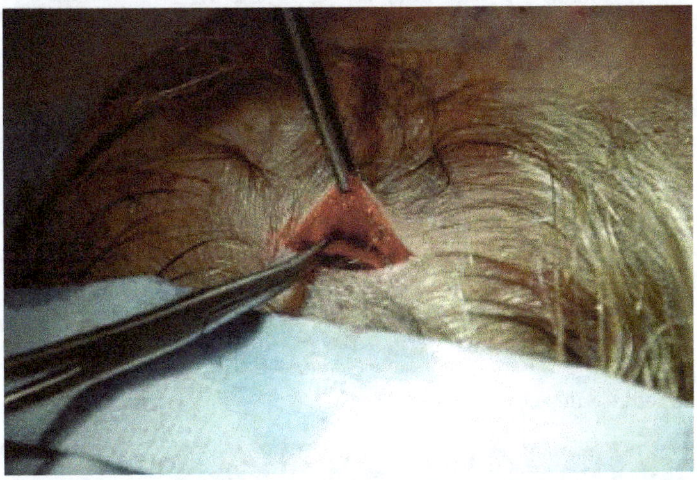

**Figure 10.** Superficial temporal fascia. The suture is placed just above the superficial temporal fascia in the subcutaneous plane.

Before passing the first Silhouette suture, the suture is placed over the face externally to determine how many cones should be left on the suture and how many (if any) should be excised. Once lifted, all cones should be positioned inferior to the zygomatic arch, to avoid tethering the zygomatic ligament, resulting in irregularities that can be difficult to correct. Usually, leaving 3-4 cones on the suture is sufficient, although this depends on the size of the patients face. The first suture is passed through the face by placing the blunt tip of the Silhouette needle subcutaneously, above STF, until the needle tip is ready to emerge through the dermis at the first exit point lateral to the nasolabial fold. The soft tissues should not be squeezed or compressed around the needle during passage to avoid irregularities. The malar fat can be lifted slightly to "present" it to the needle once the needle passes over the zygomatic arch. This maneuver also facilitates the needle to exit through the skin perpendicularly. A 16-gauge needle is used to puncture the skin over the exit point to allow the blunt-tipped needle to emerge (Fig. 11). The needle is pulled through gently. A characteristic clicking of cones is heard as they pass through the soft tissues. Care should be taken not to pull through too many cones; once they exit the skin they cannot be retracted back into the tissues. The predetermined number of cones is excised from the suture, and the suture is cut distal to the knot that lies proximal to the last cone being removed (Fig. 12). The proximal end of the suture is lifted to retract the knot back into the cheek and lift the tissues. The same process is repeated for the other sutures until all four sutures are placed in the fibrofatty malar fat pad. Although four sutures are usually placed for midface lifting, more or fewer sutures can be employed depending on the patient and indications. However, the lateral face region should be avoided since the soft tissue envelope in this region is thinner and the dermis is more adherent to the superficial musculoaponeurotic system.

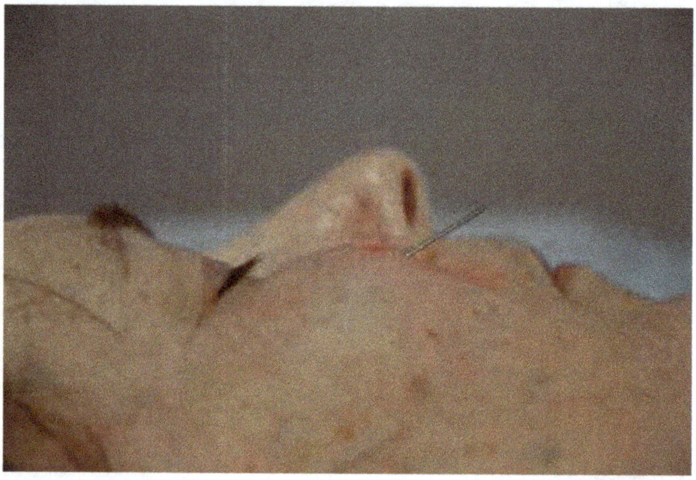

**Figure 11.** Blunt-tipped needle exits perpendicularly

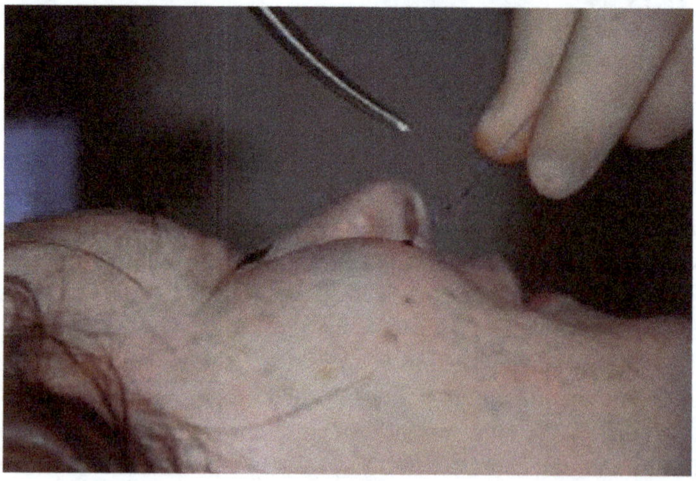

**Figure 12.** The suture is brought through and the predetermined number of cones is excised from the suture

The half-circle needle swaged to the proximal end of the Silhouette suture is passed first through the superficial temporal fascia. Then a bite of the deep temporal fascia is taken, emerging through the polypropylene mesh. Once all of the proximal needles are anchored to the deep temporal fascia and mesh in this way, the sutures are retracted gently to affect a lift on the midface (Fig. 13). The sutures are tied to one another in pairs over the polypropylene mesh. The superficial temporal fascia is closed with vicryl. Skin closure is performed with interrupted skin sutures or skin clips.

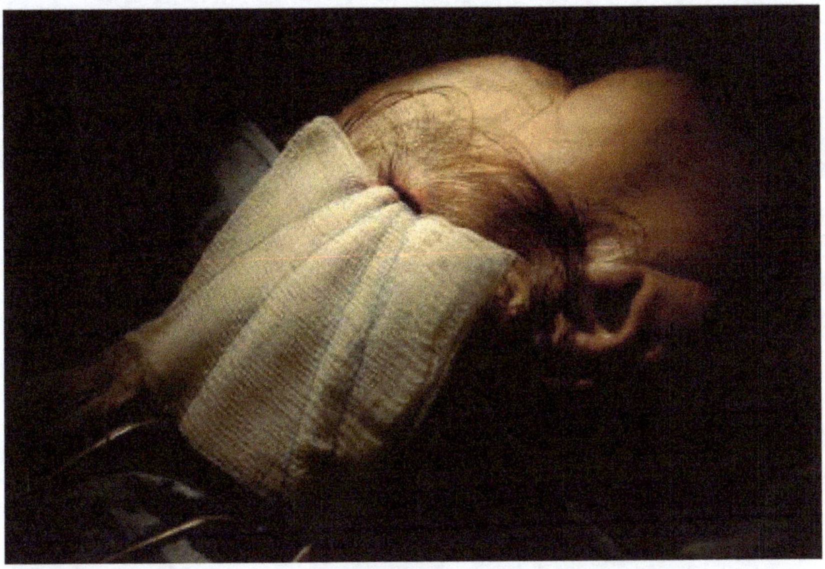

**Figure 13.** Four Silhouette sutures are used on each side to elevate the midface

## 5.2. Neck

Markings are made from an incision site at the hairline below the ear along the neck under the jawline toward the midline. Two exit points are marked on each side, before the midline (Fig. 14). Local anaesthetic is infiltrated subcutaneously along the suture paths. A 2 cm incision is made at the hairline and the cervical fascia is exposed with blunt dissection (Fig. 15). The first Silhouette needle is passed under the dermis toward the midline. Laterally, the dermis is adherent to the underlying fascia over sternocleidomastoid and more resistance is felt in this area using the blunt-tipped needle. More medially, less resistance is encountered as the needle glides through the preplatysmal fat. The dermis is punctured with a 20-gauge needle to allow the Silhouette needle exit. Most or all of the six cones on the Silhouette suture are left in place for neck lifting. In some cases, two cones are excised, leaving four on the suture to lift the tissues. Once both sutures are passed, the proximal ends are anchored by taking a bite of cervical fascia and tying the sutures down over a small pledget of polypropylene mesh. Care should be taken to avoid the mesh curling upward toward the dermis by seating it properly on the fascia. The skin is closed using 4/0 or 5/0 sutures. Moderate, transient bunching occurs laterally following Silhouette suture lifting of the neck.

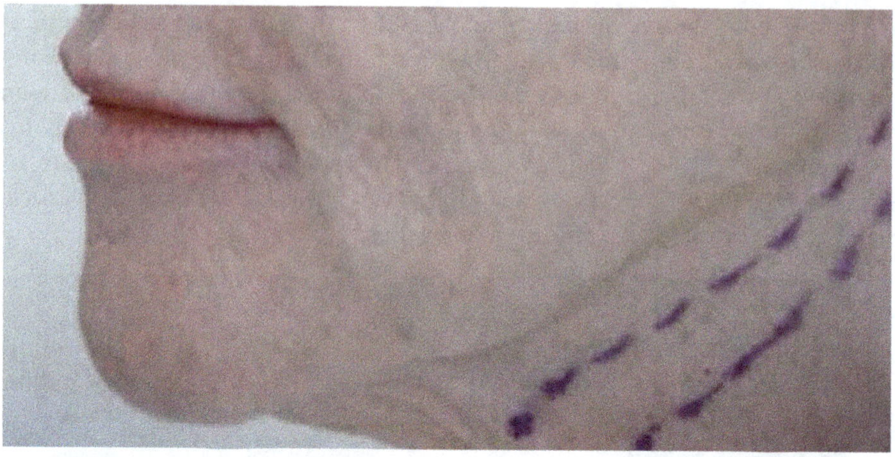

**Figure 14.** Preoperative marking for Silhouette suture neck lift. Two sutures are passed on each side from the hairline to a exit points near the midline.

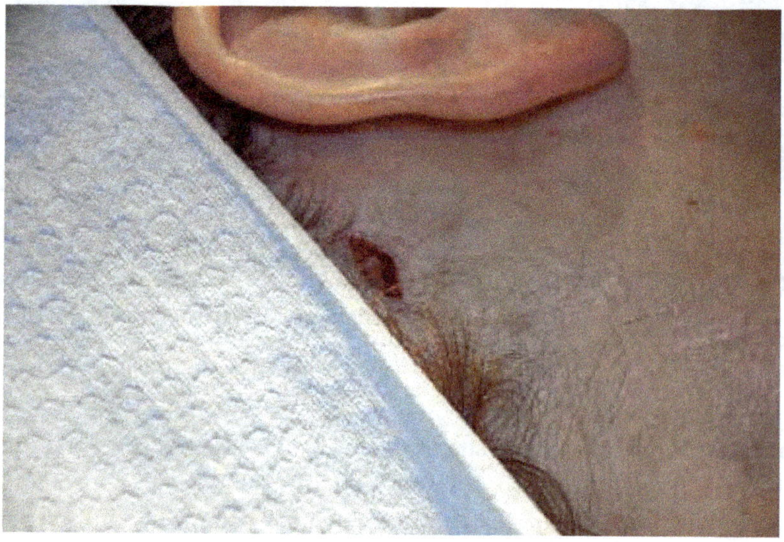

**Figure 15.** Incision for Silhouette suture lift of the neck

## 5.3. Brow

A Silhouette lift of the brow improves aesthetics by elevating the lateral aspect and tail of the eyebrow (Fig. 16). In heavy brows, elevation also reduces dermatochalasis. The author recommends chemodenervation of lateral fibres of orbicularis oculi with botulinum toxin at least two weeks prior to the suture lift to reduce downward movement on the cones.

The patient is carefully assessed to decide the best lifting points in the lateral brow (Fig. 17). The exit points and anchorage point will determine the ultimate lifting effect and shape of the brow.

Local anaesthesia is infiltrated along the suture paths, creating a hydrotomy that somewhat lifts the normally adherent dermis off the underlying frontalis. A 1 cm incision is made in the

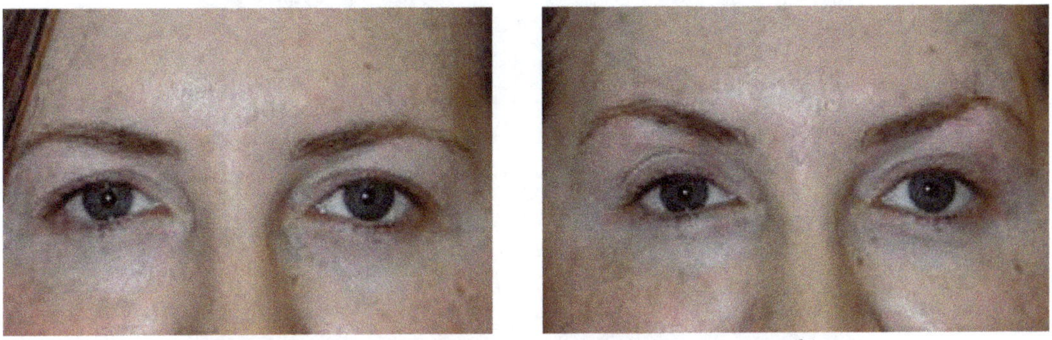

(a) (b)

**Figure 16.** a. Before, b. Immediately after Silhouette brow lift.

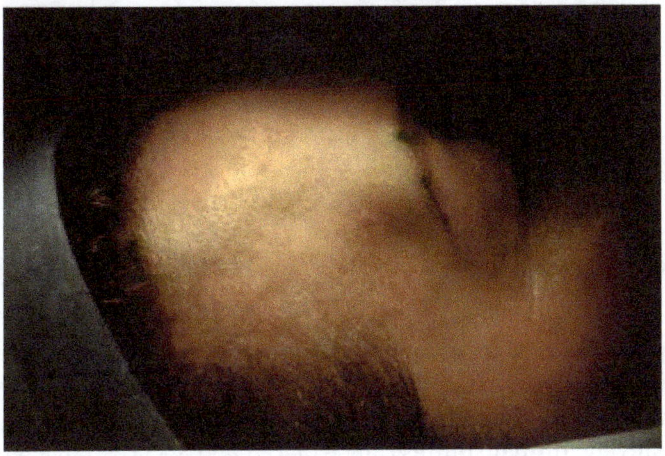

**Figure 17.** Preoperative markings for brow lift using Silhouette sutures. An incision is made at the hairline. There are two exit points at the brow.

skin at the hairline. The first Silhouette suture is passed from the incision to the exit point in the brow (Fig. 18). There is usually no need to excise any cones from the suture, leaving six cones to elevate the tissues above the brow. The second suture is passed in the same way. Each proximal end of the suture is anchored by passing the half circular needle deep to periosteum. The suture ends are tied to one another over a small pledget of polypropylene mesh, which sits on the galea. The pledget and suture ends are buried satisfactorily before the skin is closed.

Mild irregularities or bunching occur immediately following Silhouette brow lifting. This resolves and softens in a number of days.

## 6. Results

The Silhouette suture lift procedure elevates and suspends tissues providing immediate results. These minimally invasive techniques, performed under local anaesthesia, do not replace excisional surgery such as cervicofacial rhytidectomy, but are ideally suited for younger patients or those who do not want more invasive intervention. They can also be performed as a complementary procedure during open surgery.

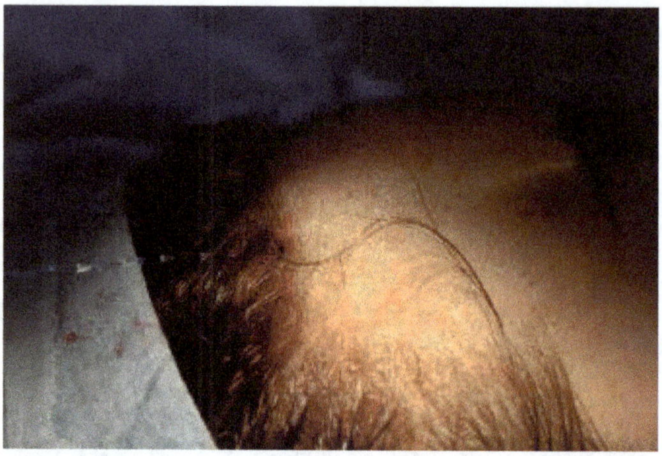

**Figure 18.** The first Silhouette suture is passed from the incision at the hairline to the brow.

Immediately after the procedure, there is usually mild swelling secondary to local anaesthesia, as well as some bunching or irregularities over the sutures. It should be explained to the patient preoperatively that it takes a few days for the tissues to smooth and soften and for the bunching to subside, particularly in the neck. The patient should not rub or massage the face or neck for several weeks. Gentle handling is important to avoid disruption of the sutures, and to allow fibrosis around the cones and knots on the sutures to occur.

After the poly-lactide cones on Silhouette sutures absorb over about 10 months, what remains are the polypropylene sutures, knots, and bundles of fibrous tissues that remain tethered to surrounding tissues. After 1-2 years, Silhouette sutures can be retightened by opening the old incision, re-suspending the proximal suture ends, and tying them down again to restore the desired lift. Alternatively, further sutures can be placed and anchored in a redo procedure.

## 7. Complications

Although complications associated with Silhouette suture lifts are uncommon, they can occur and the patient must be informed of all potential sequelae, side-effects, and risks. Normal after-effects include swelling, mild bunching and irregularities, ecchymosis, discomfort, and transient dysaesthesias. Complications are listed in table 1.

Infection should be treated with antibiotics initially. If there is evidence of infection along the suture, the sutures should be removed. Prophylactic antibiotics and sterile technique serve to minimise the risk of infection.

Whilst a small haematoma may resorb without intervention, if a large haematoma occurs, this may need to be evacuated. The presence of a haematoma also increases the risk of localized infection.

Non-absorbable sutures may extrude through the skin, even years following a suture lift. It is important to bury suture knots or seat the tied sutures or mesh deep where possible so that it is less likely to irritate the dermis. This is particularly important in the forehead with brow lifting and incision at the neck hairline with Silhouette neck lifts.

Persistent irregularities or dimples overlying sutures can usually be corrected with gentle manipulation of the tissues over the suture. If the dermis cannot be released using this maneuver, subcision may be used using a needle.

| | |
|---|---|
| Infection | Facial nerve injury |
| Bleeding | Sensory impairment |
| Haematoma | Chronic pain |
| Suture extrusion | Palpability |

**Table 1.** Complications associated with suture lifting

## 8. Conclusion

The Silhouette suture is a novel device used for minimally invasive face and neck lifting under local anaesthesia without the need for long incisions, tissue undermining, or skin excision. Retraction or suspension of soft tissues is achieved through absorbable cones distributed along the length of the suture. Silhouette sutures are most commonly employed for midface lifting, where the fibrofatty malar fat is elevated and anchored by suturing the proximal ends of the sutures to the deep temporal fascia behind the hairline. The non-absorbable polypropylene sutures allow secondary re-tightening at a later stage. Silhouette sutures are also suitable for lifting and improving ptosis in the neck and in the brows.

## Author details

Peter Prendergast
*Venus Medical, Dublin, Ireland*

## 9. References

[1] The American Society for Aesthetic Plastic Surgery: Cosmetic surgery national database statistics 2011, ASAPS website, http://www.surgery.org (accessed 1 May 2012).

[2] Kress DW. The History of Barbed Suture Suspension: Applications, and Visions for the Future. In: Shiffman MA, Mirrafati SJ, Lam SM (eds.). Simplified Facial Rejuvenation. Berlin Heidelberg: Springer-Verlag; 2008. p247.

[3] Sasaki GH, Komorowska-Timek ED, Bennett DC, Gabriel A. An Objective Comparison of Holding, Slippage, and Pull-out Tensions for Eight Suspension Sutures in the Malar Fat Pads of Fresh-Frozen Human Cadavers. Aesthetic Surgery Journal 2008; 28(4) 387-96.

[4] Prendergast PM. Danger Zones in Surgical Facial Rejuvenation. In: Shiffman MA, Erian A (eds.). Advanced Surgical Facial Rejuvenation. Berlin Heidelberg: Springer-Verlag 2012. p24.

[5] Rohrich RJ, Pessa JE. The Fat Compartments of the Face: Anatomy and Clinical Implications for Cosmetic Surgery. Plastic and Reconstructive Surgery 2007; 119(7): 2219-27.

[6] Jones BM, Grover R. Anatomical Considerations. In: Jones BM, Grover R (eds.). Facial Rejuvenation Surgery. Philadelphia 2008. p18-22.

[7] Berkovitz BKB, Moxham BJ. Head and Neck Anatomy. A Clinical Reference. Philadelphia: Taylor and Francis; 2002. p118.

# Combined Techniques - Sutures and Barbed Threads

# 12

# T3 - Soft Face Lift by Suspension Surgery

Pier Antonio Bacci

## 1. Introduction

Surgical strategy using barbed or not barbed threads is now an asserted truth with numerous and official follow-up and experiences. These strategies are named as "mini invasive aesthetic metholodologies" because provide for good results with little incisions and few complications

Today there are many different mini-invasive surgical techniques available, using different kinds of surgical suspension threads. All of these are due to four main authors: Guilleman, Sulamanidze, Serdev and Ruff.

## 2. The Guilleman technique

This is the basic technique known and published under the name of *"Curl Lift"* and is certainly the mother of all the other methods used.

It is the simplest and most intelligent method to lift the relaxed tissues with simple and everyday used surgical threads, absorbable or not. **(Fig. 1)**

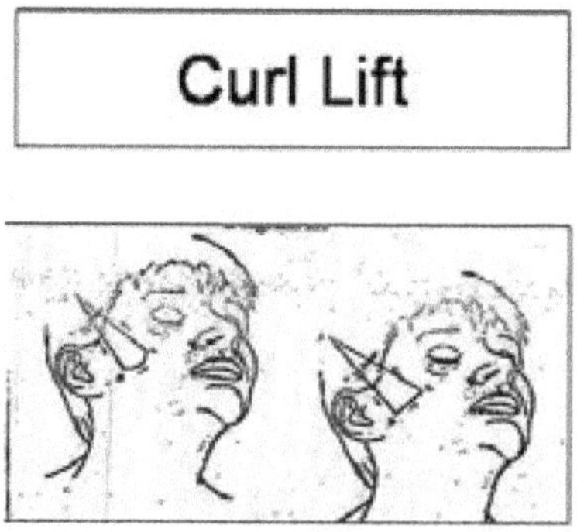


**Figure 1.** The initial idea of the Curl Lift

## 3. The Sulamanidze technique

This method uses a particular surgical thread with barbs, like opposing ears of wheat, thanks to which the threads support themselves in the tissue.

The criticism that can be made about this technique is the fact that the calibre of the needle-cannula used to introduce the thread into the tissue is greater than the thread itself, which can cause some difficulties in hooking the barbs and easy bruising. Finally, this method may be sometime as no long-lasting as the others. It can be very useful in some mini-invasive corrections of the face, such as of the eyebrows or neck. **(Fig. 2)**

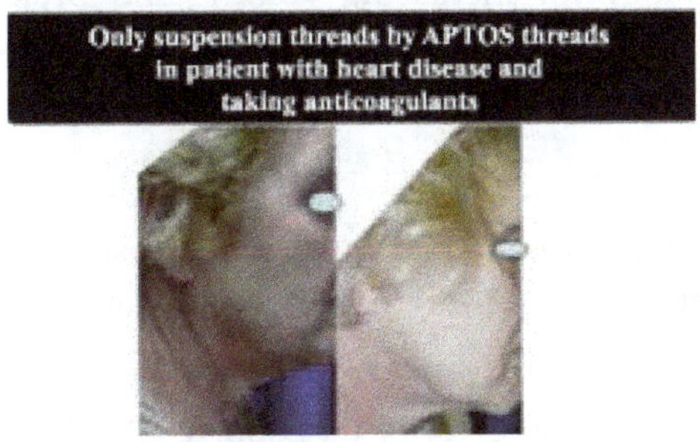


**Figure 2.** Mini invasive treatment of the neck with original Russian APTOS threads in a subject with heart disease taking Acenocumarol (*Bacci archive*)

## 4. The Serdev technique

Starting from French surgeons Galland and Clavier, the Bulgarian cosmetic surgeon Nikolay Serdev uses special semi-elastic threads with long-term absorption, along with special needles of his direct invention and preparation that are used to fix the tissues to solid or fixed structures.

In our experience this method has had almost always good results in various aesthetic pathologies, especially for outlining ill-defined cheekbones and the chin line, thanks to the possibility of creating tobacco-pouch sutures that allow us to define the outlines. **(Fig. 3-4)**

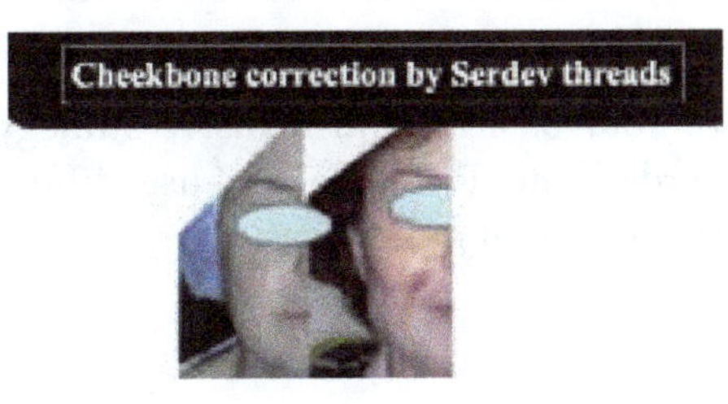


**Figure 3.** Definition of the cheekbones with Serdev threads (*Bacci archive*)

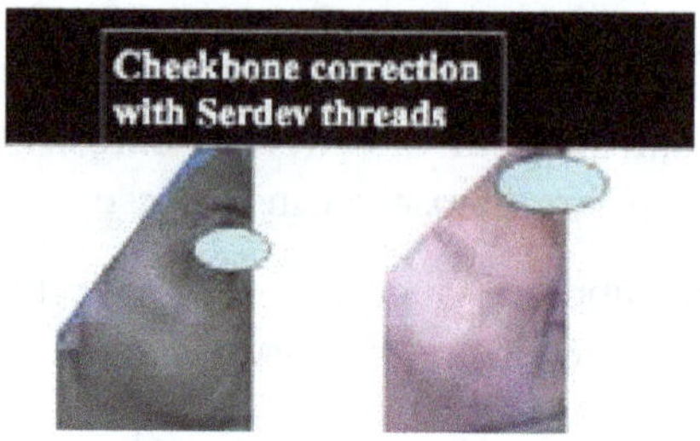


**Figure 4.** Definition of the cheekbones with Serdev threads (*Bacci archive*)

This is the ideal methodology for increasing volume and projecting the tissues without prostheses, for cheekbones, chin, breasts or buttocks, of course, in selected cases.

## 5. The Ruff method

This strategy has certainly represented a new era in cosmetic surgery as it is the first methodology officially approved by the FDA for rejuvenation of the face and neck using unidirectional barbed threads.

It is an effective mini-invasive strategy offer us good results. It uses barbed not-adsorbable one-directional threads introduced by special needles and a method that offers the concrete possibility of creating a true anchor point for the thread, thus becoming similar to a track upon which the skin slides and is anchored, thanks to the unidirectional barbs that are arranged in a spiral shape, guaranteeing its strong hold on the tissues. **(Fig. 5)**

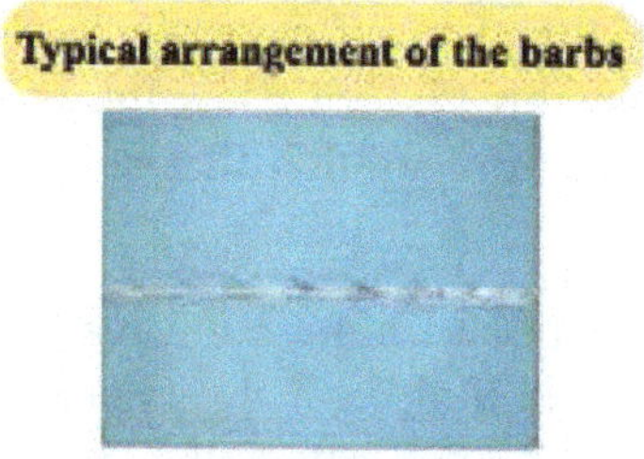


**Figure 5.** Typical spiral arrangement of the unidirectional barbs. (*Bacci Archive*)

Typical characteristic of these barbed surgical threads is the possibility to lift-up all part of the tissue, particurarly midface, neck and eyebrown, or the cutaneous layer that the adipose –muscular deep wraps.

To conclude, we have today four basical mini invasive strategy by threads, according to Guilleman, Sulamanidze, Serdev and Ruff, we can use different strategies, in integrate methodology too, on respect to different indications.

## 6. T3 - Soft Lift

In 2001 we began our first experiences with the integration of two methods, suspension threads and surgical soft lift.

We started with unidirectional, barbed absorbable surgical threads we made by hand in the operating room using a simple method with a monofilament. Our experience then developed particularly while observing their capacity to form a temporary tissue fibrosis along the thread's path in 8-12 weeks' time.

This is how we started the mini-invasive method we call *"T3-Soft Face Lifting"*, meaning *"Traction Threads Treatment"*, or a treatment that uses the traction on surgical threads to lift the tissues, avoiding more extensive dissection, in one or more sessions.

Basically, this strategy consists of two mini-invasive surgical sessions done with local anaesthesia.

- *1st session* - The purpose of this procedure is to introduce the barbed unidirectional "polypropylene" suspension threads using particular carriers that adapt to the various positioning needs of the different suspension threads. **(Fig. 6)**

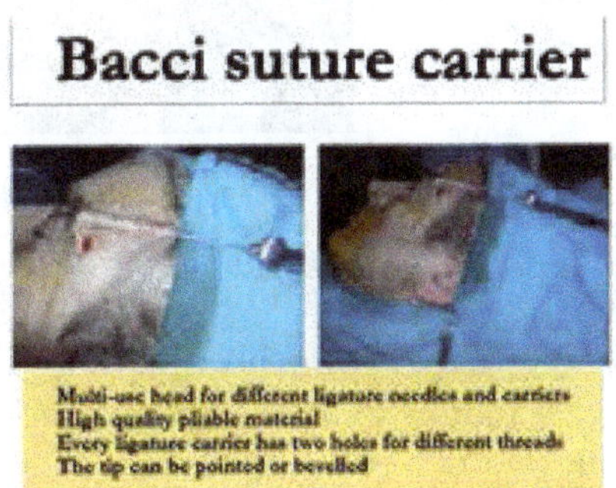


**Figure 6.** Bacci's instrument for introducing threads – (*Bacci Archive*)

Depending on need or the skin to be eliminated, an incision can also be made (as small as possible) along the classical lines in front of or behind the ear, in the frontotemporal area, then the smallest dissection necessary is done to traction the SMAS, doubling it or creating a small flap.

Then a typical vertical mini-lift is done, but using the traction of the threads, therefore avoiding tissue dissection and complications. **(Fig. 7)**

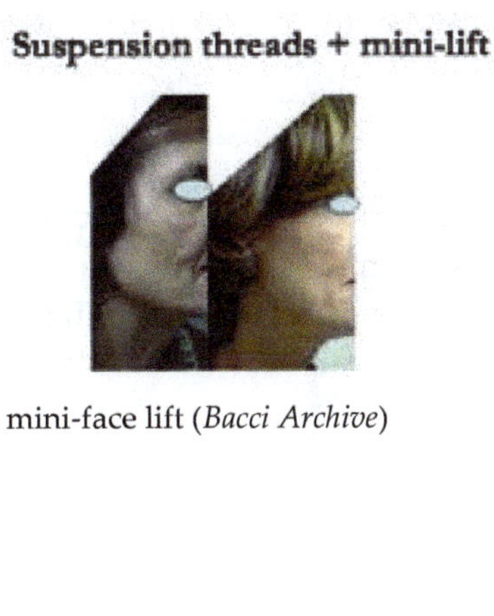


**Figure 7.** Suspension threads and mini-face lift (*Bacci Archive*)

In patients requesting or needing greater traction or greater excision of skin tissue we can also associate a more ample lift, lifting both the temporal region and the midface and neck, thus reconstructing a better triangle of youth, and still limiting dissection thanks to the use of unidirectional barbed threads or of Serdev's circular method. **(Fig. 8)**

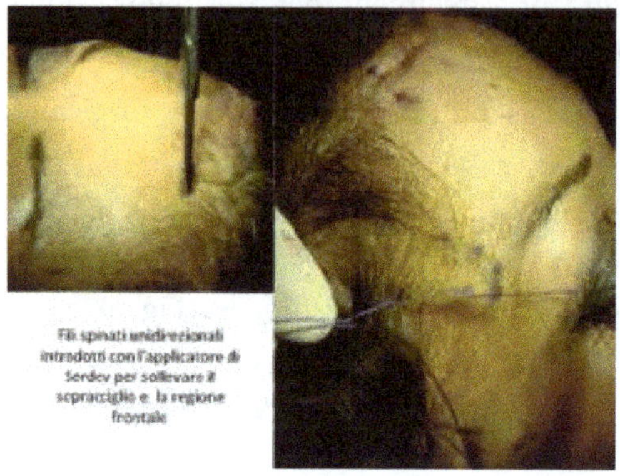

**Figure 8.** Suspension threads and superior blepharoplasty using Serdev Methodology (*Archive Bacci)*

Normally, in this first session lipofilling is associated with the suspension threads, allowing the tissue metabolism to activate thanks to the hormonal impulse given by the autologous fat tissue inserted into the tissue.

The suspension thread and fatty tissue association (*T3-Fat Lift*, or *stabilised lipofilling*) has a particular importance since it favours metabolic recovery of the tissues and vascularization of the cells of the fatty tissue injected, thus prolonging its life and active stay in the tissue.

Sometimes we also perform a superior blepharoplasty in this first session in order to increase eye brightness.

*-2nd session* -_When it is necessary, the second session is as a rule done after 2-3 years, it allows stabilization of the results and offers new traction without dissection. A small incision with local anaesthesia is sufficient to pick up, by Muller's hook for microvarices, the old thread which will be pulled and sutured to the fascia with a 5/0 nylon thread, in a new position.

**Method**

Usually, four or six non-absorbable unidirectional barbed threads are applied for side. They allow traction of the tissues, thus limiting dissection. Then a semi-circular or "S" incision is done, separating the layer as little as possible and locating the threads in place we traction on them and work the SMAS which is duplicated with suture, when it's necessary. **(Figs. 9-10 )**

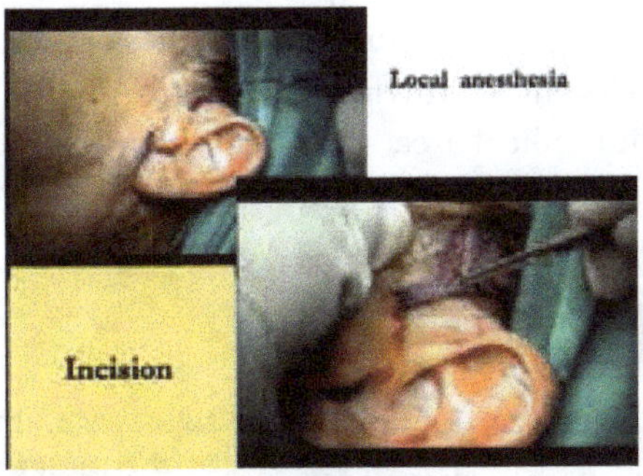


**Figure 9.** After a little local anaesthesia we traction the tissue and SMAS pulling the threads that hook onto the tissue, and then we suture. (*Bacci Archive*)

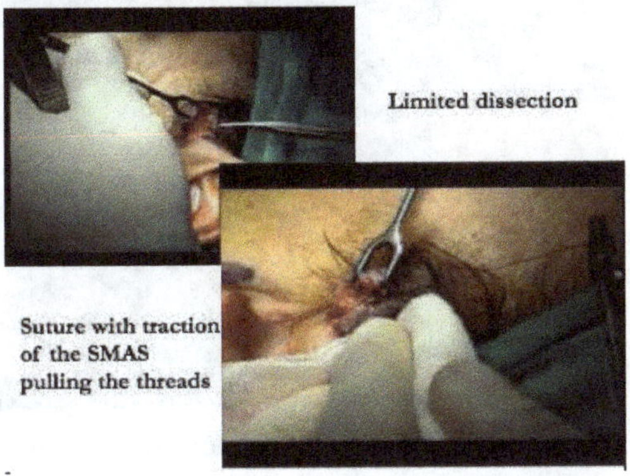


**Figure 10.** After a little local anaesthesia we traction the tissue and SMAS pulling the threads that hook onto the tissue, and then we suture. (*Bacci Archive*)

After this phase the excess skin is cut and then sutured, following the same traction path of the threads if possible and doubling the tissue for better harmony of the neck, within the same amount of operating time. **(Fig. 11)**

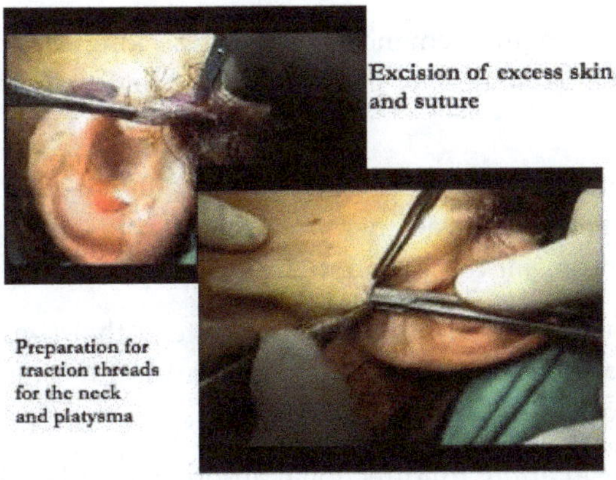


**Figure 11.** Skin excision and traction on the tissues of the neck. (*Bacci Archive*)

We then move on to reshaping the outlines and volumes of the face in the naso-labial, zygomatic areas, of the cheeks and chin with "rice grain" lipofilling, after taking fatty tissue from the abdomen and periumbilical area, where it guarantees greater resistance to possible initial deficits in vascularization. Usually this fatty tissue is reinserted directly without altering it or traumatizing it. **(Fig. 12)**

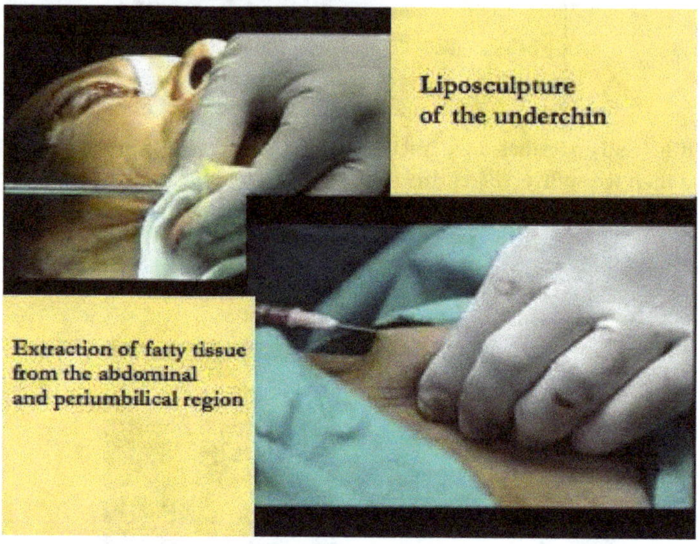


**Figure 12.** Our micro-cannulae for mini-liposculpture and for extracting fatty tissue, which can also be done with a simple needle, even if more traumatic. (*Bacci Archive*)

### Fill - traction

Today, we have more than twenty years of experience with Sulamanidze and Serdev's methods, and we have ten years of experience with unidirectional absorbable or not-absorbable barbed threads, which are used to have a new position of the tissues and to activate processes of bio-stimulation, in particular with surgical threads absorbables by hydrolytic way, such as polydioxanone (PDO). **(Fig.13)**

Currently, thanks to the changing demands of patients seeking rejuvenation of the face even before the age of 40, methodologies are greatly reduced and they are absolutely minimally invasive.

We have reduced the incisions with small lines between the tragus or hidden in the hair or behind the ear. Were reduced detachments of the skin, as results have been virtually eliminated hematoma and major complications. **(Fig.14 - 15)**

The words "Fill-Traction" means a mini-invasive strategy that uses in the same session a Prolene 2/0 not-absorbable unidirectional barbed threads for side, both in the temporal region that in the midface.

In the same session we can apply unidirectional absorbable barbed threads to maintain the position of the skin and improve the contours in the same time.

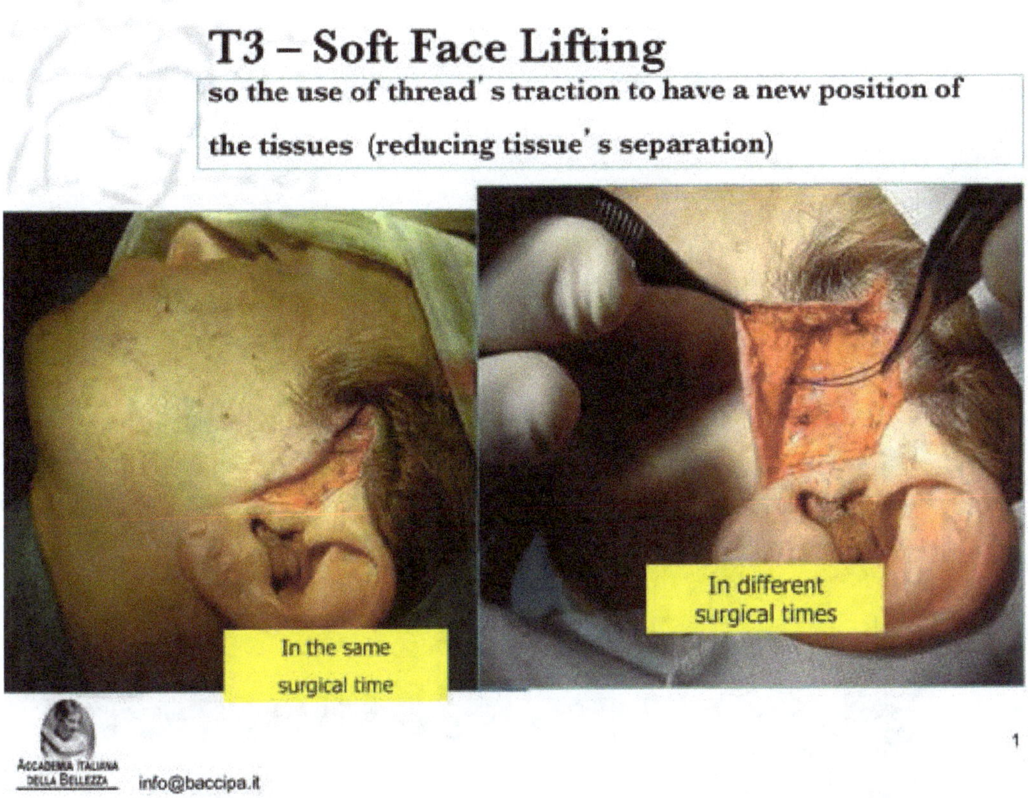


**Figure 13.** T3 –soft face lift (*Bacci Archive*)

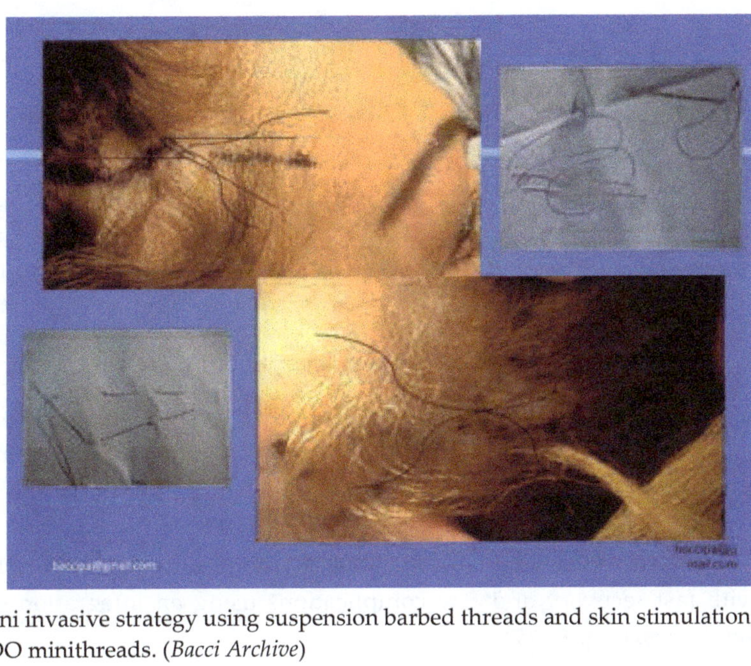

**Figure 14.** Mini invasive strategy using suspension barbed threads and skin stimulation using absorbable PDO minithreads. (*Bacci Archive*)

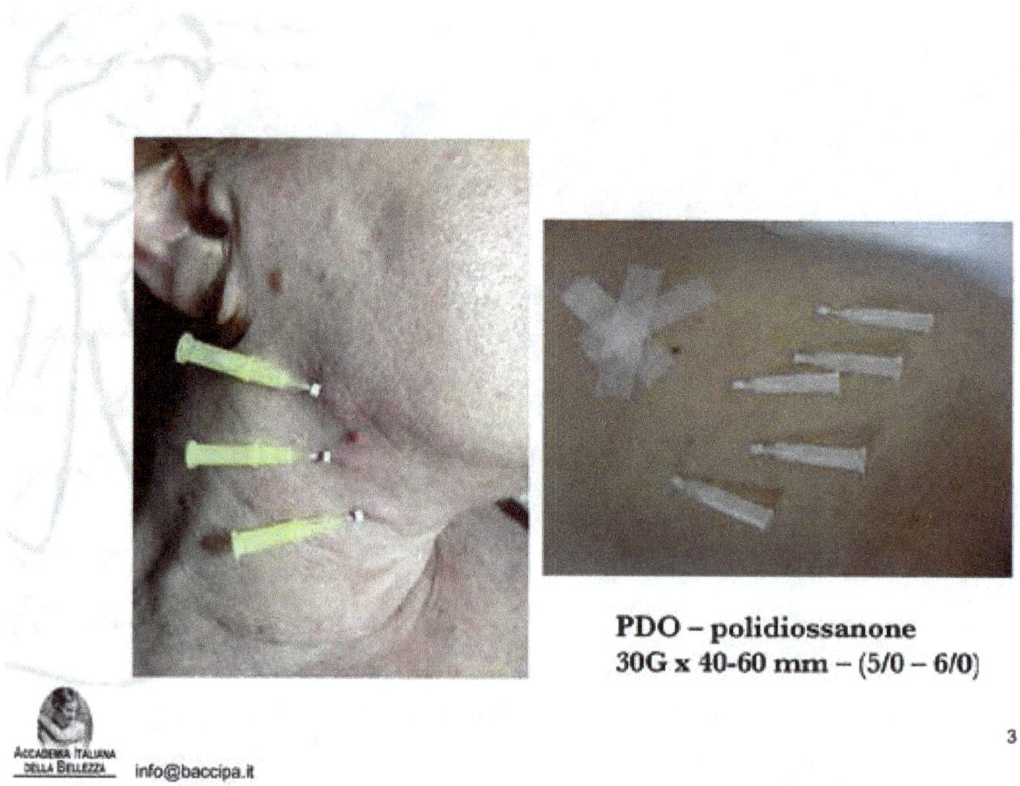


**Figure 15.** Mini invasive strategy using suspension barbed threads and skin stimulation using absorbable PDO minithreads. (*Bacci Archive*)

Also in the same session, we can use botulinum toxin or lipofiling when it is necessary.

Currently, to stimulate the tissues, we use less frequently fillers with hyaluronic acid, in fact today we can also use small threads in PDO - polydioxanone - according to the korean technique that allows us an interesting skin stimulation, in particular in the neck and in midface.

This small absorbable suture may be repeated after 6-8 months, demonstrating that we have good results with fast recovery and few complications using an integration of minimally invasive methodologies. **(Fig. 16-17)**

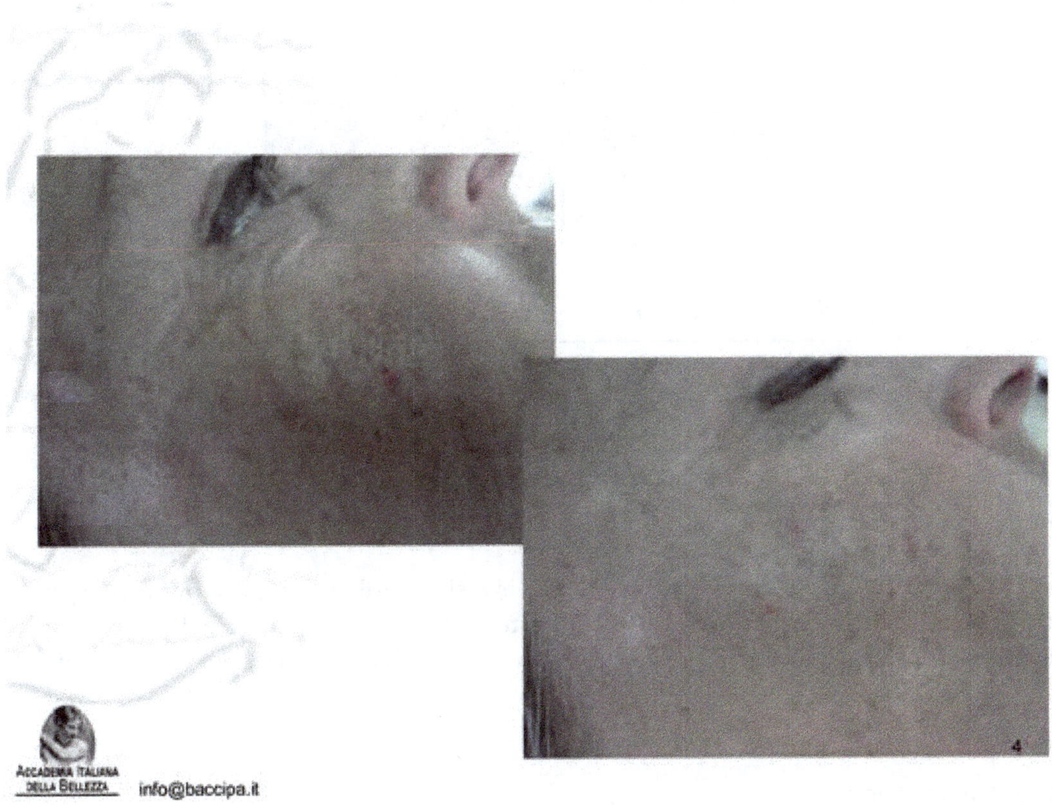


**Figure 16.** Interesting results using Fill-Traction. (*Bacci Archive*)

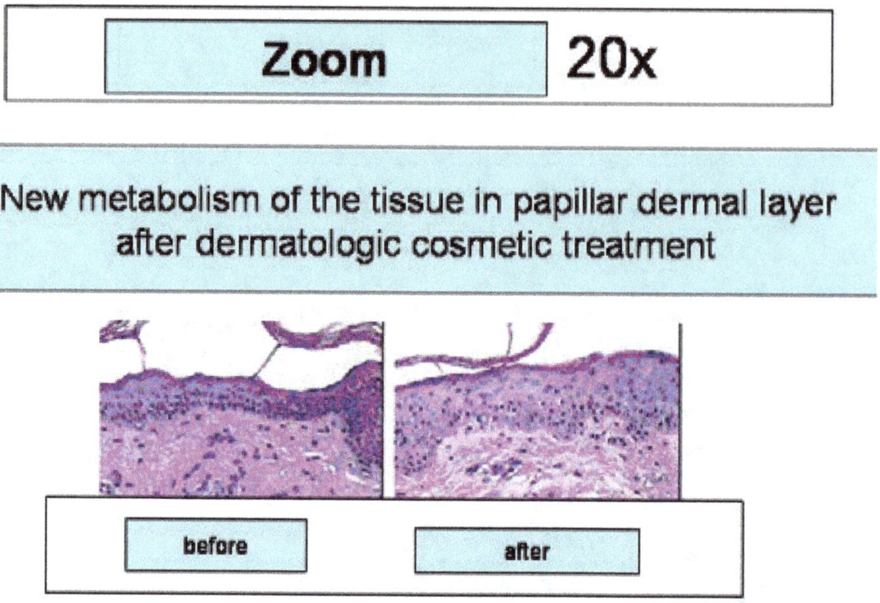


**Figure 17.** Interesting results using Fill-Traction. (*Bacci Archive*)

## 7. Conclusion

Certainly, today suspension surgery, as mini invasive aesthetic surgery by threads, is an official surgical strategy, but the best results are always lie to the precise diagnosis and in the rapport between doctor and patient, without never to have miracles or eternal results.

## Author details

Pier Antonio Bacci
*Mini invasive Aesthetic Surgery Italian Centre, Arezzo, Italy*

## 8. References

[1] Abraham R.F., De Fatta R.J., Williams III E.F.: "Thread-lift for facial rejuvenation. Assessment of long-term results". Arch. Facial Plast. Surg. 11(3):178-183; 2009.
[2] Bacci P.A.: "T3 soft face lifting and bioresurfacing". Paper presented at the Cosmetic Surgery congress, Varna, June 2003
[3] Bacci P.A.: "T3-soft face lifting". Paper presented at the Aesthetic Medicine Congress AGORA, Milan, October 2004
[4] Bacci P.A.: "T3-soft face lifting". Paper presented at the 29th World Congress of Cosmetic and dermatology surgery, Manila, February 2004

[5] Bacci P.A.: "Soft face lifting and reposition threads". Presentazione al 49th World Meeting of the International Academy of Cosmetic Surgery, Lisbona, September 17-18th; 2004.

[6] Bacci P.A.: "T3-Biolifting using absorbable fillers with a few quantity of proteins". Presentazione al World Meeting AACS, Tokyo, 2005, February 24th; 2005.

[7] Bacci P.A.: "T3 Soft Face Lifting using new Threads and fillers". Presentazione al49th World Meeting of World Meeting EMAA, Parigi, September 30th – October 2rd; 2005.

[8] Bacci P.A., Mancini S.: "Chirurgia estetica mini-invasiva: fili di sostegno (Not invasive aesthetic surgery using threads)". Minelli, Arezzo; 45–180; 2006.

[9] Botti G.: "Chirurgia estetica dell'invecchiamento facciale". Piccin Editore, Padova, 521-540; 1995.

[10] Capurro S: "The Double-Tipped Needle". Plast. Reconst. Surg. 79 n°6: 1006-7, 1987

[11] Capurro S. Jr.: "The double tipped needle". Plast. Reconst. Surg., June 1987.

[12] De Lorenzi C.L.: "Barbed sutures: rationale and technique". Aesth. Surg J. 26:223-229; 2006.

[13] Eremia S., Willoughby M.A.: "Novel face-lift suspension suture and inserting instrument: use of large anchors knotted into the suture with attached needle and inserting device allowing for single entry point placement of suspension suture. Preliminary report of 20 cases with 6- to 12-month follow-up". Dermatol. Surg. 32:335–45; 2006.

[14] Fournier P., Flores M.: "Le lifting invisible". Rev. Chir. Esthet. Langue Fr. 27(113):9–20; 2003.

[15] Fournier P.: "Historie de l'aguille a deux pointes". Rev. Chir. Esthet. Langue Fr. 28(115):19–27; 2004.

[16] Goldman M., Bacci P.A., Hexsel D., & Coll.,: "Cellulite: diagnosis and therapy". Taylor & Francis Ed., New York, : 28-74; 2006

[17] Hernandez Perez E., Abbar K.: "A percutaneous approach to eyebrow lift: the Salvadorian option". Dermatol. Surg. 29(8):852–855; 2003.

[18] Hochman M.: " Mid-face barbed suture lift". Facial Plast. Surg. Clin. North Am.15(2):201-207, 2007.

[19] Horne D.F., Kaminer M.S.: "Reduction of face and neck laxity with anchored, barbed polypropylene sutures (Contour Threads). Skin Therapy Lett. 11(1):5-7; 2006.

[20] Hudson D.A., Fernandes D.B.: "Caveats for the use of suspension sutures". Aesth. Plastic Surg. 28:170-173; 2004.

[21] Ingle N.P., King M.W., Leung J.C., Batchelor S.: "Barbed suture anchoring applicability to dissimilar polymeric materials, society for biomaterials". 29th annual meeting transactions, 26:100; 2003.

[22] Kazinnikova O.G., Adamian A.A.: "Age specific changes in facial and cervical tissue: a review". Ann. Plast. Reconstr. Surg.1:52–61; 2000.

[23] Khawaja H.A., Hernandez-Perez E.: "The Delta Lift : a modification of S-Lift for facial rejuvenation". Inter. J. of Cosmetic Surgery and Aesthetic Dermatology, Glendale USA, Mary Ann Liebert Ed., Vol.4, N.4:309-315; 2002.

[24] Lee S., Isse N.: "Barbed polypropylene sutures for mid-face elevation: early results". Arch. Facial Plast. Surg. 7: 55, 2005.

[25] Leung J.C., Ruff G.L., Megaro M.A.: "Barbed bi-directional medical sutures: biomechanical properties and wound closure efficacy study". Society For Biomaterials 28th annual Meeting Transactions 25:724, 2002.

[26] Lycka B., Bazan C., Poletti E., Treen B.: "The emerging technique of the antiptosis subdermal suspension thread". Dermatol. Surg. 30: 41, 2004.

[27] Mc Kenzie A. R.: " An experimental multiple barbed suture for the long flexor tendons of the palm and fingers". J. Bone Joint Surg.49:440-47; 1967.

[28] Rashid R.M., Sartori M., White L.E et Alii: "Breaking strength of barbed polypropylene sutures: rater-blinded, controlled comparison with non-barbed sutures of various calibers". Arch. Dermatol. 143:869–72; 2007.

[29] Serdev N.: "Own method scarless breast lift by suture and needles perforations only". Int. J. Cosmet. Surg. 1(1):1–41; 2001.

[30] Serdev N.: "Scarless Serdev suture methods in brow and face lifts". Int. J. Cosmet. Med. Surg. 3(1):9–15; 2001.

[31] Serdev N.: "Serdev suture for scarless buttock and ultrasonic liposculpture of the buttocks". Int. J. Cosmet. Med. Surg. 5(1):27–34; 2003.

[32] Serdev N.: "Scarless buttock lift using Serdev suture". International Journal of Cosmetic Surgery, Vol.3 N.3: 294-329; 2003.

[33] Serdev N.: "Scarless APTOS versus SERDEV suture lifting methods". Int. Journal of Cosmetic Surgery, vol. 4 – N. 2: 1-10; 2004.

[34] Sulamanidze M. A., Salti G., Mascetti M., Sulamanidze G. M.: "Wire scalpel for surgical correction of soft tissue contour defects by subcutaneous dissection". Dermatol. Surg. 26:146, 2000.

[35] Sulamanidze M. A., Fournier P. F., Paikidze T. G., Sulamanidze G.: "Removal of facial soft tissue ptosis with special threads". Dermatol. Surg. 28: 367, 2000.

[36] Sulamanidze M. A., Shiffman M. A., Paikidze T. G., SulamanidzeG. M., Gavasheli L. G.: "Facial lifting with Aptos threads". Int. J. Cosmet. Surg. Aesth. Dermatol. 4: 275, 2001.

[37] Sulamanidze M.A., Fournier P.F., Paikidze T.G., Sulamanidze G.M.: "Removal of facial soft tissue ptosis with special threads". Dermatol. Surg. 28:367-371; 2002.

[38] Stark G.B., Bannasch H.: "The 'Golden Thread Lift': radiologic findings". Aesth. Plast Surg. 31(2):206-208; 2007.

[39] Helling E.R., Okpaku A., Wang P.T. H., Levine R. A.: "Complications of facial suspension sutures". Aesth. Surg J.27:155–161; 2007.

[40] Lee C. J., Park J.H., You S.H., Hwang J.H. et Alii: " Dysesthesia and fasciculation: unusual complications following face-lift with Cog Thread". Dermatol. Surg. 33:253–255; 2007.

[41] Silva-Siwady J.G., Diaz-Garza C., Ocampo-Candiani J.: "A case of Aptos thread migration and partial expulsion". Dermatol. Surg. 31:356-358; 2005.

[42] Winkler E., Goldan O., Regev E. Mendes D., Orenstein A., Haik J.: "Stensen duct rupture (sialocele) and other complications of the Aptos Thread Technique". Plast. Reconstr. Surg. 118: 1468, 2006.

# 13

# Experience in the Use of Barbed Threads and Non-Barbed Serdev Sutures in Face and Body Lift – Comparison and Combination

Vilma L. Padín

## 1. Introduction

### 1.1. Barbed threads

This technique created by George Sulamanidze uses barbed non sutured monofilament polypropylene threads called APTOS (Polypropylene sutures were modified by designing many dents along their lengths. These "APTOS" threads hold tissue firmly because of the sharp edges to the dents) [1] and allows to relieve facial soft tissue ptosis when it is light or moderate. With this method is possible to lift different areas of the three thirds of the face. This is a simple technique with simple instrumentarium. We use a modification of barbed Aptos threads called Fiberlift® (Firming threads, Multifix threads, and Fiberlift threads). These threads have bidirectional cogs and multidirectional cogs to get the lifting effect of the tissue and a new collagen generation. Barbed polypropylene threads are inserted through the fat tissue with only a long and thin (21 Gx2 or 21 Gx3.5) needle as a guide. These polypropylene barbed threads may be used in face, neck and body lift. This simple and non recovery time procedure, without incisions or scars, achieves to lift and gives new volume and contour with few complications and long lasting results. They get an adequate position of the soft tissue which decreases lymphatic stasis, improves oxygenation, provides energy and stimulates the muscles recovering the normal tissue metabolism and slowing the aging process [2]

### 1.2. Serdev sutures

The use of Serdev sutures in face lift treatments allows us to lift one mobile tissue, the SMAS, and carry it to a non movable point, stable fibrotic and fascia structures, using polycaproamide Serdev sutures and a Serdev special flexible, curved and semi elastic needle. [3] These methods may be done to lift several areas of the face, neck and body. We have experience in temporal face lift, medial face lift, brow lift, chin enhancement and buttock lift with Serdev sutures. These procedures are simple without scars and uncomplicated in the postoperative time and they get aesthetic proportions, aesthetics angles and aesthetic volumes avoiding the "operated look."

Since the year 2000, we have been practicing with the procedures of mini-invasive lifting with Aptos barbed *threads* (George Sulamanidze) and *sutures* (Nikolay Serdev). In the past it was believed that such techniques were only fashionable in the field of cosmetic surgery. After using these methods for 12 years and seeing the positive results in our patients not only within my country but in foreign countries as well, it has come to my attention that "threads" are not something in vogue but are here to stay for good as an important feature in mini-invasive cosmetic surgery. Proof of clinic results, photo images, dermatological examinations and patients' approval after 5 years should establish that lifting with threads and sutures are highly effective; no surgery marks or scars, natural results without undergoing an operation or post operative. It enables the patient to return to work immediately. Through the simple method of "barbed or anchorage threads" the results that are obtained show that reaching beauty may be a simple medical procedure, non invasive, responsible, ethical, in accordance with the physical and spiritual integrity of the patient. The facial softness treatment with the application of both barbed threads or Serdev sutures or their combination allows us to fulfill the requirements that nowadays the patients ask for daily in our clinic.

### 1.3. Materials

1. Polypropylene 2.0 Barbed threads are used with converging cogs called "FIRMING THREADS" (by Fiberlift®)

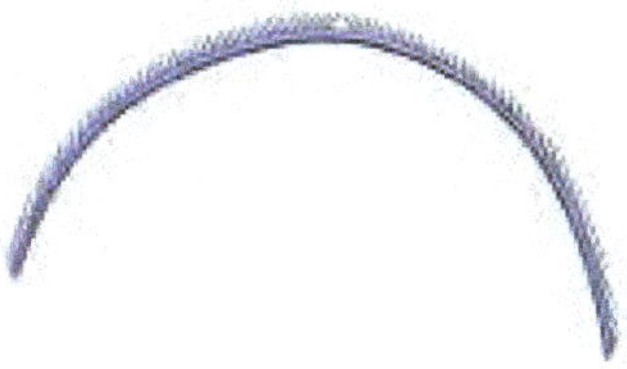

- Monofilament polypropylene 2.0
- Convergent cogs
- 6cm, 8cm, 10cm long
- 4 or 6 units pack

Source: Proesteticamed, 2003

**Figure 1.** Firming thread

2. Polypropylene 2.0 Barbed threads with multi-directional cogs, 2cm right section, and 2 cm left section called "MULTIFIX." (by Fiberlift®)

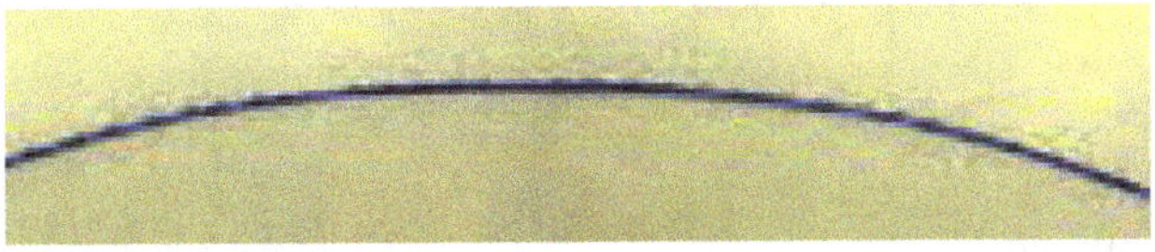

- Monofilament polypropylene 2.0
- Multi-directional cogs
- 12 cm long
- 4 units pack

Source: Proesteticamed, 2006

**Figure 2.** Multifix thread

3. Polypropylene 3.0 with diverging cogs in 2 stages, 3cm each one with one free central piece and 2 long plain ends, called "FIBERLIFT." (by Fiberlift®)

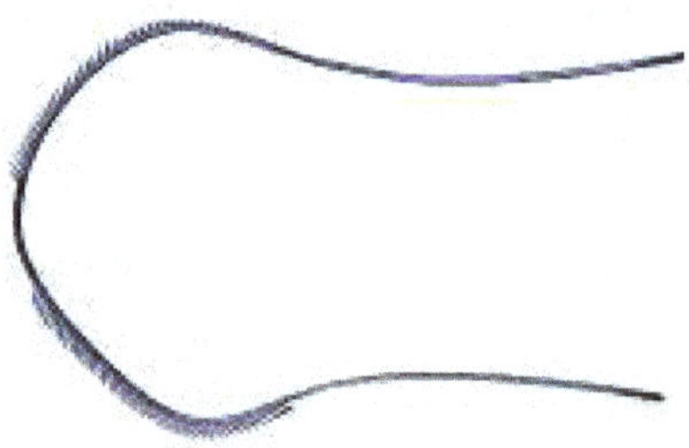

- Monofilament polypropylene 3.0
- Divergent cogs
- Center and ends without cogs
- 30 cm long
- 2 units pack

Source: Proesteticamed, 2004

**Figure 3.** Fiberlift® thread

All these barbed threads are made in Argentina as a modification of Aptos Threads, and they are sterilized abiding by the ISO regulations.

4. Serdev Sutures (Semi elastic, braided, yellow polycaproamide non barbed sutures)

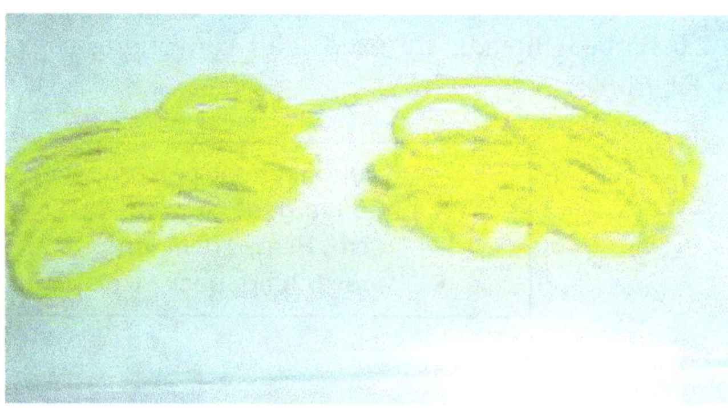

Source: Ambulatory temporal SMAS lift by sutures with or without incisions IJCS 2001; 1(4):97-106

**Figure 4.** Serdev sutures

### 1.4. Surgical instruments

- Halstead claw.
- Iris scissor.
- 21 Gx2 or 21 Gx3 needles.
- Syringe and 30 Gx½ needle for anesthesia.
- Lidocaine 2% with epinephrine.
- Special Serdev flexible needles in different sizes from a large to a mini- mini needle.

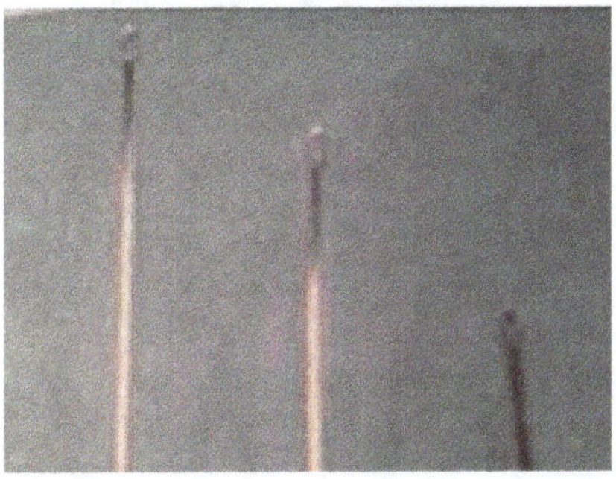

Source: Ambulatory temporal SMAS lift by sutures with or without incisions IJCS 2001; 1(4):97-106

**Figure 5.** Special Serdev elastic needles.

## 2. Procedures

### 2.1. Barbed threads in face and body lift -

#### *2.1.1. Face lift*

##### *2.1.1.1. Lower third and jawline*

The aim of this technique is to lift and improve the contour of the lower third of the face and jawlines. We insert eight polypropylene barbed (4 on each side) FIBERLIFT® FIRMING THREADS between 8 to 10cm long in a simple procedure and without recovery time.[4]

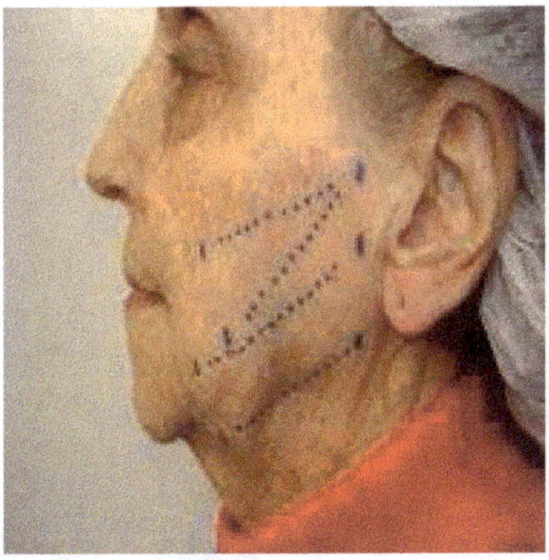

Source: Personal archive

**Figure 6.** Patient's marcation for operation

###### *2.1.1.1.1. Materials*

FIRMING THREADS: Polypropylene 2.0 barbed threads with convergent cogs.

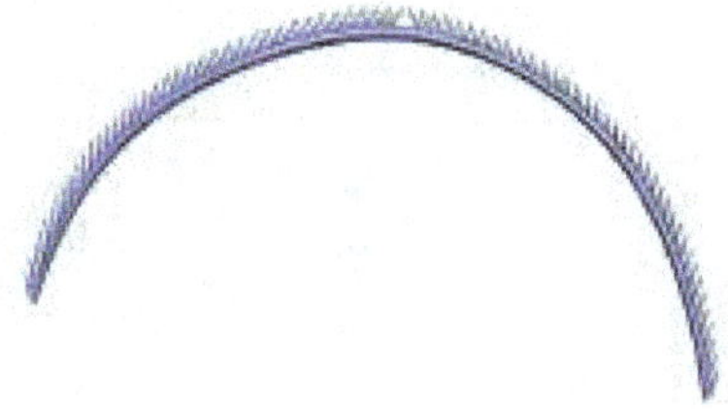

Source: Proesteticamed, 2003

**Figure 7.** Firming thread with convergent cogs

*2.1.1.1.2. Description of technique*

| | |
|---|---|
| Step 1<br>First, we must take frontal and profile photographs. | |
| Step 2<br>Feel along the patient's face with our fingers and mark it. With this, an individual sketch is obtained. | 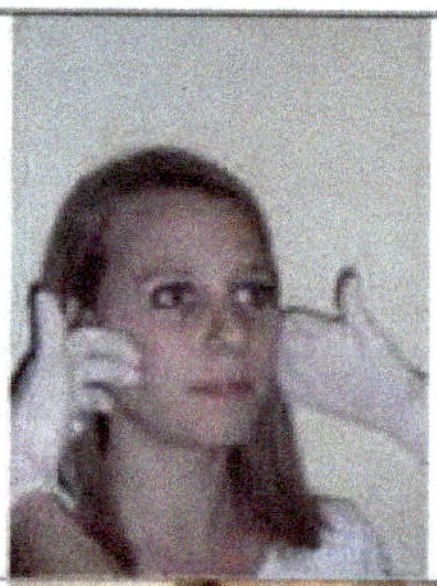 |
| Step 3<br>Mark on the face of the patient the course of the thread drawing the shape of a "Z" on the lower third of the face, in the aim of inserting 2 barbed convergent parallel threads with a third one crossed in the form of an open Z.<br>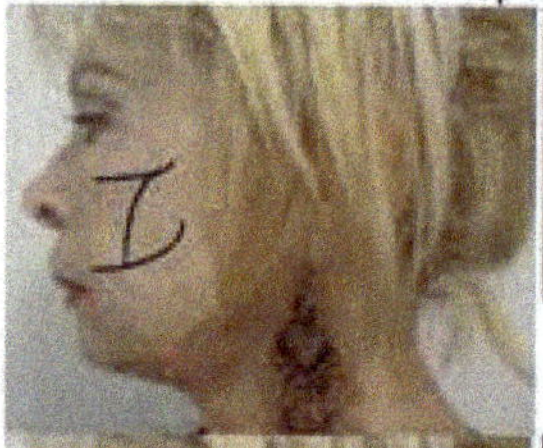 CORRECT "OPEN Z" In this way we avoid deformation of the mouth<br>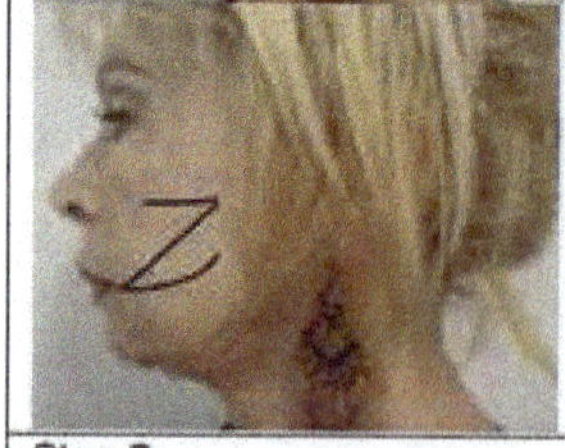 INCORRECT "CLOSED Z" In this way the mouth may be deformed | 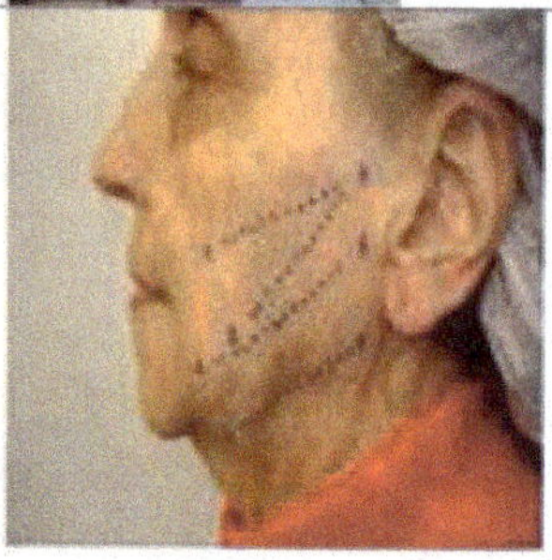 |
| Step 2<br>Paint the face with povidone. | 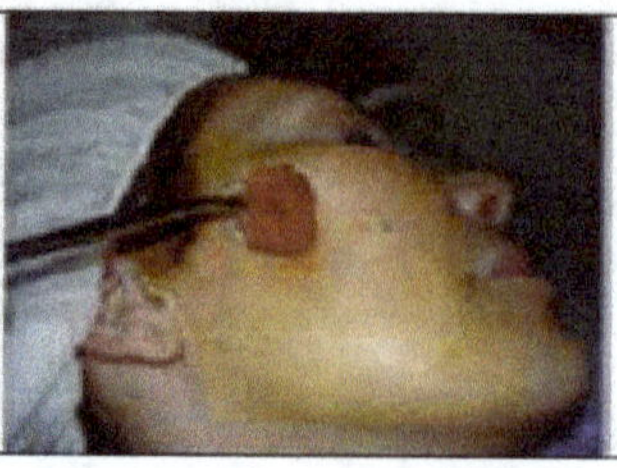 |

| | |
|---|---|
| Step 3<br>Inject the anesthesia only at the entrance and exit points. Use lidocaine 2% with epinephrine 0,5 c.c per point. | 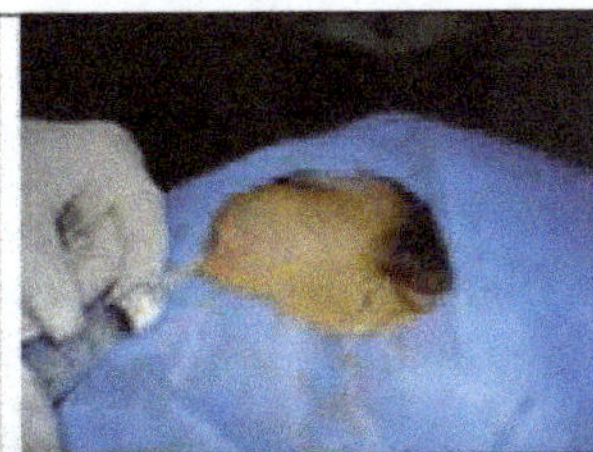 |
| Step 4<br>Tunnel from the external point to the internal one, with a 21 Gx2 needle.<br>Parallel threads must be inserted 1 cm away from the nasolabial fold to preserve the natural form of the face. | 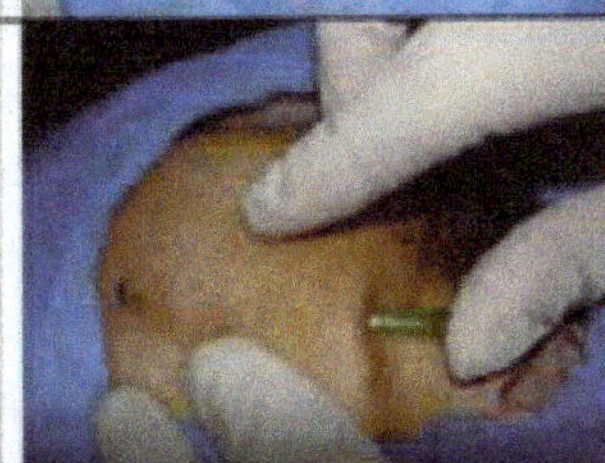 |
| Step 5<br>Thread the barbed polypropylene thread, being careful with the cogs because they are convergent, so it's very easy to thread the first half but it is a little more complicated to pass the second half because the cogs are opposite to the sense of the needle. This situation is very easy to overcome by, with the use of a thicker needle. But using a 21 Gx2 needle we assured that the aesthetic results will be excellent and without scars. | 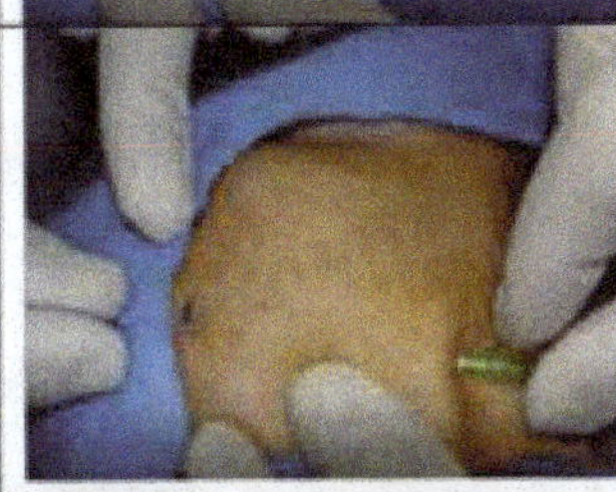 |
| Step 6<br>Check that the thread is firm. | 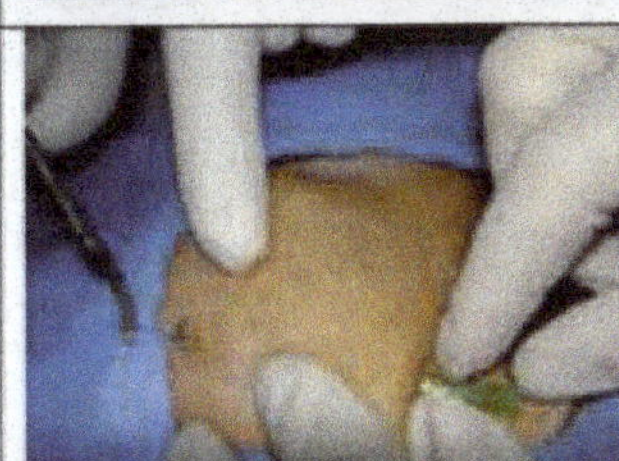 |
| Step 7<br>Remove the needle and the ends of the thread will be found outside the surface of the skin. | 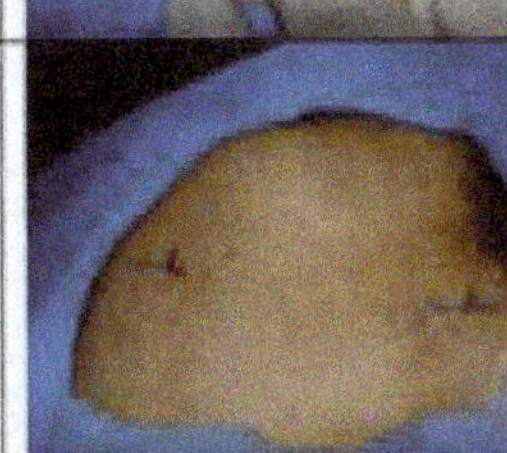 |
| Step 8<br>Cutting the thread. We must be very careful cutting the thread. The skin should be pushed down with the scissors. This simple switching enables us to cut the thread at a good position avoiding it getting long. | 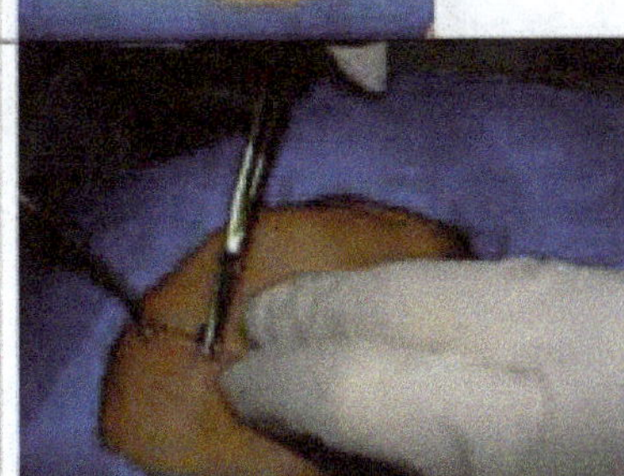 |

Source: own elaboration using pictures of personal archive

**Scheme 1.** Lower Face Lift Technique with Barbed Threads

*2.1.1.1.3. Results*

Barbed threads have two ways of acting. The first is the lifting effect given by the cogs. It is immediate. This effect is poor. The other action is delayed, due to the inflammatory reaction when the thread is placed, producing vas dilatation, increased capillary permeability, inflammatory exude that will be represented by leukocytes, erythrocytes, plasmatic proteins and fibrin which take us to the epitelization; that is: fibroblasts are generating collagen and elastine fibers.

So we can say that the barbed thread face lift has good results that change the angles of the face with an aesthetic expression, giving contour as well as improving the skin. Patients like this technique and ask for more threads. It is long lasting. Experienced doctors can insert more threads several times.

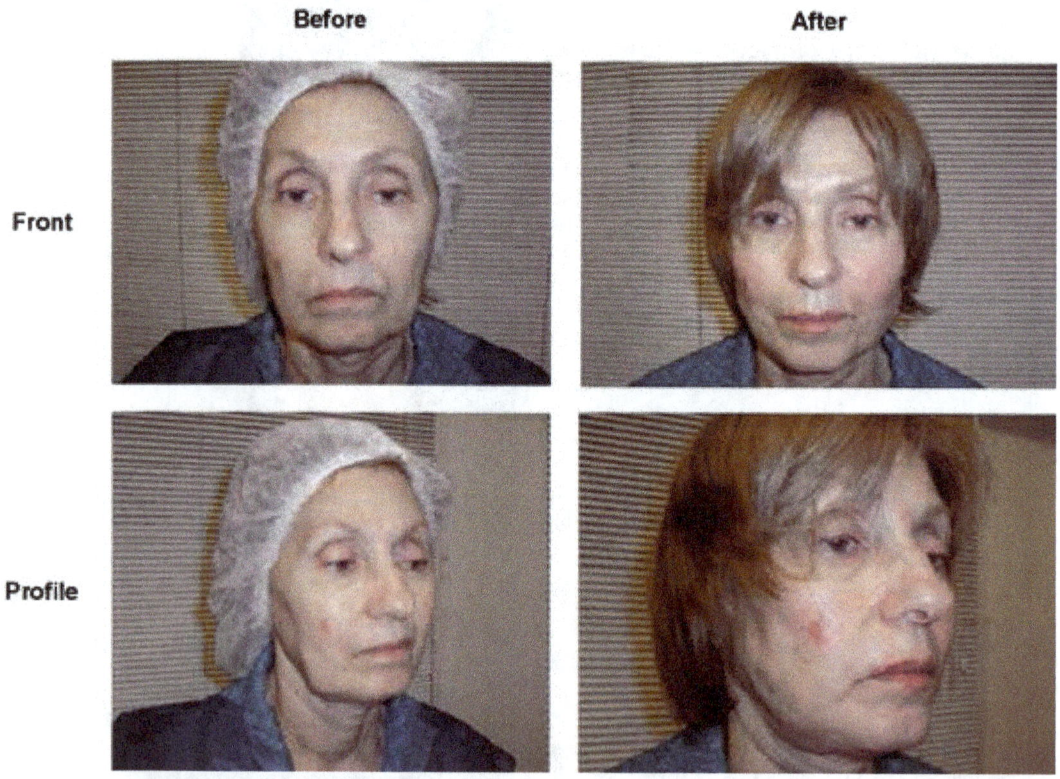


Source: own elaboration based on pictures from personal archive

**Figure 8.** Lower Face Lift Results

*2.1.1.1.4. Complications*

This technique has few complications, one of them is cutting a long thread producing it to prick from within. This is the most common complication. Another one is the migration of the thread. We have had a 3% rate in migrations. Extrusion is unusual (1% of the cases). Another authors have found thread visibility, migration, and exposure; linear bleeding along the needle course; skin dimpling; hypocorrection and hypercorrection; transient paresthesias; and a small number of cases of injury to major vessels, nerve branches, and parotid capsule/duct [5] mild asymmetry, ecchymosis, erythema, bleeding, swelling, and discomfort were the only minor. [6]

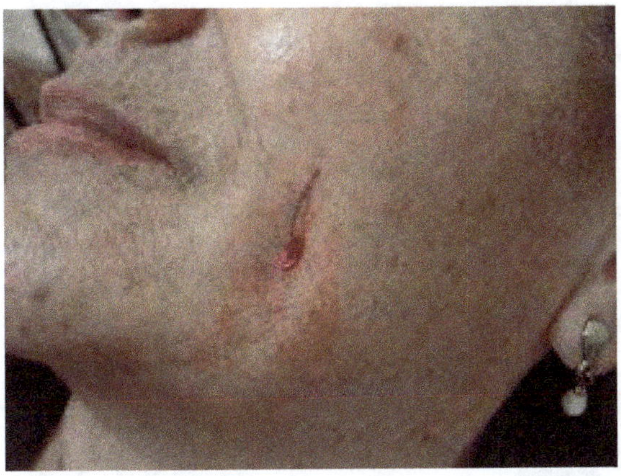

The most common complication is the thread cut long, so it pricks and we have to explore it. If the thread is anchored, we can keep it in the same place but if it is loose we have to remove and replace it.

Source: Personal archive

**Figure 9.** Thread cut long

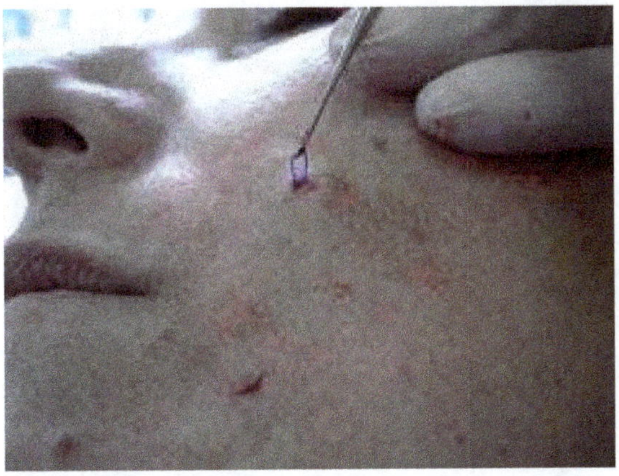

A different way to remove a migrated thread. In this case with a crochet needle

Source: Personal archive

**Figure 10.** Removing a thread

*2.1.1.2. Medial third*

The aim of this technique is to lift the cheek bone zone and indirectly also to improve the jawline and smoothing the folds. We insert one or two barbed multifixing thread of 12 cm. long, added to the above procedure in vertical form.

*2.1.1.2.1. Materials*

FIBERLIFT® MULTIFIX THREADS: Polypropylene 2.0 barbed threads with multidirectional cogs.

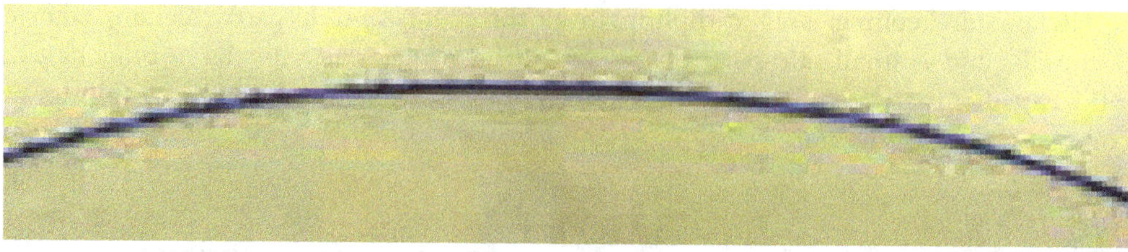

Source: Proesteticamed, 2006

**Figure 11.** Multifix thread

This procedure allows us to lift the soft tissue and reshape the cheek bone too as well as smoothing the folds and commissures.

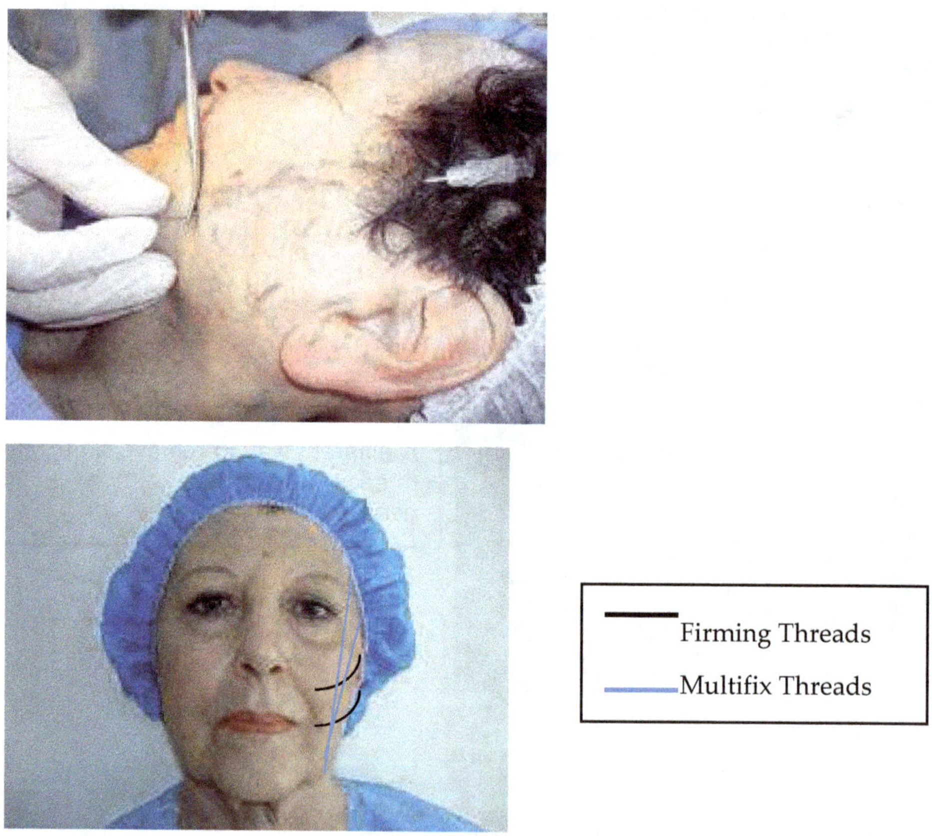


Source: Personal archive

**Figure 12.** Multifix thread located in vertical form with 21 Gx3 spinal needle

*2.1.1.2.2. Procedure*

One or two FIBERLIFT® MULTIFIX THREADS are placed in vertical form from the jawline to temporal zone with a 21 G x3 spinal needle, following the same procedure as in the case of Firming Threads.[7]

*2.1.1.2.3. Comparative study*

Between November 2006 and July 2007 we performed an 8-month study on 32 healthy patients of both sexes, ages ranging between 38 and 66 years old. On 16 of them, we had applied firming threads or anchorage threads as the only treatment. The other half of the patients was treated in the same form except for the extra plus combination of multifix threads. The following was observed:

The patients treated with multifix threads combined with firming threads or anchorage threads presented better results, longer lasting time span, a more important lift effect and a lower number of migrations and extrusions compared to those treated with only one technique. We think due to the multi-directional cogs because they do a more important anchorage surface.[5]

*2.1.1.2.4. Results*

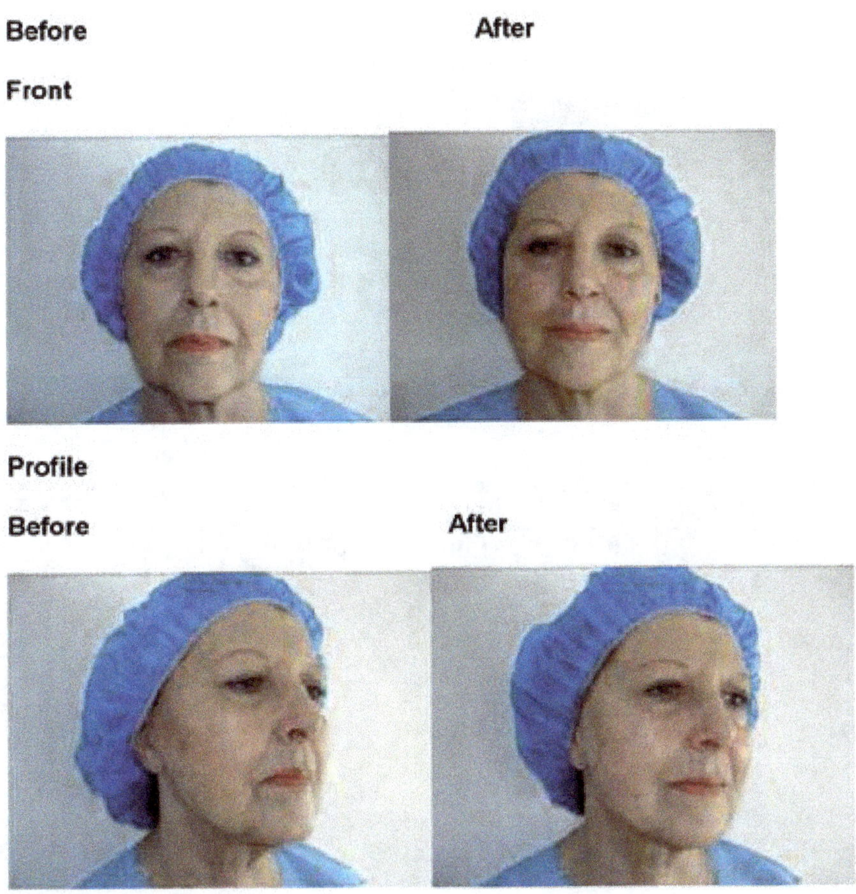


Source: own elaboration based on pictures from personal archive

**Figure 13.** Multifix threads plus Firming threads. Results

*2.1.1.3. Neck lift and double chin*

*2.1.1.3.1. With firming threads*

We can improve the aging neck by using 2 or 3 barbed Firming Threads 10cm's long on both sides of neck. We prefer to place them 2cm away from the midline because we have seen a lot of extruded threads when placed from the midline to the sides. This treatment is good for the neck and double chin. It is simple and only local anesthesia is used, therefore improving 35% of the contour. It is ideal for those patients who elude operations and for those who are knowledgeable on the results attained by this technique. Firming threads are inserted with a 21 Gx2 needle. Entering at point two fingers below the edge of the mandible and below the earlobe, above the sternocleidomastoid muscle to a point located in the same line, 1 or 2cm outside the outer border of the central band of platysma.

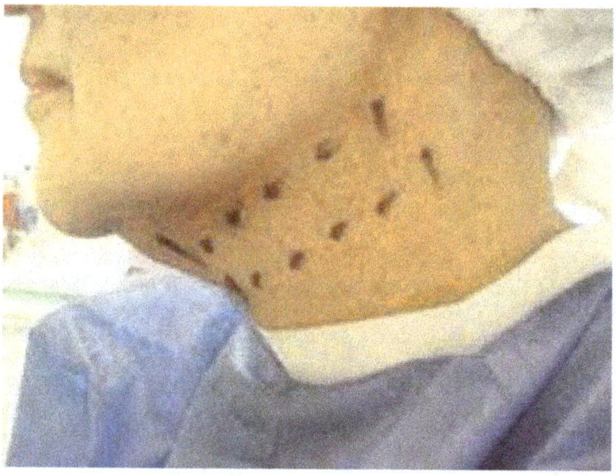

Source: Personal archive

**Figure 14.** Marcation on the patient's neck

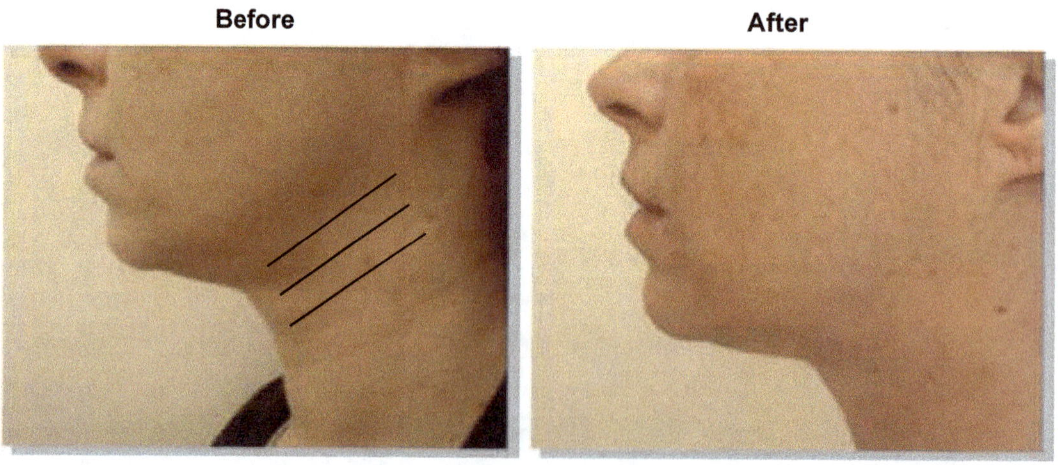


Source: Own elaboration based on pictures from personal archive

**Figure 15.** Neck Lift and Double Chin with barbed threads Results

### *2.1.1.3.2. With fiberlift®*

FIBERLIFT THREAD (By Fiberlift®) is a barbed polypropylene 3.0, with divergent cogs. It is not an autosustentation thread but an anchorage one, 30cm long, with two parts each consisting of 3cm with divergent cogs separated by a smooth area and two smooth ends.

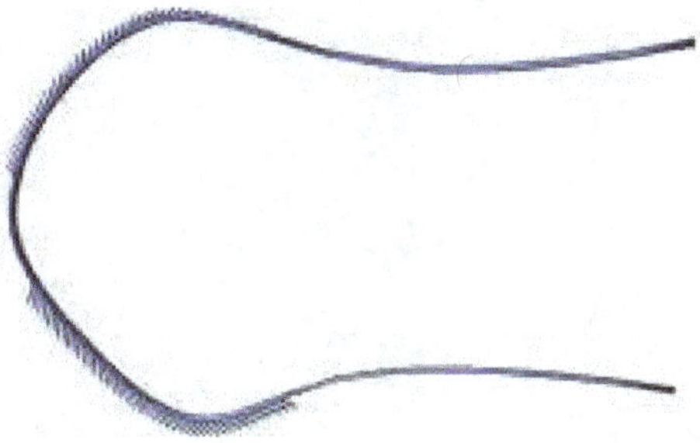

Source: Proesteticamed, 2004

**Figure 16.** Fiberlift® thread

This method is simple and allows us to lift the neck in a better way than in the FIRMING LIFT. The procedure is done with local anesthesia, using the 21 Gx2 needle, by entering the mastoid zone making a small incision of 1cm. The aim is to introduce the thread in the shape of a "V." Firstly, we enter through one side of the incision and exit on the internal point out of the platysma band, once more holding the needle and entering again on the other side of the incision, secondly, exiting at the same anterior point and out through the platysma band. The results are very good, on the other hand some complications have arisen such as persistent folds and pain. Only one case has been registered of a torn thread.

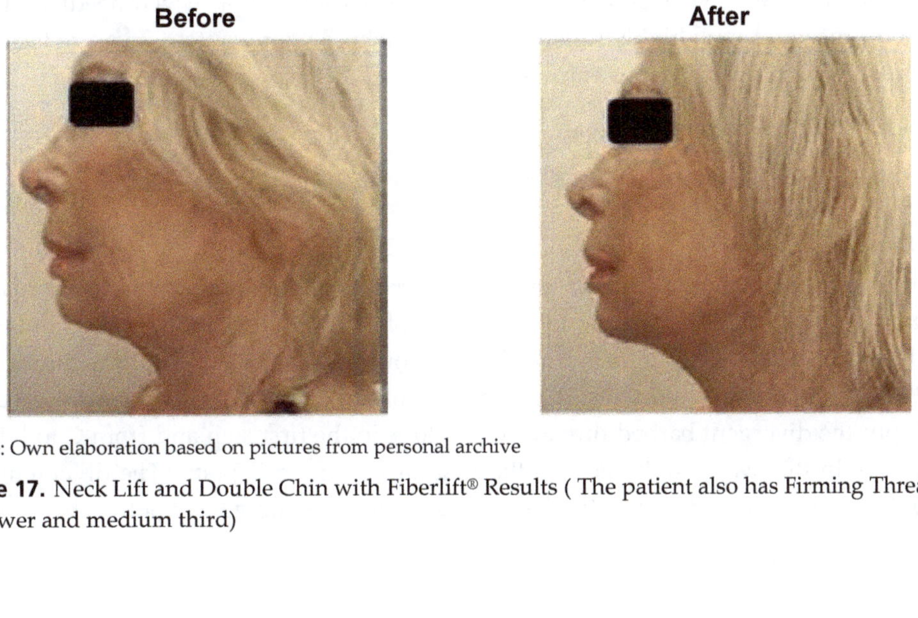


Source: Own elaboration based on pictures from personal archive

**Figure 17.** Neck Lift and Double Chin with Fiberlift® Results ( The patient also has Firming Threads at the lower and medium third)

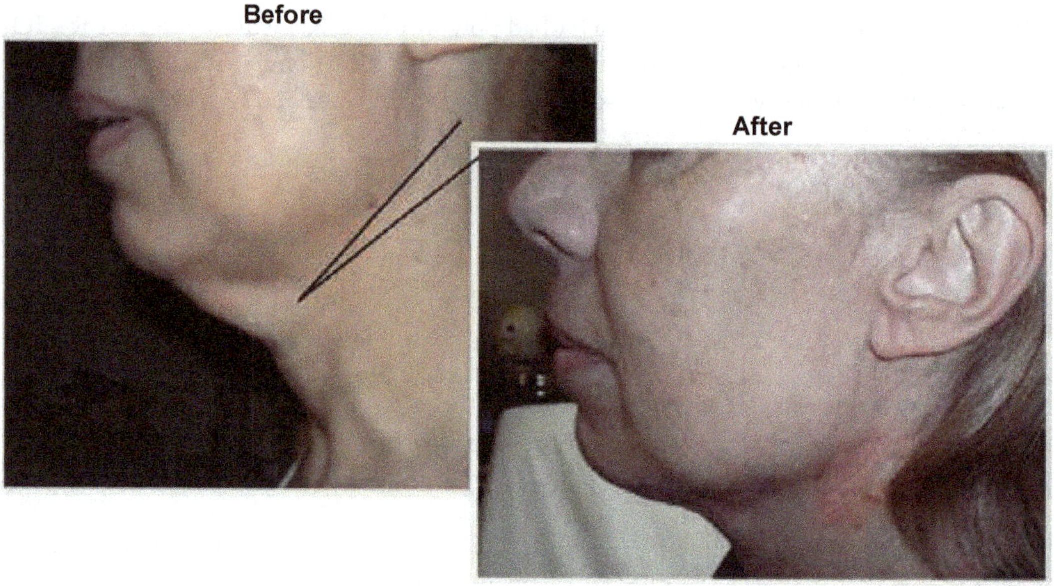


Source: Own elaboration based on pictures from personal archive

**Figure 18.** Neck Lift and Double Chin with Fiberlift® Results

*2.1.1.4. Upper third*

*2.1.1.4.1. With firming threads*

Brow lift may be done with one or two 6cm convergent barbed threads being very careful with the blood vessels. Work on frontal zone is made easier with a curved needle. This is a very good procedure with highly satisfied patients, who do not want an invasive technique and this one is performed in a few minutes.

**COMPLICATIONS:** only hematomas.

**RESULTS** are good and long lasting. Patients are very happy.

*2.1.1.4.2. With fiberlift®*

Fiberlift® is a triple anchorage polypropylene 3.0 30cm divergent barbed thread that is used to lift the eye brow tail. The technique is very simple with only a small incision of 0.5 to 1 cm. at the coronal line. Fiberlift is a procedure of double entrance and triple anchorage. We use a 21 G x2 needle and enter twice. The first entrance of the needle is AC and the second is BC. We put the divergent barbed thread from C to A in the first step and from C to B in the second step. In this way the thread has the first anchorage in C point. The divergent cogs picture the second anchorage and the last one is given by a sub-galea knot in the temporal zone. This method is very good to lift the eye brow, opening the eyes and smoothing the periorbital lines. Patients like it very much. Initially, we have seen few complications. Pain and persistent folds are improving with practice.

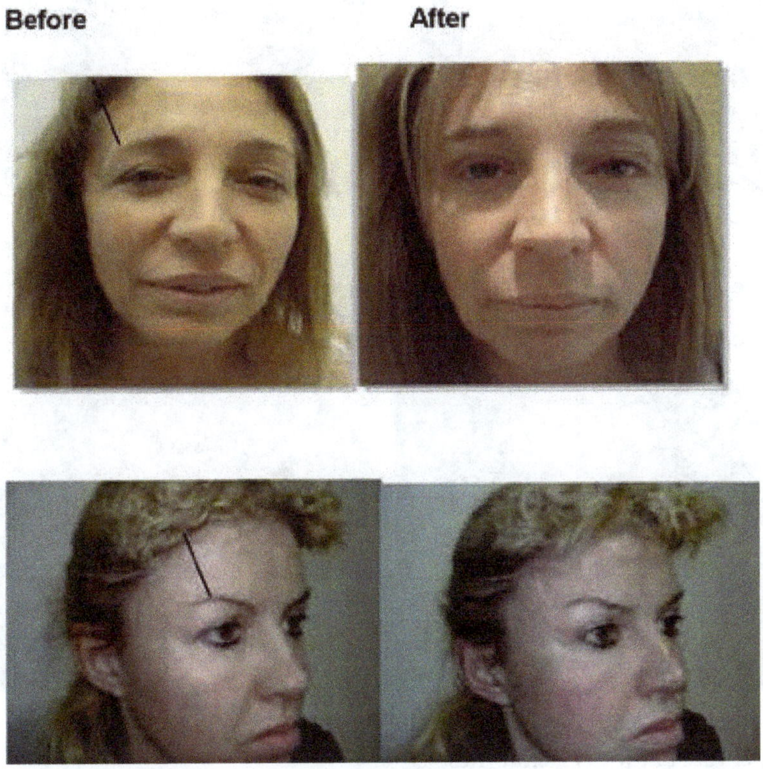


Source: Own elaboration based on pictures from personal archive

**Figure 19.** Direction of the Firming thread to lift the eye brow. Results

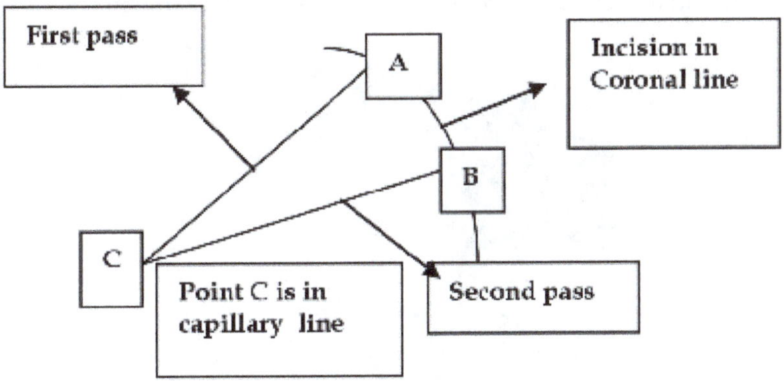


Source: Own elaboration

**Scheme 2.** Placement of Fiberlift®

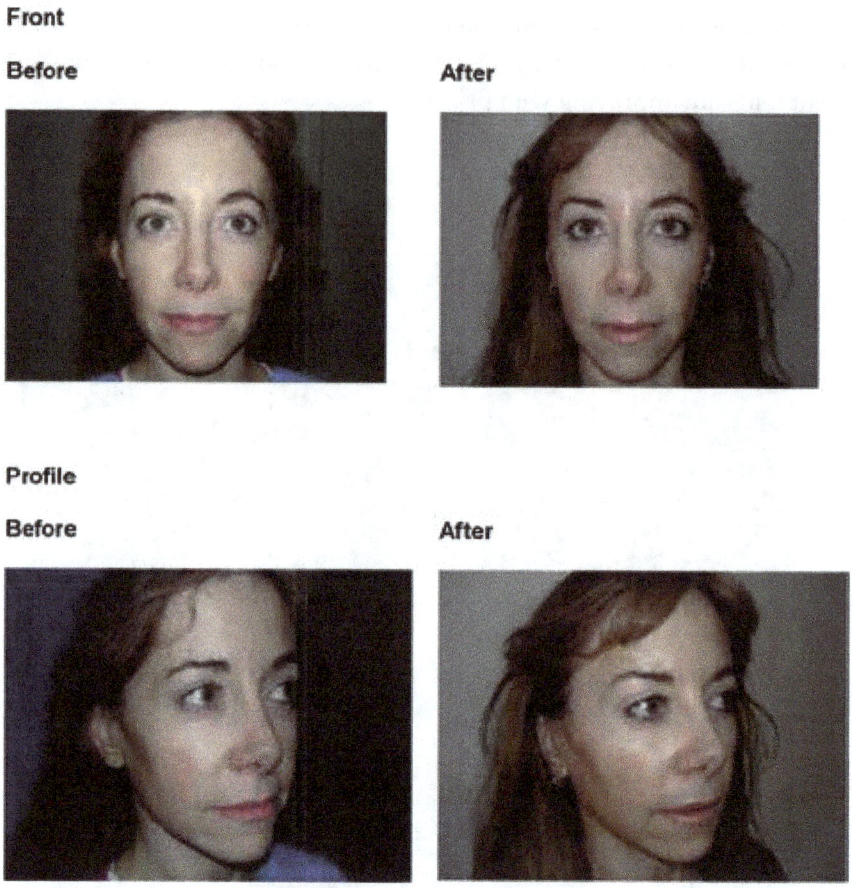


Source: Own elaboration based on pictures from personal archive

**Figure 20.** Upper Face Lift with Fiberlift® Results

*2.1.1.4.3. Complications*

In two cases we found a decubitus ulcer that needed surgical treatment.

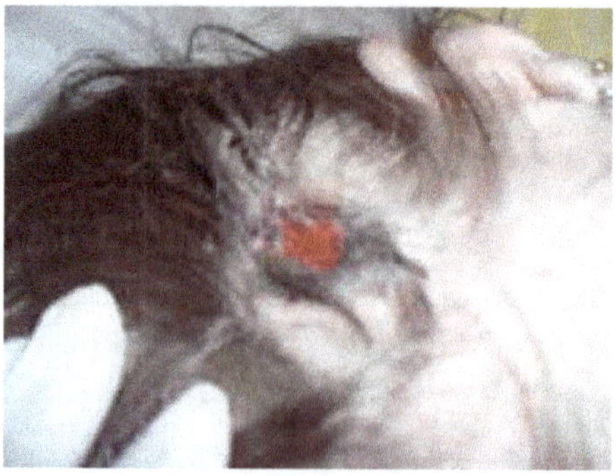

Source: Personal archive

**Figure 21.** Decubitus ulcer

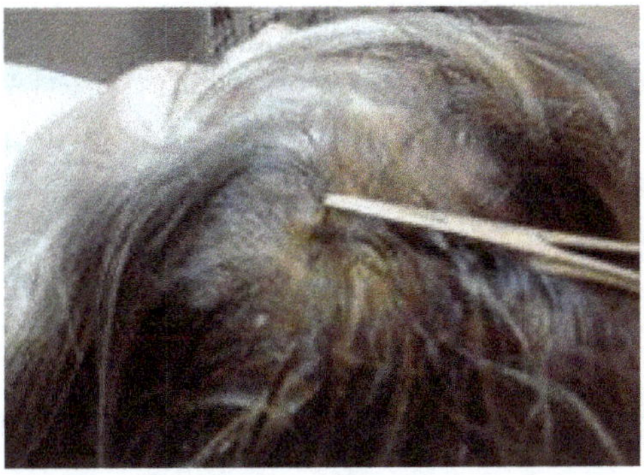

Source: Personal archive

**Figure 22.** Extrusion of Fiberlift® thread

## 2.2. Serdev sutures – Serdev methods: Temporal face lift, eye brow lift, medial face lift and chin enhancement

These techniques, created by Nikolay Serdev use semi-elastic polycaproamide, long term absorbable (2-3 years), braided, antimicrobial, Bulgarian materials, called Serdev Sutures. With Serdev's methods we can lift one mobile tissue and carry it to a non movable point.

### *2.2.1. Temporal face lift without incisions*

The Temporal face lift with Serdev sutures not only lifts the soft tissue of the upper face and the zygomatic zone but it also reflects a lifting of the lower face. The results cover in a complete way 'lifting' without an incision. It is significant to know the location of the temporal zone to prevent damage to the temporal branch of the facial nerve. It is very important for us to outline the temporal zone.[8]

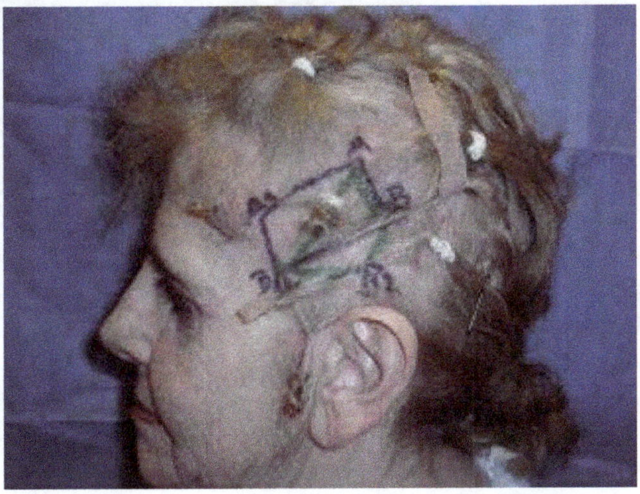

Source: Personal archive

**Figure 23.** Marcation for temporal face lift

In this outline we have marked with green a second lift treatment, in the same temporal zone to optimize the result. In this case there were another four passes (AB1, B1B2, B2B and B2B)

*2.2.1.1. Technique*

Insert the suture with a special, curved, semielastic, small or mini Serdev's needle with a tip hole. The passes are A-A1, thread the suture and leave. Go B1A1, thread the suture and leave, then BB1 thread the suture and leave and finally AB, thread the suture, knot it and cut. The passes AA1 and BB1 are sub-galea, the pass A1B1 is sub-dermic, and the last AB is sub-fascia. In this way the SMAS is lifted and fixed to the temporalis fascia.

*2.2.1.2. Results*

We can see an improvement in the aspect of the face: the eye brows, the skin and the eyes with a change in the tired expression of the face with no traces of an operation. The results of this technique are immediate and the patient's satisfaction is high.

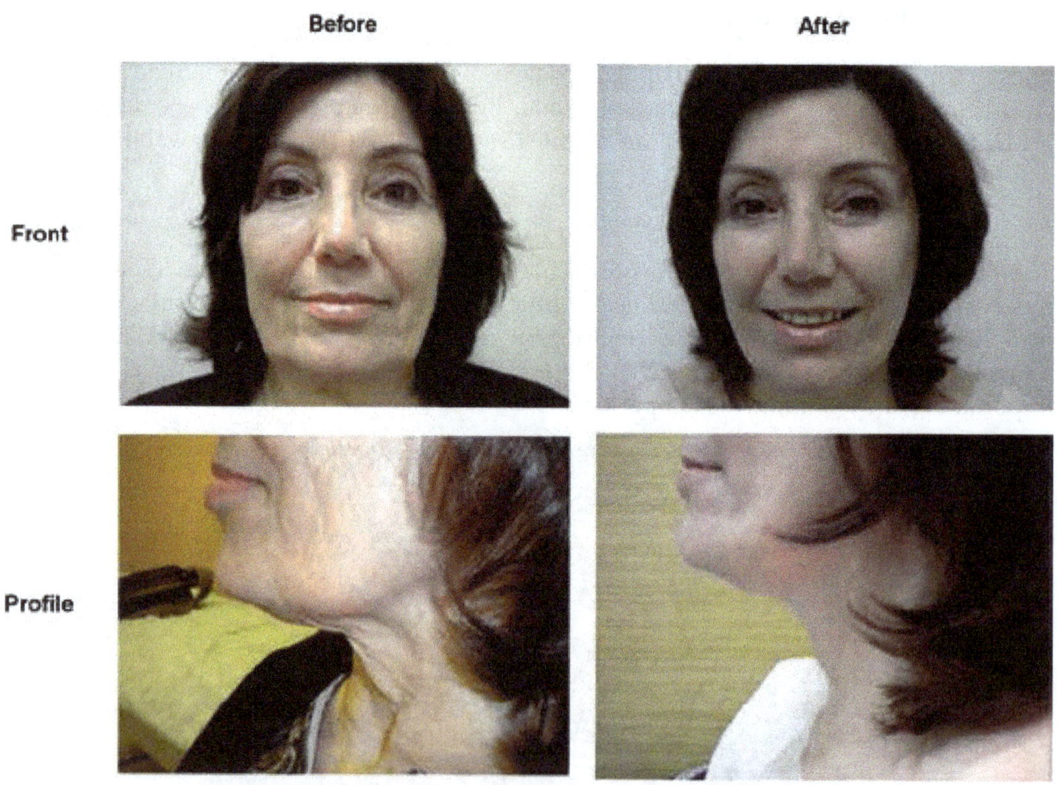


Source: Own elaboration based on pictures from personal archive

**Figure 24.** Temporal Face Lift with Serdev Sutures Results

*2.2.1.3. Complications*

Initially, we have seen skin dimpling, pain, edema of the upper face, hematoma below the eye. Skin dimpling is treated with one branch of the "mosquito" claw (Serdev). Pain is tolerable and patients can take analgesics. The edema and hematomas were produced by mistake in the surgical plane of needle puncture and suture insertion. Today, with the experience of 6 years of daily practice with this technique, complications are not significant.

### 2.2.2. *Eye brow lift with Serdev sutures and Serdev method*

This method is very simple and fast. It was described by Nikolay Serdev in 1994, [9] without incisions, only a needle perforation between the eye brow hairs. Thus, it is possible to carry

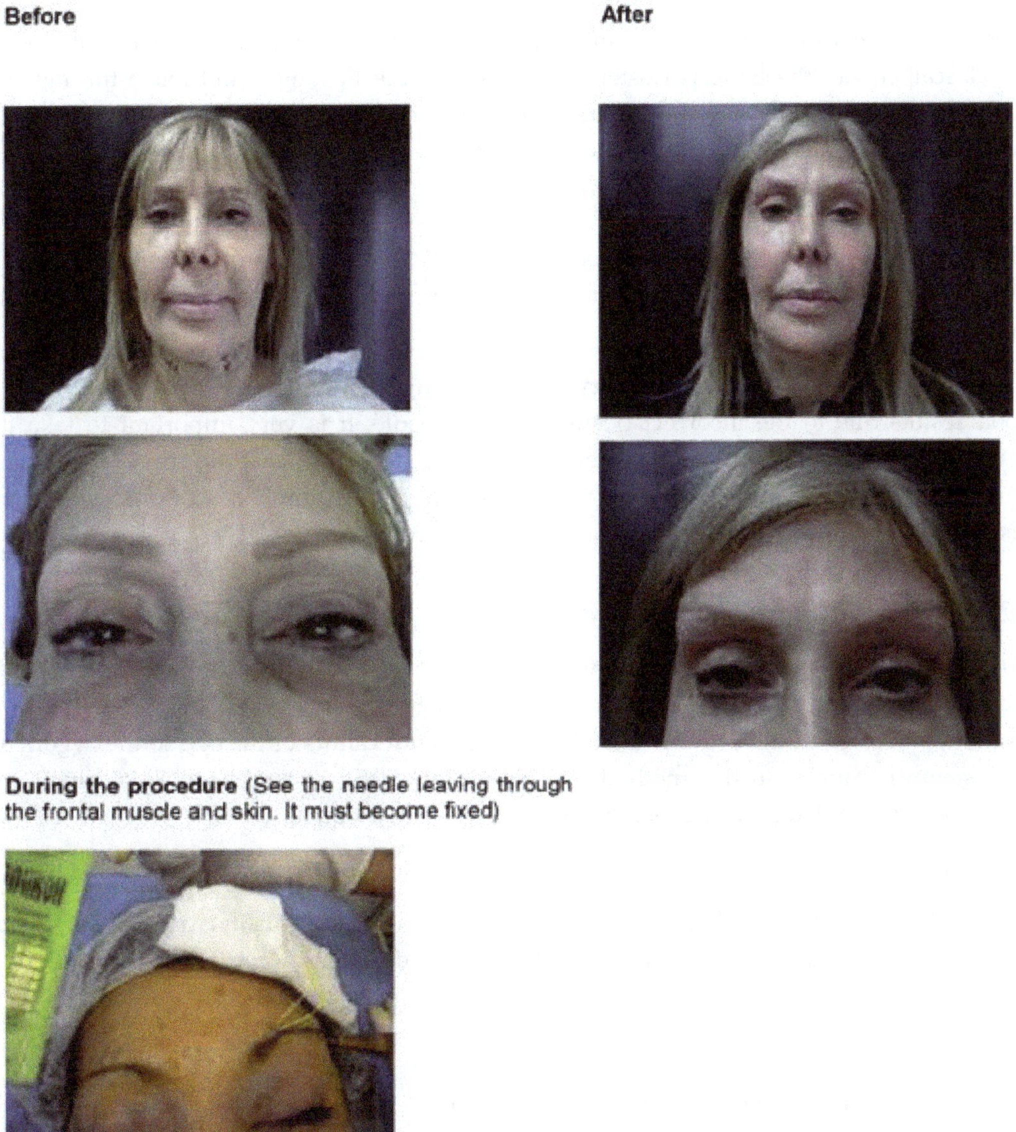


Source: own elaboration based on pictures from personal archive

**Figure 25.** Eye brow lift with Serdev Sutures and Serdev Method Results

the subdermal tissue to the bone periosteum and fix it, using a Serdev suture and a special semi elastic small (mini-mini) needle with a tip hole. The secret for success is not to be afraid of being aggressive in fixing the subdermal tissue to the bone periosteum (Serdev's 2007 Course in Sophia on Serdev Techniques.)

The procedure consists of two steps; using lidocaine 2% with epinephrine in each of the two points that we'll use (positioning previously 1cm above of the orbital rim).

*2.2.2.1. First step*

Enter in point A with semi elastic, mini Serdev needle. The incision is made with the tip of a Nº 11 scalpel. Get the bone periosteum with the needle tip down and leave through the frontal muscle and skin with the tip up; needle must become fixed, if it is not fixed it could be improperly located in a wrong plane. Thread the suture and remove the needle.

*2.2.2.2. Second step*

The 2nd needle pass is superficial, it goes through the lower dermis from point A to point B. Then a knot is made with medium tension. The dimpling is removed with a branch of the mosquito claw.

It is a very interesting method with very good and long lasting results. Initially I didn't have good results due to the incorrect position of the needle. It is very important to take the periosteum with the tip down and then turn the needle with the tip up. In 5 years I have only had one complication with a knot extrusion. In that case the suture used was a Nº2 instead of a Nº0. It was removed and replaced by the correct one.

### *2.2.3. Medial face lift with Serdev sutures*

I use only one of the several alternatives that Serdev describes for this method. It is to lift loose medial SMAS and to fix it to the stable zygomatic periosteum. Point A (entrance and fixation) is located in the zygoma 1 cm below the lateral cantus of the eye so the zygomatic periosteum is caught. In this method a Serdev semi elastic, curved needle size small and Serdev elastic braided antimicrobial polycaproamide are used.[10]

*2.2.3.1. First step*

The needle enters in point A through the bone periosteum and exits in a parallel line beside the nasolabial fold in one of three points that Serdev describes according to the age of the patient.

*2.2.3.2. Second step*

The needle enters in point A and passes superficially through the soft tissue and exits in point B describing a circle around the zygoma and zygomatic SMAS extension. Then, a knot is made with medium tension. In this way it gives new volume to the cheek bone. It is a good ambulatory method, with good results but at first patients sometimes don't accept it due to the formation of dimples. I haven't seen complications except for some dimples that patients didn't like and there has been only one case of asymmetry. The dimples disapeared in two weeks and the asymmetry, caused by exaggerated tension, was corrected by removing and replacing the suture.

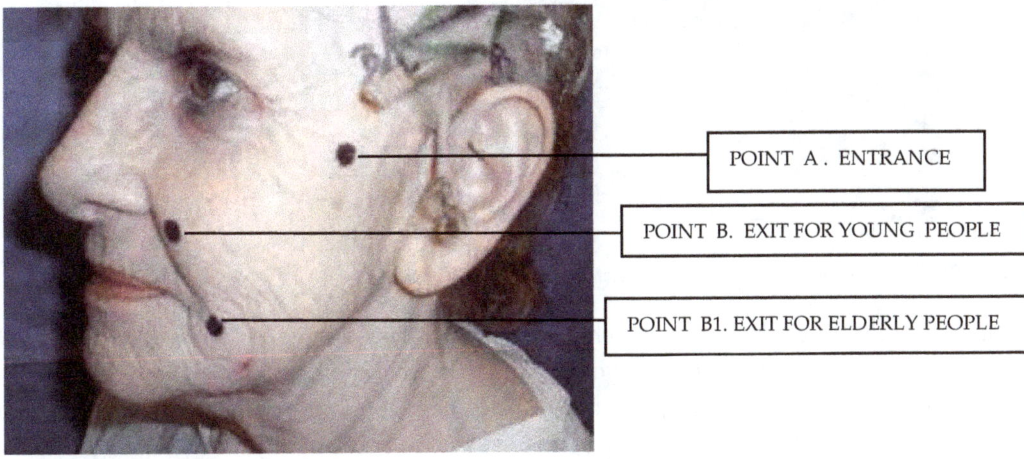


Source: Personal archive

**Figure 26.** Medial Face Lift Technique with Serdev Sutures

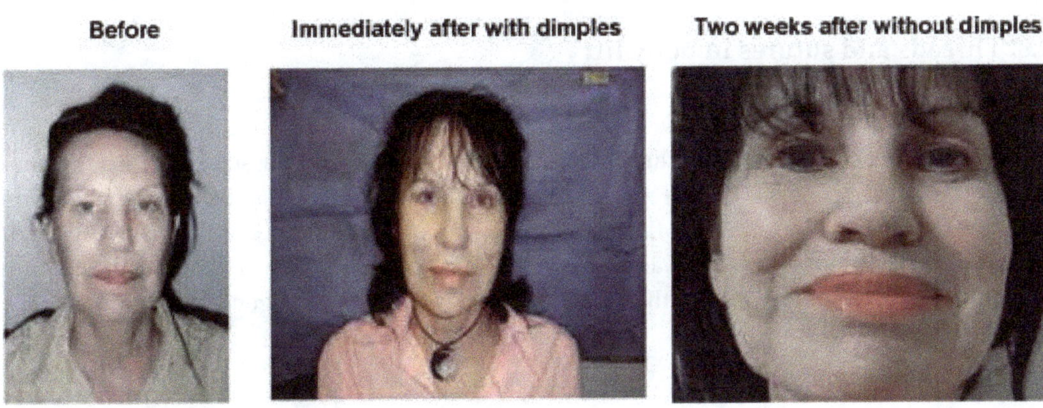


Source: Own elaboration based on pictures from personal archive

**Figure 27.** Medial Face Lift with Serdev Sutures Results

### *2.2.4. Chin augmentation using Serdev sutures*

The form and position of the chin is very important in the correct and harmonic face proportions and beauty features. It is common to see chin disproportions such as micrognathia aging, asymmetries, etc. Nikolay Serdev proposes a simple technique using non barbed suture to correct these chin disharmonies. The procedure is simple using a small semi-elastic, curve needle with a tip hole and a thin Serdev suture. The entrance may be in point A or B and the exit in the other.

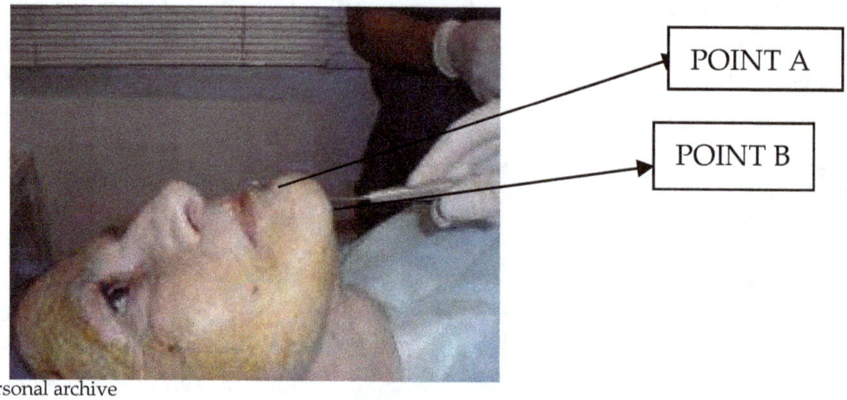


Source: Personal archive

**Figure 28.** Chin augmentation technique with Serdev Sutures

The aim is to create a circle around the chin's soft tissue, there are two steps to follow. The first pass is depth, entering in point A, going along the mandibular line, exiting in point B, threading the suture and removing the needle.[11] The second pass is done by entering point A but in a more superficial way by going under the skin and leaving through point B in the skin. The knot is done here. If there is dimpling in the skin, it is corrected with the mosquito branch (Serdev). The results are excellent and fast. The patients are satisfied. No complications.

## 2.3. Threads and sutures in body lift

### *2.3.1. Barbed threads in body lift*

The objective of these techniques are to give a lift effect to the soft tissue of the arms, inner thigh, abdominal zone and outer thigh when there have been sequelae with liposuction effects. They are good for treating flaccid or aging areas. All methods are performed without incisions and without scars. They are simple and fast, obtaining good results, with medium and long term duration due to the new collagen fibers that are generated around each thread and each cog of them.

#### *2.3.1.1. Arm lift*

##### *2.3.1.1.1. Materials*

We use MULTIFIX THREADS, multifix 12 cm nonabsorbable 2.0 polypropylene with multidirectional cogs. We insert them under the skin in the fat tissue. 4 threads or more can be inserted depending on the size of the arm.

##### *2.3.1.1.2. Procedure*

Begin with the marcation three fingers below the axilla. Prior to procedure inject lidocaine 2% with epinephrine in the skin, just 0.5cc in each point is enough.

Do the insertion with a 21 Gx3 needle (spinal needle) beginning from the external point to the internal one, repeating the same procedure many times as necessary. The thread is

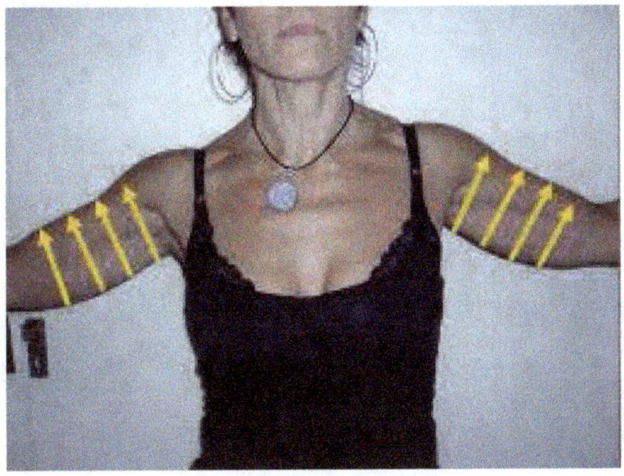

Source: Personal archive

**Figure 29.** Arms lift

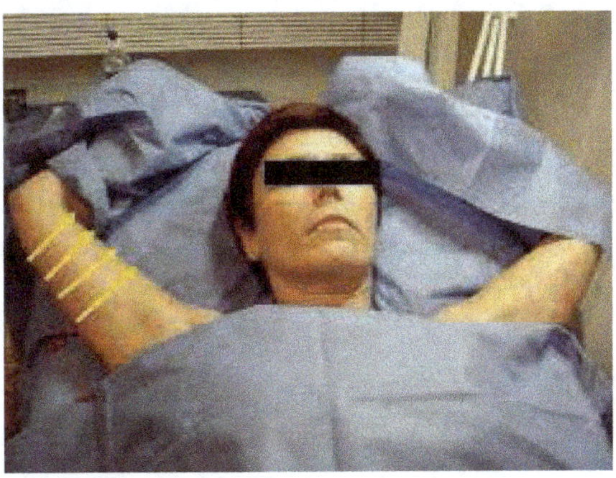

Beware of the humeral artery

Source: Personal archive

**Figure 30.** Arms lift – Procedure

positioned and anchoraged with a simple and delicate movement with the hand using a Halsted claw and pulling gently in both directions. Then we cut the ends of the thread by pushing the skin down to uncover the thread's end, avoiding a long thread. We use bandages or tight sleeves for 10 days. Nsaids and analgesics are indicated for three days.

**RESULTS** are good, it is a fast and long lasting procedure.

*2.3.1.1.3. Complications*

Pain and edema, have been seen. Sometimes a bump under the skin because of the length of the thread. We have had some extrusions in three patients. Bumps under the skin are the most common complications and are corrected by cutting the end of the thread. If it is in the correct position (fix and anchorage), it's not necessary to remove it, if that is the case only cut the end. If the thread is loose it would be convenient to remove it.

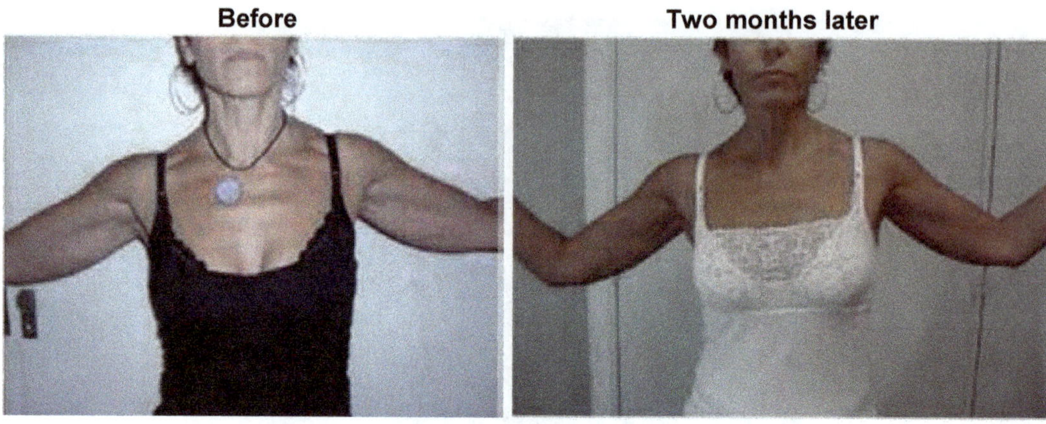


Source: Own elaboration based on pictures from personal archive

**Figure 31.** Arm Lift with Barbed Threads Results

### *2.3.1.2. Inner thigh*

The inner thigh is a flaccid and aging area that may be improved with 2.0 polypropylene multifix barbed threads with multidirectional cogs. It is a simple application done with a long 21Gx3.5 needle in the fat tissue thickness. We must be careful with the femoral artery and vein as well as with the saphen intern vein. The femoral artery can often be palpated through the skin in the inner thigh at the mid-inguinal-point, halfway between the pubic symphysis and anterior superior iliac spine. [12]

#### *2.3.1.2.1. Procedure*

Application of at least 4 threads for each side, from external (A) to internal (B) point using a 21Gx3.5 needle (spinal), being careful when cutting the ends and using an elastic compression for a week.

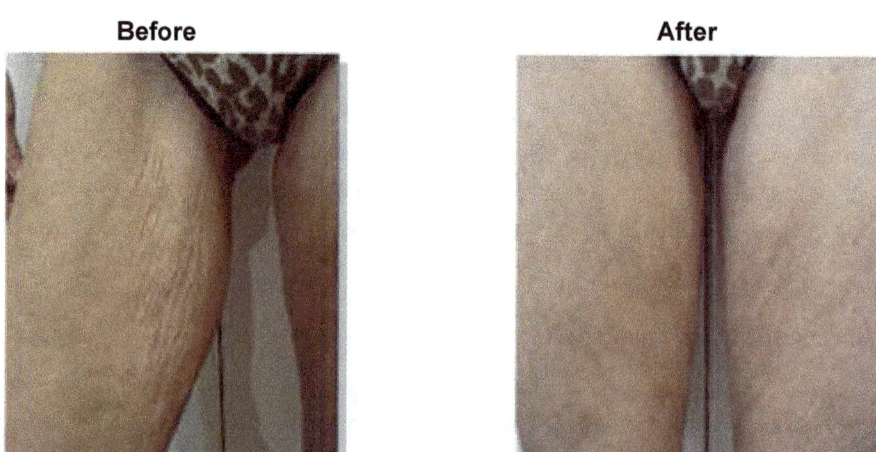


Source: Own elaboration based on pictures from personal archive

**Figure 32.** Inner Thigh Lift with Barbed Threads Results

*2.3.1.2.2. Results*

Results are very interesting, patients accept this technique. It allows them to see themselves better as well as returning immediately to their social activities. It is very important to see the changes in the general physiognomy of the skin, produced by the stimulation of collagen formation. This method is easy, fast and with a long lasting time span. In accordance with my experience, I believe the inner thigh is the best place to insert barbed multifix threads in body lift treatment.

*2.3.1.3. Front and upper face of the knee*

*2.3.1.3.1. Materials*

The upper and anterior face of the knee share with the inner thigh as the best places to lift with barbed threads. I usually use 2.0 polypropylene antimicrobial multifix barbed threads with multidirectional cogs, 12 cm length and 2.0 polypropylene antimicrobial Firming barbed threads with bidirectional cogs, 8 or 10 cm length. Multifix are inserted in a vertical form and Firming (bidirectional cogs) is used on a horizontal line.

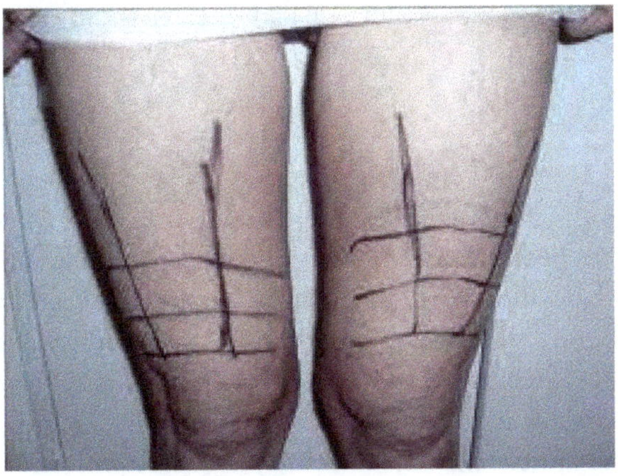

Source: Personal archive

**Figure 33.** Marcation for front and upper face of the knee lift

*2.3.1.3.2. Procedure*

It's a simple procedure, using only local anesthesia (lidocaine 2%with epinephrine) at the entrance and exit points; 0.5cc in each one. The insertion is carried out with two kinds of needles a 21 Gx2 is used to insert Firming threads and a 21 Gx3.5 is used to insert Multifix threads. This technique consists of two steps. In the first step insert Firming threads in parallel lines and in a horizontal position place the fat tissue of the anterior thigh 3 or 4 fingers above the knee. In the second step Multifix threads are inserted in diagonal form crossing over the Firming threads. As we finish we have to be careful cutting the threads in order to avoid long threads pricking from within. The use of an elastic compression or tight panties is suggested for a week.

**RESULTS** are very good. Patients are satisfied with the change in the skin and the improvement of irregularities in the tissue caused by flaccidity.

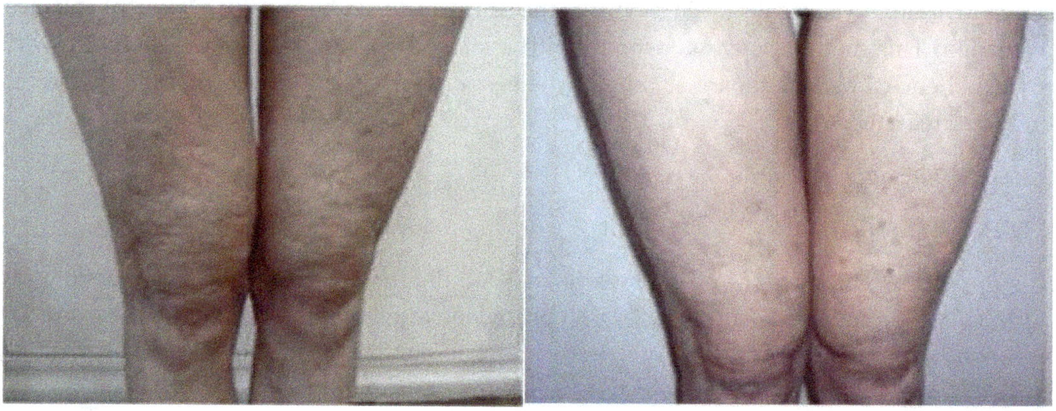


Source: Own elaboration based on pictures from personal archive

**Figure 34.** Front and upper face of the knee lift with Barbed Threads and Multifix Results

## *2.3.2. Serdev sutures in body lift*

### *2.3.2.1. Buttock lift*

I have experience in buttock lift with Serdev sutures and Serdev's technique. It is a very interesting method to lift buttocks that are flaccid. This is a mini invasive procedure without scars and with a short postoperative. A description of the subject was made by Nikolay Serdev in 2003, in Sophia, Bulgaria. It is an ambulatory procedure and it achieves the reposition of the buttock's subdermal fat tissue by lifting it and increasing its volume and anteroposterior diameter using only a suture that grasps the deep fibrous tissue and fixes it to the upper zone in the gluteus maximus fascia in its sacrum insertion. [13]

We prefer to use the Argentine modified Serdev technique (J. Ferreira, Buenos Aires 2004) due to the gluteus shape of Argentine women. [14] This technique has 3 steps as in the original Serdev's method:

First step: with the patient in a sitting position I mark the lower limit.

Second step: with the patient in ventral decubitus I draw the internal and lower points some centimeters above the inferior limit and 2 or 3 cm from the anus. There is another lateral point, the same as in liposuction. The higher point or sacrum point is in the middle line at the begining of the gluteal fold.

Third step: we then proceed to measure and to check the symmetries, drawing a print line between the three points to give the rounded desired form. It's important for me to draw the inferior limit so as to avoid a long term post-operative pain.

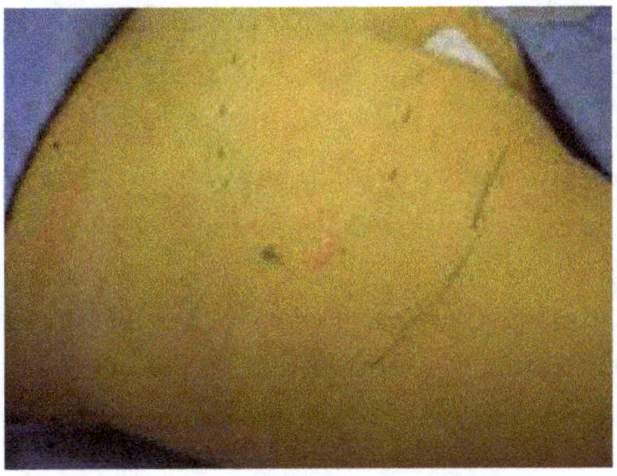

Source: Personal archive

**Figure 35.** Buttock lift. Marcation

*2.3.2.1.1. Procedure*

Antisepsis is done, the perianal zone is covered by a sterile gauze. Anesthesia with lidocaine 2% with epinephrine in each point where small incisions between 3 to 4mm will be perfomed with a number 11 scalpel blade. Klein solution is injected with a 2mm cannula into the deep fat tissue which lies on the superficial surface from the maximus gluteus fascia. A way is marked where the path of the Serdev needle will proceed.

We work with a hollow protector in lateral and inferior incision points to avoid taking superficial skin with the needle thus producing a "dimple" on the surface.

The procedure is carried out with a special needle developed by Nikolay Serdev. It is 20 cm, flexible and semi-curved with a top orifice, it is also a polycaproamide, elastic, antimicrobial Bulgarian suture. A liposuction is previously performed on the outer thigh to reduce the volume and weight of the gluteus.

First pass: from external incision to medial or a sacrum one in the shape of an arch with a Serdev needle. We thread the suture and remove the needle leaving out the ends of the suture. Second pass: from inferior perianal incision to the lateral one. Thread the suture and remove the needle.

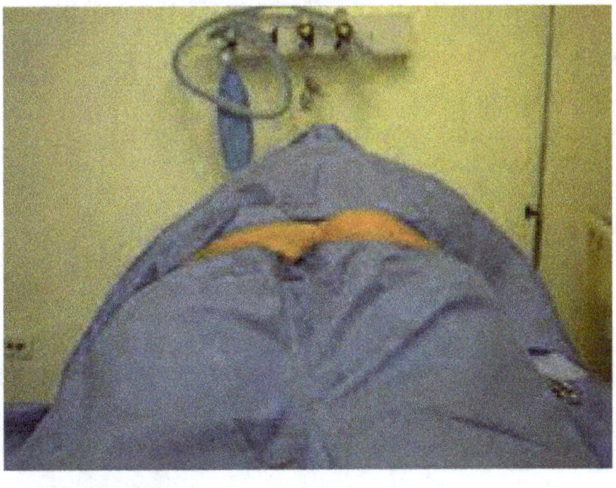

Buttock lift of only one side done

Source: Personal archive

**Figure 36.** Buttock lift only one side done

Finally we go from the sacrum incision to the inferior internal point and thread the suture, then we remove the needle and we can observe both ends of the suture in the sacrum incision. Adjust the suture to give it the desired form and height and make some surgical knots. Finish by closing the skin with a nylon 5.0 and a micropore.

*2.3.2.1.2. Results*

The results are very interesting and patients are satisfied. I have performed 104 procedures; 103 were women and only 1 man. The patients were between 20 and 65 years old. A 40% of these were combined with liposuction of the outer thigh. All patients were satisfied with the results.

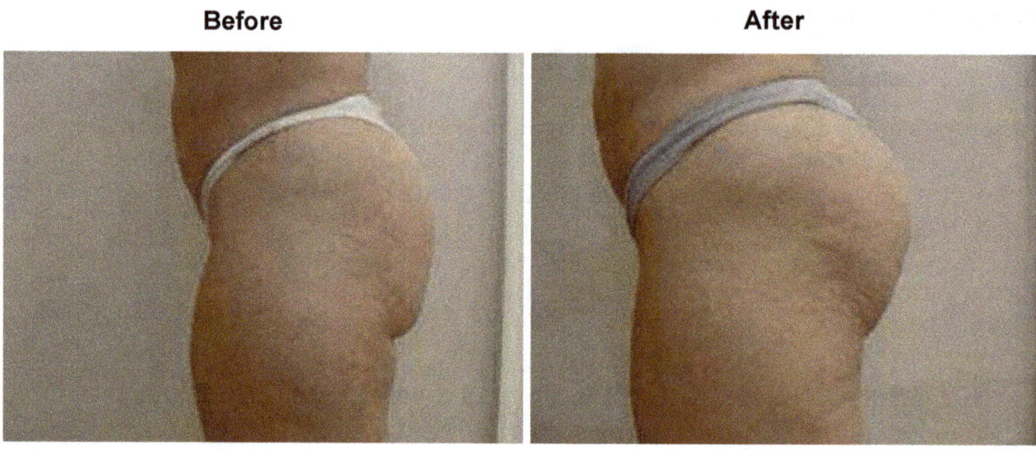


Source: Own elaboration based on pictures from personal archive

**Figure 37.** Buttock Lift Results

*2.3.2.1.3. Complications*

There are few complications; such as skin dimples or assimetries due to different tensions found in both gluteus. Pain was the most frequent undesired effect. It had a duration of 15 days and it was treated with Nsaids and analgesics. Every patient had been prescribed with antibiotics. There were neither infections nor hematomas.

*2.3.2.1.4. Comparison of both methods, barbed threads and non barbed Serdev sutures*

Both methods, barbed threads and non barbed Serdev sutures, are excellent for mini invasive techniques. Patients are satisfied with both of them. Complications are rare and the lifting effect range from good to excellent.

We have found –after 10 years of barbed thread experience and 6 years of Serdev sutures–, that lifting effect is higher with Serdev sutures, patients recover forms, angles and the tissue is repositioned without "operated look." They also improve adding a higher volume and contour. The collagen and elastic fibers generation are very important with barbed threads, improving the skin of the face, giving it light and a glow.

In an experimental study of the morphological changes in tissue with barbed threads carried out by Sulamanidze and co-writers (2002) in order to clarify the mechanism of tissue ptosis correction, it was seen in rats when polyprpopylene barbed threads were inserted subdermally and were compared with non barbed polypropylene in control rats with serial skin biopsies. It was noted that the barbed threads had elicited an earlier inflammatory response followed by a vascular proliferation and fibroblastic reaction thus creating a new collagen generation along the threads and along each barbs. In the case of non-barbed threads in rats it was found (Truswell 2008)[15] that there was neither found a collagen generation nor a vascular proliferation nor an inflammatory response nor a fibroblastic reaction.

Volume and contour were seen with Serdev suture and barbed threads in a less degree. "Z" insertion of Firming and Multifix threads has generated a new and better cheek bone.

The improvement in 1 year is important for both methods as well as the patient's satisfaction. Both methods have no post-operative recovery time. Pain is minimum in both procedures. In the field of complications we can mention that with barbed threads we've seen some cases of migration and some extrusions of the end of the thread. With Serdev sutures we have sometimes seen pain in the temporal zone.

| | BARBED THREADS | SERDEV SUTURES |
|---|---|---|
| LIFTING EFFECT | ++ | ++++ |
| COLLAGEN GENERATION | +++ | + |
| VOLUME | + | +++ |
| CONTOUR | ++ | +++ |
| IMPROVE IN ONE YEAR | +++ | +++ |
| PATIENT SATISFACTION | +++ | +++ |
| POSTOPERATIVE RECOVERY TIME | —— | —— |
| PAIN | + | + |
| COMPLICATIONS | + | + |

Source: Own elaboration

**Table 1.** Comparative chart Barbed Threads vs. Serdev Sutures

*2.3.2.1.5. Combined techniques*

It is very interesting to combine both methods using barbed threads in the lower third and temporal face lift with Serdev sutures. With this combination we can get fantastic results of the lifting effect and collagen generation. To optimize the contour with temporal face lift with sutures and barbed threads in the neck zone, improving the smoothing effect too. In my daily practice I usually perform a combined formula with temporal face lift and barbed threads insertion in the medium and in the lower third and neck. I can also add one barbed thread in each eyebrow tail.

*2.3.2.1.6. Complementary methods*

The combination of these methods is very important, with the use of barbed threads and non barbed sutures, and other rejuvenation and beautification techniques as BOTOX, Fillers, IPL, Peelings, Laser, Oxygenesis and Mesotherapy. It's specially interesting Botox application treatment in the lower third as complement of threads. We inject the botulinum toxin in both platysm bands and jawline. Also may be injected into the orbicularis angle depressor muscle to elevate the commisures [16].

## 3. Discussion

Since the beginning of mankind men and women have always seeked ways to preserve beauty and the fountain of youth. Beauty has always been portrayed through art where you will find the most beautiful features which are in harmony with perfect proportions. In such natural and beautiful forms, why should harmony be altered? There are numerous methods to treat the aging face. Surgical techniques with cuts, pain, edema, scars, long postoperative time, often are used as a matter of surgeons satisfaction who do not even consider the genuine needs of their patients. Already in 1970 R Guillemain published on Curl Lift [17] but at the time the lift with cuts was well regarded by the patients who happily wore their scars. Today the patient ask for mini invasive procedures without scars nor pain and they want to return immediately to their activities. Aging treatments with threads and sutures are chosen for our patients, because they provide a natural effect.

## 4. Conclusion

In spite of having seen some extrusions, some migrations, some cases of pain or edema, whereas the simplicity of these procedures, the good and natural results that may be seen, the long lasting, the no post-operative time, the few complications and the high satisfaction of the patients we think that threads and sutures are a great answer to our patient's modern life exigencies and their wish: "don't cut". Patient's understanding of these techniques is very important. We are convinced that these procedures are a very good way path in the current cosmetic surgery and the most requested among our patients.

## Author details

Vilma L. Padín
*CEMEC (Center of Aesthetic Medicine and Surgery), Buenos Aires, Argentine Republic*
*AIMERA (International Association of Aesthetic Medicine), Argentine Republic*

## Acknowledgement

I would very much like to thank Professor Nikolay Serdev for allowing me to write this chapter. Dr. Serdev introduced me and opened the way to the fascinating field of the mini-invasive techniques of facial and body lifting.

## 5. References

[1] Sulamanidze, M. et al., "Removal of facial tissue ptosis with special threads", *Dermatological Surgery* 28 (2002):367-371.

[2] Bacci, P., *Cirugía Estética Mínimamente Invasiva con Hilos Tensores* (Caracas; Amolca, 2008).

[3] SERDEV, N., "Scarless 'APTOS' & 'SERDEV SUTURE' Lifting Methods", *International Journal of Cosmetic Surgery* 4 (2004); 1-10.

[4] Sulamanidze M., Sulamanidze G.,"Avoiding Complications with Aptos Sutures" Aesthetic Surgery,...,2011

[5] Lycka B. et al., "The emerging technique of the antiptosis subdermal suspension thread", *Dermatological Surgery* 30 (2004): 41-44.

[6] Padin, V., "Tratamiento de la Flaccidez Facial con Aplicación de Hilos", *Revista Argentina de Rinología y Cirugía Facial* 1 (2005): 35-44.

[7] Serdev, N., "Ambulatory Temporal SMAS Lift by Sutures with or without Incisions", *International Journal of Cosmetic Surgery* 1 (2001); 97-106.

[8] Serdev, N., "A Suture Method for Scarless Brow Lift", *International Journal of Cosmetic Surgery* 1 (2001); 1-15.

[9] Serdev, N., "Serdev Suture Method for Ambulatory Medial SMAS Face Lift", *International Journal of Cosmetic Surgery* 2 (2002); 1-13.

[10] Serdev, N., "Chin enhancement and form correction using a suture of the soft tissue", *International Journal of Cosmetic Surgery* 2 (2002);16-25.

[11] Padin, V.," Dermosustentación con hilos en miembros inferiores" (presented at the II International Simposium of mini invasive procedures in Flebology, Buenos Aires, Argentina, October 2009,Medicine Faculty, Buenos Aires University).

[12] Serdev, N., "Buttock Lifts. Part I: Ambulatory Buttock Lift Using a Suture Without Incision Scars", *International Journal of Cosmetic Surgery* 2 (2002); 1-7.

[13] Ferreira, J. and Padin, V., "Lifting Glúteo con Tensores Naturales. Hilos Reafirmantes: La Gran Solución No Quirúrgica", *Portal Medestética,* 2005, accessed April 16th 2012 http://www.medestetica.com.ar/informes/informehilos.pdf

[14] Truswell, W. Surgical facial Rejuvenation: A Roadmap to Safe and Reliable Outcomes, October 25, 2008 | ISBN-10: 1588904911 | ISBN-13: 978-1588904911 | Edition: 1

[15] Padin, V. and Lopez Mecle, V., "Mejores Prácticas mínimamente invasivas para el tratamiento del tercio medio e inferior del rostro y el cuello", in Mejores Prácticas en Rejuvenecimiento Facial, ed. Allergan Academy (Buenos Aires: Allergan Press, 2011), 88-113.

[16] Guillemain, R. Le "Curl Lift" :, le Profession Medical,chirr. Plast.E Recon ;Mars 1970

# Permissions

All chapters in this book were first published by InTech Open; hereby published with permission under the Creative Commons Attribution License or equivalent. Every chapter published in this book has been scrutinized by our experts. Their significance has been extensively debated. The topics covered herein carry significant findings which will fuel the growth of the discipline. They may even be implemented as practical applications or may be referred to as a beginning point for another development.

The contributors of this book come from diverse backgrounds, making this book a truly international effort. This book will bring forth new frontiers with its revolutionizing research information and detailed analysis of the nascent developments around the world.

We would like to thank all the contributing authors for lending their expertise to make the book truly unique. They have played a crucial role in the development of this book. Without their invaluable contributions this book wouldn't have been possible. They have made vital efforts to compile up to date information on the varied aspects of this subject to make this book a valuable addition to the collection of many professionals and students.

This book was conceptualized with the vision of imparting up-to-date information and advanced data in this field. To ensure the same, a matchless editorial board was set up. Every individual on the board went through rigorous rounds of assessment to prove their worth. After which they invested a large part of their time researching and compiling the most relevant data for our readers.

The editorial board has been involved in producing this book since its inception. They have spent rigorous hours researching and exploring the diverse topics which have resulted in the successful publishing of this book. They have passed on their knowledge of decades through this book. To expedite this challenging task, the publisher supported the team at every step. A small team of assistant editors was also appointed to further simplify the editing procedure and attain best results for the readers.

Apart from the editorial board, the designing team has also invested a significant amount of their time in understanding the subject and creating the most relevant covers. They scrutinized every image to scout for the most suitable representation of the subject and create an appropriate cover for the book.

The publishing team has been an ardent support to the editorial, designing and production team. Their endless efforts to recruit the best for this project, has resulted in the accomplishment of this book. They are a veteran in the field of academics and their pool of knowledge is as vast as their experience in printing. Their expertise and guidance has proved useful at every step. Their uncompromising quality standards have made this book an exceptional effort. Their encouragement from time to time has been an inspiration for everyone.

The publisher and the editorial board hope that this book will prove to be a valuable piece of knowledge for researchers, students, practitioners and scholars across the globe.

# List of Contributors

**Nikolay Serdev**
New Bulgarian University, Sofia, Bulgaria

**M. B. Des Fernandes**
Renaissance Surgical Clinic, Cape Town, The Renaissance Body Science Institute, South Africa
Department of Plastic Surgery, Groote Schuur Hospital, University of Cape Town, Cape Town South Africa

**Meity Hidayani and Dali Amiruddin**
Dermatovenereology Department Medical Faculty of Hasanuddin University Wahidin Sudirohusodo General Hospital Makassar, Indonesia

**Syarief Hidayat**
Dermatovenereology Department Mintohardjo Navy Hospital Jakarta, Indonesia

**Ronald Feiner**
Minimally Invasive Cosmetic Surgeon "Cosmetica Medical Aesthetic Clinic" Shire Central Building, Sydney, Australia

**M.A. Sulamanidze, I.S. Vozdvizhenskiy, G.M. Sulamanidze, K.M. Sulamanidze, E.G. Azizyan and A. Kadzhaya**
Clinic of plastic and Aesthetic Surgery and Dermatocosmetology, Total Charm, Moscow (Russia), Tbilisi, Georgia

**Chedly Bouzouaya**
Occuloplastic Surgeon Belvedere Centre, Tunis

**A.A. Adamyan, M.A. Sulamanidze, N.D. Skuba and Z.R. Khusnutdinova**
Clinic of Anaplastic and Aesthetic Surgery Total Charm, Moscow, Russia - Tbilisi, Georgia

**Peter Prendergast**
Venus Medical, Dublin, Ireland

**Pier Antonio Bacci**
Mini invasive Aesthetic Surgery Italian Centre, Arezzo, Italy

**Vilma L. Padín**
CEMEC (Center of Aesthetic Medicine and Surgery), Buenos Aires, Argentine Republic
AIMERA (International Association of Aesthetic Medicine), Argentine Republic

# Index

www.ingramcontent.com/pod-product-compliance
Lightning Source LLC
LaVergne TN
LVHW062231200926
848484LV00006B/1513